Risk, Safe~~ty, and~~
Clinical Practice
Health care through the lens of risk

Risk, Safety, and Clinical Practice
Health care through the lens of risk

Bob Heyman

Monica Shaw

Andy Alaszewski

Mike Titterton

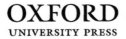

OXFORD
UNIVERSITY PRESS

OXFORD
UNIVERSITY PRESS

Great Clarendon Street, Oxford OX2 6DP

Oxford University Press is a department of the University of Oxford.
It furthers the University's objective of excellence in research, scholarship,
and education by publishing worldwide in

Oxford New York

Auckland Cape Town Dar es Salaam Hong Kong Karachi
Kuala Lumpur Madrid Melbourne Mexico City Nairobi
New Delhi Shanghai Taipei Toronto

With offices in

Argentina Austria Brazil Chile Czech Republic France Greece
Guatemala Hungary Italy Japan Poland Portugal Singapore
South Korea Switzerland Thailand Turkey Ukraine Vietnam

Oxford is a registered trade mark of Oxford University Press
in the UK and in certain other countries

Published in the United States
by Oxford University Press Inc., New York

British Library Cataloguing in Publication Data

Data available

Library of Congress Cataloging in Publication Data

Data available

Typeset in Minion by Cepha Imaging Private Ltd., Bangalore, India
Printed in Great Britain
on acid-free paper by
The MPG Books Group

ISBN 978–0–19–856900–8

10 9 8 7 6 5 4 3 2 1

For Ruth, Alan, Helen, and the volunteers and
service users of HALE

Contents

Introduction *1*
Bob Heyman and Mike Titterton

1 The concept of risk *15*
Bob Heyman

2 The social construction of health risks *37*
Bob Heyman

3 Values and health risks *59*
Bob Heyman

4 Health risks and probabilistic reasoning *85*
Bob Heyman

5 Time and health risks *107*
Bob Heyman

6 Information about health risks *123*
Andy Alaszewski

7 Health risks and the media *137*
Monica Shaw

8 The regulation of health risks *171*
Monica Shaw

9 Health risk and the patient safety agenda *195*
Monica Shaw

10 A case study of swine flu and concluding remarks *213*
Bob Heyman, Monica Shaw, and Andy Alaszewski

References *225*

Author Index *247*

Subject Index *253*

List of figure, tables, and boxes

Figure

Figure 0.1   Proportions of papers with 'coronary' in the research title also referring to 'risk' 1958–2007 *4*

Tables

Table 1.1   Two views of risk elements (Adapted from Heyman, Henriksen, and Maughan, 1998) *21*

Table 3.1   Difficulties associated with the concept of expected value *66*

Table 4.1a   First trimester screening for chromosomal anomalies such as Down's syndrome. (Bindra *et al.*, 2002) *94*

Table 4.1b   First trimester screening for chromosomal anomalies such as Down's syndrome: Summary screening statistics. (Bindra *et al.*, 2002) *94*

Boxes

Box 2.1   Processes involved in the consolidation of risk categories *44*

Box 2.2   A pharmaceutical example of commercial entrenchment *54*

Box 3.1   Unconscious preferencing and the matched guise technique *61*

Box 3.2   The essential steps in cost-benefit analysis *66*

Box 3.3   The aims of forensic mental health services: An example of implicit consequence selection *68*

Box 5.1   The time-framing of the UK smoking cessation programme *112*

Box 7.1   The representation of health risks in the 'old' media *144*

Box 7.2   The accuracy of internet health information *145*

Box 7.3   Convergence between 'old' and 'new' media representations of breast and prostate cancer on the internet (Seale, 2005) *147*

Box 7.4   Definitions of concepts used in media analysis *148*

Box 7.5   Local TV news reports on deaths and accidents in Los Angeles (McArthur *et al.*, 2001) *149*

Box 7.6   Newspaper portrayals of mental illness related to social class *150*

Box 7.7   Media framing of MRSA (adapted from Washer and Joffe, 2006) *152*

Box 7.8   Media coverage of heroic nurses *154*

Box 7.9   Media representations of Beverley Allitt *156*

Box 7.10   The Cleveland sex abuse scandal and media treatment of Dr. Marietta Higgs *157*

Box 7.11   The reception of television medical narratives (Davin, 2003) *160*

Box 7.12   Women's responses to a news story linking alcohol with risk of breast cancer (Thirlaway and Heggs, 2005) *161*

Box 7.13   The health risk of handheld mobile phones: Trust and credibility on the Internet (Richardson, 2003) *163*

Box 8.1   The Bristol Royal Infirmary *174*

Box 8.2   UK Government definitions of clinical governance (Adapted from Gray and Harrison, 2004) *178*

Box 8.3   NHS Litigation Authority (2009) risk standards for acute trusts *184*

Box 8.4   Excerpts from the 'Safety First' summary statement (Department of Health, 2006c) *186*

Box 9.1   Official analysis of adverse events occurring in the NHS (Department of Health, 2000c) *197*

Box 9.2   Coping with organizational deficiencies (Tucker and Edmondson, 2003) *200*

Box 9.3   Mortality rates related to heart surgery at the Oxford John Radcliffe Surgery Unit 2001–04 *203*

Box 9.4   Maladministration of drugs: Who is to blame? (Anderson and Webster, 2001) *205*

Box 9.5   A patient suicide attempt on an acute medical ward: Retrospective analysis of errors (Meurier, 2000) *207*

Box 9.6   Perceptions of managers and professionals of error reporting in a joint NHS and Social Care Trust (Adapted from Alaszewski and Coxon, 2007) *209*

Introduction

Bob Heyman and Mike Titterton

Aim

To outline the scope and structure of the book.

Objectives

1. To introduce the 'lens of risk'
2. To raise the idea of risk literacy
3. To locate the present book in the social science of risk
4. To outline the structure of the book.

Something old and something new

A man aged 65 visits his general practitioner concerning a minor ailment. Looking through his file after this matter has been dealt with, the doctor points out that the patient has not yet been screened for the risk of coronary heart disease. After asking questions about lifestyle and family history, she advises her patient to undergo a cholesterol test. The results indicate that his risk of experiencing a coronary event over the next 10-years is greater than 20%. This probability exceeds the cut-off for initiating risk reduction measures specified in the guidelines which the doctor is following. She therefore tells the patient that he is at high risk of coronary heart disease, and recommends statins, which he begins to take on a life-long basis.

This now routine healthcare[1] transaction illustrates a number of issues which the present book addresses. Something new and something old have happened. Coronary heart disease, a major killer, has long been treated as a

---

[1] The term 'health care' will be used to encompass all of the purposeful activities which people undertake in order to manage health. The word 'healthcare' will be employed more narrowly, to refer to the health-promoting activities of paid service providers.

major clinical problem, particularly in developed countries. But its representation as a risk invokes a historically novel mode of thought. Although they might be labelled 'patients', those offered this form of 'treatment' as prophylaxis will not usually have reported any related illness. In most cases they will not even have requested screening which, instead, their doctor proposes. As discussed in Chapter 2, a health risk is often identified by locating patients in a category of which a relatively high, but sometimes absolutely low, proportion are expected to experience the adverse outcome under consideration. Statins may confer an overall net gain in life expectancy by reducing the risk of coronary heart disease in the population (Roberts, Guallar, and Rodriguez, 2007). But this treatment introduces new risks, including muscle weakness and liver damage (Kiortsis *et al.*, 2007). Some patients who experience side-effects would not have suffered from heart problems if they had not taken statins. However, what might have happened to an individual if preventive measures had not been activated can never be known.

By offering this intervention the doctor draws attention to a particular health issue which has to have been both **selected** and **categorized** before it can be managed. (The highlighted topics will be further discussed in subsequent chapters.) The demarcation of risks is by no means straightforward. For example, McCormack, Levine, and Rangno (1997) define 'cardiovascular events' as including *angina, unstable angina, myocardial infarction or death from coronary artery disease*. The targeting of a particular health risk category requires **value judgements** about its undesirability. Such judgements may seem obvious. But they will sometimes be contested, for instance with respect to the desirability of preventing the birth of children with disabilities. The patient whose imaginary case was presented above might be informed that he faced a greater than 20% risk of coronary heart disease over the next 10-years. Numerical risk assessments of this form are based on **probabilistic reasoning**. They provide the basis for bifurcation into high and low risk categories, since an intervention may be either given or withheld, which requires a dividing line to be selected. Despite the aura of precision carried by numbers, the thinking behind this form of reason is not clear-cut. In addition, probabilities cannot be quantitied unless confined to a **time frame** which may be set differently, changing the probabilities on which clinical decision-making is based. In this case, the risk of congestive heart disease (CHD) after more than a decade has been routinely excluded from consideration.

This and many forms of health risk management are located in wider social contexts. They are arranged around **the organized processing of information**, and are influenced by the wider **societal representation** of health and illness. For example, the iconic patient with coronary heart disease is an unfit, overweight man. Health professionals do not select health problems entirely spontaneously. Their choices are influenced by **regulatory systems** which distribute incentives and sanctions. For instance, patients may not appreciate that UK general practices are paid for achieving nationally targeted screening rates. Regulatory systems focus on **patient safety**, which they are designed to enhance. Finally, these and other processes fit together, not always coherently, in socially organized packages of purposeful **risk management**. As discussed in the next chapter, risk management should not be thought of as an activity undertaken only by professional experts on behalf of clients. Instead, it should be considered to involve all of those who respond to a particular health problem in terms of risk. The stakeholders include the public, patients, carers, practitioners, service managers, and policymakers.

The lens of risk and the risk epidemic

The title of this section recycles two borrowed phrases which provide a starting point for reflecting critically about risk and health care. The often-used term *lens of risk* (e.g. Hunt, 2003) draws attention to an interpretive framework which risk managers adopt, usually without conscious reflection. Rose (1998b) labelled this way of looking at the world *risk thinking*. The optical metaphor implies that a biomedical or psychological phenomenon will appear different when viewed through the lens of risk. Moreover, the impact of looking through this metaphorical optical device involves far more than perception. Actions taken from a risk perspective have the potential to change the biomedical phenomena which they address, often creating new risks, as illustrated above.

The second borrowed phrase, *risk epidemic*, was invented by Skolbekken (1995). He wished to convey not that the world had become more dangerous (although it certainly has through the looming threats of climate change and resource depletion), but that medicine was becoming increasingly dominated by risk thinking. Skolbekken documented this trend by analysing the use of risk language in medical journals. An updated illustration is offered below, in Figure 0.1.

The chart was developed by finding papers identified by the academic search engine Google Scholar for 5-year periods between 1958–62 and 2003–07. Counts were obtained for papers containing the word 'coronary', and for those both 'coronary' and 'risk' in the title. The displayed percentages portray the extent to which risk was considered sufficiently important to be included in the title of papers concerned with coronary heart disease at different periods in recent history. The chart illustrates two trends. Firstly, it documents steady and cumulatively massive publication growth in this field over the period covered.

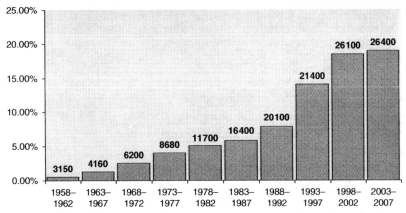

Figure 0.1 Proportions of papers with 'coronary' in the research title also referring to 'risk' 1958–2007 (totals at tops of bars).

Secondly, it points to a historical increase in the proportion of papers which included 'risk' in the title. Use of this term accelerated particularly rapidly in the 1990s, and appears to be tailing off in the 21st century. A less stringent test produces an even more striking comparison. In 1963–67, 8% of 12 700 papers containing the word 'coronary' anywhere in the text also included the word 'risk'. By 2003–07, this proportion had increased 10-fold, to 83% of 160 000 papers. Similar trends can be found for many health issues. Readers can confirm this assertion for themselves by carrying out a comparable analysis for any medical subject which interests them. In most cases, the trend will be perfectly ordered, with the proportion of 'risk' papers on any clinical topic increasing for each later period. (Search engines provide an invaluable tool for digging into the recent archaeology of knowledge!)

Researchers, including the present authors, appear to have been tugged by an unnoticed but gradually strengthening force which induced them collectively to don metaphorical risk spectacles. It might be argued that the trend documented above results merely from linguistic changes. From this perspective, organized responses to perceived health problems have remained constant, but are now likely to be discussed in terms of 'risk'. Skolbekken and many other writers have maintained that a more fundamental shift has occurred. He documented collective, unconscious distortions generated by the risk epidemic. These biases include: lack of attention to iatrogenic risks, caused by medicine itself; particular overrepresentation of risk thinking in medically dominated clinical arenas such as obstetrics; and use of a narrow vocabulary which largely excludes related but distinctive concepts such as 'uncertainty', 'danger', and 'vulnerability'. This novel form of thinking detects problems by locating them in populations, frequently creating new risks, generated by responses to the prior concern, potentially *ad infinitum*.

The present book draws upon the social science of risk. It will start from the assumption that a fundamental transformation has taken place. For better or worse, the world in general, and health in particular, look different when seen through the lens of risk. This tendency affects all aspects of health care, not just the academic publication production line which the above chart dissects. National Governments throughout the developed world have established official bodies, such as, in the UK, the Patient Safety Agency and Care Quality Commission, which prioritize risk management. Services have been transformed by risk thinking. The safety agenda aims to minimize iatrogenic risks, such as hospital-acquired infections and medical errors. Health promotion campaigns attempt to persuade individuals to abandon immediate pleasures by promising to reduce their risk of developing long-term conditions. By deciding whether or not to take up screening, reduce their dietary fat intake, or require condom use, members of the public who do not consider themselves ill become health risk managers. Health service providers seek to help patients to navigate complex risk management decision trees about screening and treatment, or to reduce the risk of patients with mental health problems harming themselves or others. They aim to minimize professional risks, such as being subject to litigation or accused of misconduct. Although risk avoidance often tends to predominate in practice, health professionals do sometimes promote positive risk-taking (Titterton, 2005), and seek to help service users to find optimum balances between safety and autonomy (Heyman and Huckle, 1993; Heyman, Huckle and Handyside, 1998).

The lens of risk has not retained a fixed shape during the relatively brief period during which it has occupied centre stage in developed societies. Power (2007) has argued that risk thinking has *increasingly shifted from the science of risk analysis itself, and its epistemological debates, to the organizational systems in which it is embedded.* In the healthcare domain, this shift was marked, in the UK at least, by the establishment of formal clinical governance systems during the 1990s. The global financial collapse of 2007 is stimulating a fundamental change in attitudes to risk regulation which spills out well beyond the failed banking sector. The protective power of regulatory systems is no longer taken for granted. The question of who will guard the guards has re-emerged in relation to all forms of risk management. The bank meltdown has also shown that the biggest risks may remain unnoticed because they are too large to be seen. It might be fancifully suggested that risk itself evolves. The culturally shared, taken-for-granted presuppositions which underpin risk thinking do not

themselves remain constant. The apparent oddness of talking about risk changing arises out of a ubiquitous tendency to view risks as natural phenomena
which possess measurable properties, rather than as interpretive devices.

Risk literacy

The authors of the present book have attempted to produce a guide to thinking
critically about health risks and their management. Readers will be invited to
explore behind news headlines and official pronouncements about risks.
The present book does not offer solutions to specific health risk management
problems. Instead, the authors seek to promote 'risk literacy'. They have
endeavoured to articulate and question the assumptions on which any form of
health risk management must be based. Subsequent chapters will seek to demonstrate that risk managers cannot avoid engaging with difficult issues concerning the nature of reality, goodness, chance, time, information, and social
order. These questions have been debated for thousands of years. Practising
risk managers cannot be expected to solve them. Nor can the present authors.
But their implications for health risk management need to be considered.

Some health professionals may feel that excessive reflection will impede
them from taking forwards their mission of benefiting patients. However,
peering into Pandora's box, rather than keeping it resolutely closed, can venti-
late some stuffy areas of health care practice. The book offers a critical guide to
risk thinking, a function not dissimilar to that of a guidebook. Travellers cannot afford to visit all of the potentially interesting sites in a particular locality,
and do not have the time to read up all the relevant information. Guidebook
writers attempt to select and comment on the most significant landmarks.
They deliberately adopt an opinionated stance, knowing that readers will readily
reject views which they do not agree with.

This book provides a guide to risk thinking itself, as applied in health care
contexts, rather than to the social science of risk. A number of recent texts
reviewed in the next chapter have performed this task well enough. Instead,
the book will draw upon the many interesting ideas which can be discovered in
this literature. A social science based guide to risk thinking will introduce the
field, facilitate critical scrutiny, and encourage deeper exploration. Much of
the academic literature is aimed at fellow members of particular disciplines,
sub-disciplines, and schools of thought. It does not offer easy reading.
Conflicting ideas are rife. An introduction to risk thinking which starts from
the concept itself provides one way of cutting through this rich but chaotic
resource, hopefully tempting readers to explore further.

The remainder of this Introduction will discuss the background and origins
of the book, differentiating it from other texts about risk. The sequence of the
chapters which follow will then be outlined.

The social science of risk

Anybody hunting for a quick fix on the social science of risk in the early 1990s could have been forgiven for concluding that little was available. Sociology and psychology textbooks did not even index references to the topic. Only a few social science texts on risk had been published (e.g. Krimsky and Golding, 1992; Adams, 1995). Risk thinking did not resonate with traditional concerns of psychology, sociology, and anthropology such as individual differences, social inequality, and comparisons between cultures, respectively. By 1995, a substantial divide had opened up between the lack of focus on risk in the social sciences and its expanding role in other discourses. For example, the daily news contained wide-ranging references to risks. The language of risk connected diverse domains, including sport, business, weather, the environment, crime, politics, and health. Social scientists started to orient themselves to this important trend.

Few generic social science of risk texts existed in 1995. However, a disparate range of disciplines had long engaged with the analysis of risk and related concepts such as chance and uncertainty. Some threads of scholarship, particularly debates about the nature of probability, have continued for centuries (Hacking, 1975). Major original contributions, now integrated into the social science of risk, have come from a wide range of disciplinary sources. Relevant texts include, among others: *The Economic Theory of Entrepreneurship* (Knight, 1921); *The History of Probability* (Hacking, 1975); *Judgements Under Uncertainty: Heuristic and Biases* (Kahneman, Slovic, and Tversky, 1982); *The Use of Heuristics to Simplify Decision-Making* (Gigerenzer, Todd, and The ABC Research Group 1999); and *Risk and Blame* (Douglas, 1992). Sociologists have analysed risk thinking in relation to the intensifying global ecological crisis (Beck, 1992) and growing societal system complexity (Luhmann, 1993). Although not using the specific term 'risk', Foucault's concept of 'governmentality' (Foucault, 1991) was soon applied to its analysis (Dean, 1999). This approach treats risk thinking as a new means of social control, through which individuals are encouraged to regulate themselves responsibly, guided by scientific evidence.

These and many other ideas have heavily influenced the current social science of risk. But a coherent knowledge base has not yet developed, and perhaps never will. Contention and divergence are only to be expected in relation to the analysis of such a complex concept. Scholars who are heavily immersed in particular disciplines may not even know about the contributions of others. Psychologists and sociologists in particular tend, on the whole, to interact no more constructively than cats and dogs! Outsiders to this academic mélange may feel overwhelmed. However, social scientific concepts do provide a useful resource for the analysis of health risk management. They can be drawn upon eclectically.

Since 1995, the availability of social scientific analyses relevant to health risk management has been transformed from famine perhaps even to glut. A specialist journal, *Health, Risk & Society*, launched in 1999, catalysed the consolidation of a new academic sub-discipline. Anybody who, as of 2009, wishes to maintain a comprehensive collection of books relevant to health care risk management will need a large bookcase. Generic texts on risk have been written from the perspectives of single disciplines such as sociology (Zinn, 2008) and psychology (Breakwell, 2007). Some books have brought together multiple disciplines (Mythen and Walklate, 2006), or developed a multidisciplinary approach (Renn, 2008). Others have homed in on risk-related topics, including chance (Gigerenzer, 2002), risk regulation (Power, 2007) and risk in everyday life (Tulloch and Lupton, 2003). A rarer sub-breed of risk books has focussed on conceptual issues. A text edited by Lewens (2007) asks much needed philosophical questions. One edited by Ericson and Doyle (2003) probes the crucial but neglected issue of the relationship between risk and morality. Another variant offers social and healthcare professionals practical advice about how to manage risks (Titterton, 2005). A further strand has reviewed the risk literature in relation to the needs of particular professions such as social work (Parsloe, 1999) and nursing (Godin, 2006). These texts, all recommended, and many others, offer a detailed resource for further study of risk social science.

The present authors seek to distinguish their text from the pack in two ways: by focussing specifically on health-related matters; and by attempting to combine critical sophistication with accessibility. In relation to the first issue, the book will concentrate on health risk management, albeit from an analytic rather than a directly practical perspective. Many existing social science texts attempt to cover the whole span of risk applications. However, health risk thinking possesses at least two distinctive features which will be addressed in later chapters. One is the centrality of its engagement with moral issues. People are generally regarded as valuable in themselves, although fetuses inhabit an intermediate zone in which their destruction can be contemplated. In contrast, for instance, capitalist societies are supposed to allow unfit firms to die (even if the survival of the fittest principle does not apply to large financial institutions). Risk thinking concerned with people, regarded as ends-in-themselves, will take on a moral character not found when expendable entities are being managed. Generic approaches to the social science of risk have sometimes given insufficient emphasis to this difference.

A second distinctive feature of health risks involves the nature of their evidence base. When the lens of risk is pointed at human-beings, it focusses on the most complex organized entities presently known to inhabit the universe.

Because of this complexity, health outcomes mostly cannot be predicted in individual cases. On the other hand, a large number of people are available to be observed. All but the rarest diseases manifest themselves many times in large populations. Enumerating how frequently a specified outcome occurred in the past provides a limited source of guidance about the future. In contrast, for example, analysts concerned with the safety of nuclear power plants can at least hope to make a runaway chain reaction very unlikely by modelling and predicting how an individual reactor should behave. But they cannot test their strategy by observing large numbers of cases.

The presence of features distinguishing health risks from other forms justifies their separate consideration. A second claim to divide this book from the social science of risk pack is stylistic. The authors have attempted to make the book as accessible as possible whilst doing justice to the complexity of its subject matter. It is designed for health care practitioners, researchers, and others who are interested in the management of health risks. The authors have endeavoured to steer a course between the twin rocks of unexamined assumptions and impenetrability, both of which are illustrated below. Inevitably, a balance has to be struck between readability and doing justice to the difficult issues embedded in risk thinking. To this end, technical vocabulary, otherwise known as jargon, has been avoided as far as possible. Citations have been used sparingly to illustrate rather than fully represent the points being made. A limited number of 'ugly' technical phrases will be used because of their central importance to health risk thinking. These include 'contingency', 'risk virtual object', 'inductive probabilistic reasoning', and 'time-framing'. They will be discussed more fully at their points of use.

Unexamined assumptions and impenetrable social science

The following chapters will challenge implicit presuppositions underpinning clinical risk management. Authoritative accounts sometimes uncritically transmit the assumption that health professionals know best about risks. For example, Paling (2006) has written a practical guide to risk communication for health professionals which has been endorsed by the British Medical Association. In this book, patients are depicted as prone to *assess risks primarily on emotions rather than facts*. Doctors are described as *so focused on evidence-based decision-making that they see their main task as being better at communicating the key numbers to their patients*. The stated contrast between emotional patients and rational doctors is not necessarily endorsed by the above writer, but reflects a widely held view. This contrast begs many questions about the limits of evidence and its relationship to values. The mystique of science can easily create a tyranny of numbers without addressing methodological or value questions. Social scientists are interested in the emotions which lurk concealed beneath number crunching.

The social sciences offer extensive resources that can be drawn upon to facilitate critical thinking about health risk management. Unfortunately, much of this material is produced for fellow members of academic sub-disciplines, often in an abstruse style. The writing is not aimed at practitioners who can be faced with a choice between the uncritical and the incomprehensible. Instead of making fun of a piece of heavy sociology, the first author will target himself. He was asked by an irritated hospital consultant to explain the following quotation drawn from a paper concerned with women's understandings of prenatal chromosomal screening for conditions such as Down's syndrome (Heyman *et al.*, 2006):

> Probabilistic induction from populations to individuals requires heuristic acceptance of the ecological fallacy that aggregate properties of a category appertain to its members.

The writer sent a 1-page apologetic expansion of this cryptic statement to the aggrieved consultant who replied that he now understood and agreed with the argument. (The issue presented telegraphically in the quotation will be discussed in detail in Chapter 4.) One person's jargon is another's technical vocabulary. The present authors have had to struggle with their own immersion in the social sciences. They have tried to make the book accessible to readers whose needs and backgrounds will vary considerably, whilst avoiding oversimplification.

The study of risk and the study of risks

Drawing a distinction between the study of 'risks' and the study of 'risk' (Heyman, 1998) provides one useful starting point for constructive critical analysis of risk thinking. Particular risks are considered mainly for practical reasons such as improving outcomes, calling for increased resources, or establishing retrospective accountability for adverse events. The analyst has enough problems getting to grips with the biomedical, statistical, organizational, legal, and moral complexities of the risk in question without having to worry about the nature of risk itself. In contrast, students of risk, the focus of the present book, seek to investigate the properties of risk thinking. However, they can only probe this interpretive framework by exploring the ways in which social actors manage particular risks. The student of risk therefore needs to look for common patterns across different clinical domains. This requirement will be met in the present book through the consideration of diverse examples, although the range of clinical contexts covered is inevitably limited by the authors' knowledge and experience.

Structure of the book

The chapters which follow offer an introduction to the critical analysis of health risk management. The next chapter will consider the definition of 'risk', an issue which tends to be taken for granted in many texts. The discussion will introduce important related issues, including: the central importance of contingency, which frames thinking about alternative futures; the nature of the 'existence' of risks; the location of risk in a wider family of terms; the distinction between taking a risk and being at risk; and the concepts of risk management, risk manager, and risk owner. This definitional labour will result in risk thinking being decomposed into four primary elements: categorizing, valuing, uncertain expecting, and time-framing. It will be argued that anyone thinking about a particular risk brings together these four components, although often unreflectively. The social sciences draw attention to the assumptions, usually taken for granted, on which risk thinking is based.

Each component of risk thinking will be analysed in a separate chapter (Chapters 2–5). Chapter 2 will work through the argument that risks cannot 'exist' unless the complexity of the real world is simplified through categorization, which can be achieved in many different ways. The third chapter will explore the unavoidable role of valuing in risk analysis, examining risk selection and the moral ingredient, often concealed, of risk judgements. Chapter 4 will argue that the calculation of quantitative probabilities requires tacit acceptance of the simplifying rule of thumb assumption that individuals personally 'carry' outcome probabilities estimated through observation of constructed categories. It will be maintained that this simplifying step has important implications for clinical practice which can be detected in the interactions between health professionals and patients. The final chapter in this sequence of four will focus on the role of time interpretation in risk management, particularly the inevitable but often unreflective adoption of particular temporal horizons such as 5-year survival.

The second part of the book (Chapters 6–9) will locate health risk management in a wider cultural and health service context. The topics covered include risk and information, risk and the mass media, risk regulation, and the safety agenda. The two parts of the book are connected by the following crucial argument. Risk statements describe an individual's **relationship** to a categorized outcome. In contrast to disease, pain, and death, risks never 'exist' independently of observers' knowledge, beliefs, and values. They refer to what an observer thinks might happen, or might have happened, rather than directly to the material world. In consequence, a person may be considered to have been 'at risk' even though nothing untoward actually occurred. But responses to risks cannot be socially organized unless risk managers orient themselves to the same entity. This coordination of perceptions is achieved by excluding observers' active interpretive roles from conscious scrutiny. Communal interpretation is projected onto the risk which comes to be experienced as a naturally existing object. However, these projections remain open to challenge, making the social orders on which they are based inherently fragile.

Chapter 6 will consider 'encoded' risk knowledge, as exemplified by clinical guidelines and health promotion messages. It will be argued that the encoding process provides a lever for societal control over individual behaviour. But this approach tends to fall down on account of its lack of attention to the crucial roles of social context, trust, and emotion. Chapter 7 addresses the role of the mass media in constructing and selecting risks for societal attention. The complex and little understood processes through which the media bring certain risks to centre stage, often temporarily, whilst ignoring others, will be reviewed, as will the active interpretive role of media recipients. Chapter 8 will raise crucial questions about the critical role of healthcare regulatory organizations, such as the Care Quality Commission for England. These bodies are supposed to manage risks arising from healthcare itself on behalf of the public. Like bank regulators, they have attempted to do so mostly by indirect means, relying heavily on the testimony of provider organizations. The global banking fiasco of 2007/2008, followed closely in the UK by the exposure of grotesque parliamentary quasi-corruption, have forced doubt about the adequacy of indirect risk regulation to centre stage. Chapter 8 will address this issue in relation to healthcare systems. It will be argued both that risk regulators have been cast as the guardians of the social order in secular risk-based societies, and that they are structurally incapable of playing this role. It is now apparent that alternatives to centrally driven systems which attempt to command and control health risk management are urgently needed. Chapter 9 will complete a circle from health risk to health safety by reviewing recent Government attempts to promote and enforce the latter. It will be argued that these initiatives tend to conflate adverse events such as medical interventions causing deaths with clear-cut avoidable errors like wrong-site surgery. Instead, an approach will be advocated in which the limitations of healthcare risk management are acknowledged, and the potential for front-line multidisciplinary teams to improve clinical outcomes is harnessed more effectively. Chapter 10 will draw together the themes discussed in the book through an illustrative case study of the UK response to the 2009 swine flu pandemic.

Four authors have worked together to produce this book. They share a commitment to bridging the worlds of healthcare and social science in the field of risk studies. The chapters have been written by named individuals, as indicated in the text. The responsibility for views expressed in particular chapters rests solely with their writers.

Conclusion

In this introductory chapter, it has been argued that the social sciences provide a valuable resource for practitioners, researchers, and others who seek to think critically but constructively about managing health risks. The authors aim to promote the development of 'risk literacy' by steering a course between an oversimplified natural attitude to risk and impenetrability. The book will delve a little more deeply than some other texts into the concept of risk itself, and locate health risk management in a wider societal context, drawing out implications for clinical practice.

Chapter 1

The concept of risk

Bob Heyman

Aim

To critically analyse the concept of risk.

Objectives

1. To define risk
2. To map the concept of risk onto that of contingency, establishing its 'virtual' status
3. To locate risk in a wider linguistic context with respect to related but distinctive terms, such as danger, uncertainty, and safety
4. To distinguish between taking a risk and being at risk
5. To introduce the concepts of risk management, risk manager, and risk owner.

Introduction

This chapter will address the crucial issue of defining risk, locating the concept within a wider family of terms. As documented below, this definitional task has been somewhat neglected even in the critical social science literature. Relative silence about the meaning of the term risk stands in sharp contrast to its extended usage in every sphere of modern life. Much effort is put into thinking about particular risks, far less into reflecting upon the concept itself. Risks seem to have become so important in modern societies that the framework of meaning in which they are located has been obscured. In this sense, people who manage particular risks may 'know not what whereof they speak'. A visitor from another planet might be struck by the amount of energy invested by some of its inhabitants in managing a phenomenon which they cannot define. Health professionals may feel that such philosophical niceties merely distract them from their difficult practical mission of benefitting patients. However, patients cannot make informed choices unless they fully understand the risks which they are invited to co-manage. In turn, it is not possible to think clearly about risks without understanding the concept of risk.

The present chapter will review extant definitions of risk, and put forward a working formulation. The relationship of risk to the broader idea of contingency will then be outlined, and linked to the notion of risks as virtual entities. Risk will be related to the wider vocabulary in which it is embedded. The superficially similar but fundamentally different states of 'taking a risk' and 'being at risk' will be distinguished. Finally, the meanings of the terms risk manager, risk management, and risk ownership will be reviewed.

The definition of risk

Does the concept of risk retain any meaning?

The term risk is used in such a diversity of domains that attempts to generate a single clear definition may be doomed to failure. Power (2007) has argued for this pessimistic view, noting that:

> Philosophers tell us that nouns are misleading because they suggest that a clear object exists when this is often not the case. In the case of 'risk' and 'risk management' we would do well to heed their advice. However, this book takes as its point of departure the surely uncontestable fact that the noun has grown in use and significance in organizational life.

This quotation invokes a characteristic social scientific manoeuvre. It suggests, in effect, that risk can mean whatever people thinking about particular risks take it to mean. By implication, researchers and scholars should analyse how the terms 'risk' and 'risk management' are actually used to organize social life. They should not naively assume that the presence of a word reflects the existence of an entity. Similarly, Garland (2003) has eloquently raised the question of whether risk discourses share any common attributes. He outlines the wide range of substantive social domains in which risks are discussed, e.g. sport, insurance, negligence litigation, finance, public health, lifestyle, the environment, and war. This range, he argues, is cross-cut by a variety of approaches to risk which can be applied in any domain:

> Today's accounts of risk are remarkable for their multiplicity and for the variety of senses they give to the term. Risk is a calculation. Risk is a commodity. Risk is a capital. Risk is a technique of government. Risk is objective and scientifically knowable. Risk is subjective and socially constructed. Risk is a problem, a threat, a source of insecurity. Risk is a pleasure, a thrill, a source of profit and freedom. Risk is the means by which we colonize and control the future. 'Risk society' is our late modern world spinning out of control.

Finally, another major contributor to the social science of risk, Hansson (2005) dismisses as the *first myth of risk*, the idea that risk *must have a single, well-defined meaning*. It can be argued that the term 'risk' may now be used so ubiquitously that it has lost any shared meaning. It could even be maintained that the meaning of the term has become so imprecise that its use militates against clear thinking. However, this position flies in the face of popular opinion, which implicitly presupposes that phenomena linked by a shared conceptual label share common attributes, however loosely. The present book is based on the assumption that the shared use of risk vocabulary in diverse domains does reflect linking themes, as elaborated below.

Social scientific definitions of risk

Many books about risk do attempt a definition, but these efforts are often cursory. Anyone comparing these offerings might well agree with Rosa (2003) who identified *an intentional silence about defining risk at all* in much of this literature. Luhmann (1993) refers to *carelessness in concept formation*. One reason for reticence and sloppiness may, as already argued, be that because the concept of risk is used so frequently, and in such a wide variety of contexts, its meaning has come to be taken for granted even by critical social scientists.

Familiarity can breed blindness to presuppositions. A story illustrating the absurdity of the notion of culturally fair intelligence tests has a small Scottish boy who lives in a remote rural area puzzling over a picture of a cow. Worried about his apparently low intelligence quotient (IQ), the tester prompts the boy to guess what the picture represents. After considerable thought, he replies that he thinks that it is an Aberdeen Angus. Risk, like cows to farmers, has become so familiar that its conceptual underpinnings have been lost to conscious scrutiny. Asking what the term means has a slightly disruptive impact, gently shaking the cultural foundations of late modern society.

All too often, foundational work stops before 'risk' has been placed under more than superficial scrutiny. For example, *Risk: Philosophical Perspectives* (Lewens, 2007) provides a ground-breaking contribution to the *sparsely populated* field of risk philosophy. The Introduction leaps into a discussion of decision-making about *risky options* without any debate about what makes an option 'risky'. If even philosophers do not ask conceptual questions about risk, what hope is there for clinically focused practitioners and researchers?

Renn (2008) anchors his definition of risk in the idea of contingency:

> All concepts of risk have one element in common: the distinction between possible and chosen action ... Philosophers call this contingency ... If the contingent nature of our actions is taken for granted, the term 'risk' denotes the possibility that an

> undesirable state of reality (adverse effects) may occur as a result of natural events or human activity.

Despite noting that the key notion of contingency raises philosophical issues, Renn does not probe this idea further. Contingency is mentioned on the first page of his book, without any accompanying analysis, and does not reappear. The offered sketch of contingency homes in on causes such as natural events. But it does not articulate the relationship between what actually happens and the alternative outcomes. A second shortcoming with this definition is that it does not give centre stage to the role of probability in risk discourse. The definition as written would apply equally to a seer who predicts certain doom unless sinners mend their ways.

Three further definitions of risk offered by major figures will be reviewed below in the section concerned with the term's linguistic family. As will be seen, Douglas, Luhmann, and Castel all defined risk in relation to danger, but in very different ways. Douglas (1992) regarded risk as a modern synonym for the much older term 'danger'. Luhmann (1993) defined risk and danger in relation to the presence and absence, respectively, of contingency. For Castel (1991), risks appertain to statistics derived from populations, whilst dangerousness belongs to individuals. Such differences in formulating the distinction, if any, between risk and danger reflect considerable conceptual disarray in current social science analyses of risk.

A definition of risk

The definition set out below is not offered as a definitive answer to the conundrum of risk. It provides a working specification which is intended to provide a clear starting point for the analysis that follows. The definition is founded on two principles. Firstly, as further argued below, only human-beings (or other cognate entities) who understands the concept can 'take a risk'. This definitional condition excludes the apparently comparable activities of non-human animals and babies. Similarly, only an observer who has adopted a risk framework can judge others to be 'at risk'. Secondly, as noted above, the definition offered below is based on the assumption that the concept of risk contains a core of common meaning across the wide range of domains to which it is applied.

The notion of risk offered in the present book reframes a widely quoted definition. The Royal Society (1992) defined risk as:

> the probability that a particular adverse event occurs during a stated time period, or results from a particular challenge.

This formulation was designed to justify the quantification of risk. But it can also be used to bring out the complexity of the concept. The definition points to four components which are folded into risk judgements, namely categorization of events, value judgement about their negativity, expectations about their occurrence, and location in a temporal framework. Reframing these four elements so as to emphasize the importance of the observer's interpretation of a risk generates a less pithy but more accurate definition of risk as:

> The projection of uncertain expectation, viewed in terms of randomness, about the occurrence of a negatively valued outcome category within a selected time frame.

The phrase *viewed in terms of randomness* has been chosen in order to indicate that the lens of risk encourages its wearers to think about events **as if** they occurred randomly. For example, whether the patient survives major surgery might well be determined by the interactions of a large number of complex processes. An observer in possession of vastly more scientific knowledge than is currently available might be able to predict the outcome with near certainty. Risk managers, at present, cannot achieve anything like this degree of prognostic accuracy in most clinical circumstances. They can, instead, gain some modest predictive leverage by drawing upon knowledge of the past, for example, in this case, about the outcomes of previous operations. This knowledge can then be applied to individuals who are assigned the rate observed in a group. The crucial steps of conflating complexity with chance and applying collective rates to individuals come at a price. For instance, many probabilities of the same outcome can reasonably be derived from observation (Suppes, 1994). These matters are discussed in Chapter 4.

The term *negatively valued outcome* has been selected in order to indicate that risk thinking includes a focus on adversity. Purposeful risk-taking entails taking into account potential benefits as well as possible costs. It tends to encompass multiple contingencies, the anticipated pleasure of eating cream cake as well as the perceived extra risk of heart disease. However, even thrill seekers such as mountaineers who enjoy the experience of taking risks for its own sake do not usually seek to fall down a crevasse. Some engagement with adversity, reframed more accurately as negative valuing, is built into the architecture of modern risk thinking. As Shakespeare's *Merchant of Venice*, quoted by Bernstein (1996), neatly put it, at the start of the period in which modern science, commerce, and risk thinking began to develop:

> My ventures are not in one bottom trusted,
> Nor to one place; nor is my whole estate
> Upon the fortune of this present year;
> Therefore, my merchandise makes me not sad.
>
> (Act I, Scene I, *Merchant of Venice*)

In relation to multiple consequences, a useful distinction, discussed in Chapter 3, can be drawn between outcome-independent and outcome-contingent risks (Butler, 2008). The former should as far as possible be avoided. The *Never Events* policy developed by the National Patient Safety Agency (2009a) for the UK lists eight selected events such as wrong-site surgery which should never occur, but still continue to happen. In relation to outcome-contingent risks, the inherent negativity of risk thinking needs to be balanced against consideration of the positive benefits of risk-taking (Titterton, 2005). For example, an adult with learning disabilities might be 'allowed' various degrees of licence to travel solo (Heyman, Huckle, and Handyside, 1998). Using a metaphorical local passport, this person perhaps risks becoming involved in a traffic accident, or being abused. On the other hand, personal mobility allows them to enjoy some degree of independence. An obviously optimal solution to this type of dilemma cannot be found. Instead, risk managers need to consider various balances between safety and autonomy, taking into account service user and carer preferences.

The definition offered above is fairly similar to the one quoted below (Rosa, 2003) which defines risk as:

> a situation or event where something of human value (including humans themselves) is at stake and where the outcome is uncertain.

Rosa's definition, in contrast to the one given by the Royal Society (1992), quoted above, brings the observer to centre stage. It does so by referring to value and uncertainty rather than adversity and probability. The latter merely project interpretations onto the external world, obscuring the potential for different perspectives. The definition offered in the present book retains this clear interpretive focus. It adds two extra elements to the risk compound, categorization and time-framing, giving four in total.

These four elements of risk thinking tend to be **projected** onto the external world. A person considering a risk plays an active judgemental role which can sometimes be obscured by habit and social consensus. This projection process can be seen most clearly in relation to value. An observer cannot attribute adversity, or benefit, to outcomes without making implicit or explicit value judgements, as discussed in Chapter 3. Viewing adversity as an intrinsic property of outcomes displaces values from acts of interpretation to events, making challenges to underlying but unstated assumptions more difficult to mount. For example, classifying sadness as depression, an illness, makes it easier to take its undesirability for granted (Robertson, 2008).

Although not as pithy as the Royal Society definition, the alternative outlined above offers a more complex understanding of risk in which the observer plays a central role. The risk observer needs to:

1. Categorize outcomes before they can become a selected focus of risk analysis

2. Make value judgements, positive and negative, about the multiple consequences seen to arise from taking a risk

3. Develop expectations about the likelihood of an adverse outcome occurring, using the past as a guide to the future

4. Place temporal boundaries around a risk before any kind of risk calculation can be undertaken.

Each of the above elements of risk thinking can be framed in a way which excludes or includes the risk observer, as shown in the top part of Table 1.1.

The projection process shifts these four ingredients of risk thinking from the right to the left column, generating the terms used in the Royal Society definition. Managers of specific risks may adopt the *natural attitude* (Schutz, 1962), viewing risks as existing physically and possessing measurable attributes. Students of risk seek to uncover the interpretive processes, often habitual, unarticulated, and societally validated, which underpin all understandings of risks. The bottom half of Table 1.1 lists some components of risk management which will be considered mainly in the second part of the book.

Table 1.1 Two views of risk elements (Adapted from Heyman, Henriksen, and Maughan, 1998)

Risk viewed as referring to natural phenomena	Risk viewed as referring to interpretive phenomena
RISK CONSTRUCTION	
Event	Category
Adversity	Value
Probability	Uncertain expectation
Time period	Time frame
RISK MANAGEMENT	
Service delivery	Service organisation
Evidence-based practice	Practice encoding
Information giving	Information representation
Regulation and safety	Control

Contingency and risk virtual objects

Using the lens of risk entails the construction of contingencies, as argued by Luhmann (1993) and Renn (2008), both mentioned above. This mode of thought derives from the visualization of two or more alternatives, defined so that one and only one must occur. An individual might or might not die before the age of 65, be treated for a mental disorder during their lifetime, or experience a cancer relapse within 5-years of being treated, for example. Nature does not produce identical events. Hence, classificatory activity is required in order to locate outcomes in categories, the topic of Chapter 2.

Human-beings who have acquired language can represent the world symbolically. Their powerful ability to generate mental constructions, both a blessing and a curse, enables them to imagine alternative futures. From this perspective, one or another type of outcome **might** occur. Identifying contingency makes it possible to 'observe' an outcome 'not happening'. This way of understanding the world is found in all human cultures. But risk thinking provides only one, historically recent, approach to visualizing alternative futures. For example, members of a culture who believe that only followers of the true faith will be saved, and that all others will suffer eternal damnation, are thinking contingently. They envisage two alternative trajectories, one and only one of which must occur, and operate a belief system concerning the control of these possible futures. But they do not look through the lens of risk.

By definition, only one of the multiple outcome types specified by a given contingency will actually occur in individual cases. Nevertheless, the others continue to exist as possibilities until one of them is observed to have come to pass. In every case, a set of envisaged alternative futures eventually narrows down into a single historical fact within the frame of the categorization system in use. Once an outcome is known, it can no longer turn out differently. It ceases to be a risk for that individual. The solidly alive patient who takes certain risks by undergoing surgery is now, unfortunately, dead. Alternatively, the same patient makes a good recovery. The stark reality of the outcome contrasts with the conjectural status of the risk. The previously envisaged possibilities reside in the human social mind, not in nature. This location gives contingencies, and therefore risks, the ethereal but also real character of 'virtual objects', as argued by Van Loon (2002):

> The problem with risk is that it does not exist without representation ... It's presence is thus always necessarily deferred. Risk is a potential coming-into-being, a becoming-real. Hence the 'presence' of a risk can never be completely objective but has to be mediated in some form.

Van Loon derives the concept of virtual object from the work of Law (1996) and Hilgartner (1992). The required consensus without which social life could not be organized around virtual objects is easily undermined. The process of 'deletion' (Law, 1996) protects these fragile but influential entities from such challenges, at least temporarily, by excluding the processes through which they were created from societal discourse.

The creation, protection, and dissolution of virtual objects can be found in any culture. Without these processes, societies could not simultaneously self-organize and respond to change. The virtual status of risks and other forms of contingency arises because they reference not what is, but what might be, or might have been. Prospectively, risks do not manifest themselves except as indicators of possible trouble ahead. By definition, the risked outcome in question has not yet happend. Retrospectively, risks can be considered to have 'existed' even if the adverse event under consideration did not actually occur. In this case, an observer who was not looking through the lens of risk would notice nothing. In contrast, as noted above in relation to all contingency thinking, a person who was thinking about a risk would 'see' an adverse outcome 'not happening'. For example, parents who leave a young child home alone for a long period whilst they go abroad on holiday are not absolved from culpability merely because the child came to no harm. They will be deemed to have committed a criminal offence of neglect. The presence of a risk cannot be disconfirmed through observation, at least in single cases.

Although risks do not map directly onto individual events, they become observable at the level of aggregation. Whilst most individuals survive major surgery, for instance, a proportion will die. Hence the hypothetical status of this risk for individuals is counterbalanced by apparent solidity when a substantial number of cases is taken into account. However, this appearance of substantiality at the aggregate level depends upon categorization, itself a mental act. As discussed in Chapters 2 and 4, observers may categorize outcomes in many different ways, each generating its own form of aggregation and distinctive risk virtual object. For example, the aggregate risk of dying during major surgery will depend upon the nature of the operation, characteristics of patient populations, the quality of care provided, and many other factors. Each of the many possible configurations will generate a different set of probabilities.

Because contingencies are concerned with possibilities, an indefinite number might be envisaged. But only a small selection can even be contemplated, let alone managed. Those contingencies which have not been thought of cannot be responded to. The following example illustrates this clinically important truism. The Butler Report (Home Office/Department of Health and Social Security, 1975) stimulated the development of medium-secure forensic mental health units in the UK. The report was initiated in response to the case of Graham Young. Whilst confined to a high secure institution, Young actively pursued his interest in poisoning, for which he had been incarcerated, borrowing library books on this topic. After being released, he promptly resumed his career as a poisoner. This tragic but blackly comic example provides a striking example of risk blindness. Risk managers can only respond to contingencies which they imagine. In turn, the selection of contingencies depends heavily on the direction of organized social life. Physically and socially remote from wider society, staff working in high-security institutions may have become oriented towards internal risks such as patients harming themselves or others on the ward. They simply did not visualize an outcome which appeared glaringly obvious from outside the social system in which they were immersed.

Contingencies which have not been conceptualized cannot be managed. On the other hand, the very mention of a previously unconsidered risk conjures it into an initially fragile existence as a virtual object. In 2009, an email was circulated to forensic mental health service providers concerning possible risks from compact discs (CDs) and digital versatile discs (DVDs). A patient had pointed out that they could be turned into sharp weapons, a contingency which service providers had never previously considered. Colleagues had thought about banning these items, but rejected this risk management response as a knee-jerk reaction, noting that no incident had ever been recorded at the unit in question. The email requested information from elsewhere as to whether others shared their concern, or knew of actual cases. This example illustrates the risk management implications of the virtual, ethereal status of contingency quite vividly. Until the risk was envisaged, it could not be managed. Once articulated, it gave rise to concern which was not alleviated by recognizing that no cases had been locally recorded. Their absence did not preclude adverse events happening in the future. Moreover, such incidents might have taken place elsewhere without information about them having spread, or might occur in the future[1].

In summary, the lens of risk provides one particularly modern way of thinking about contingency. A contingency is invoked whenever an observer considers that one outcome out of a number of envisaged alternatives will occur. Since contingency refers to what might happen, its presence cannot be disconfirmed by individual events. Contingencies, and therefore risks, do not exist as material entities. But once their presence has been recognized by a social group, contingencies generate substantive responses. This combination

---

[1] Subsequently, another email discussion concerning the risks arising from patients possessing ball-point pens took place. Once the possibility of patients using everyday objects as weapons was raised, it could be generalized indefinitely.

of immateriality with motivational potency can be represented by thinking of risks as virtual objects.

Risk's linguistic relatives

In everyday life, the term 'risk' may be chosen from a wide lexical repertoire. Alternatives, in English at least, include 'hazard', 'danger', 'threat', 'vulnerability', 'safety', 'protection', 'security', 'chance', 'probability', and 'uncertainty'. Selection of particular words draws differently nuanced attention to possible future adverse events. As noted in the Introduction, Skolbekken (1995) has perceptively observed that the language of medical research draws upon a narrow vocabulary which involves heavy usage of the term 'risk'.

The social scientific literature on risk offers a somewhat haphazard and not very illuminating mapping of this linguistic family. A major source of confusion arises from a propensity to attempt to map terminological variations against presumed intrinsic differences. This hunt for essential distinctions obscures the pragmatic force of language which subtly combines description with communication of attitude, seeking to influence as well as to describe. The same phenomenon can be labelled in different ways, depending upon the language user's stance. For example, depicting a frail older person as 'vulnerable' brings questions about their capabilities to the fore, suggesting that a **person** has a *need for protection* Fenge (2006). In contrast, expressing concern for an individual in terms of 'safety' draws primary attention to their **environment**. For instance, Vincent (2006) equates patient safety with the minimization of harm arising from medical errors. Such apparently trivial verbal choices implicitly slant the representation of risks in different ways.

The following two sub-sections offer a brief analysis of two crucial distinctions, risk-danger and probability-uncertainty. In each case, an analysis which attempts to uncover an essential distinction between phenomena will be rejected. Instead, an approach which emphasizes variations in attitude will be recommended. It will be argued that the same outcome can be described as a risk or as a danger, depending upon the speaker's stance towards it. Similarly, an outcome may be depicted as having a degree of uncertainty or of probability. But the choice of word conveys a view about the risk in question.

Risks and dangers

Some writers treat 'risk' and 'danger' as synonyms, alternating between the two merely for the sake of stylistic variety. Douglas (1992, present author's comment in parentheses) has gone further, arguing that *the idea of risk is* [i.e. ought to be] *transcribed simply as unacceptable danger*. This transcription is appropriate in modern societies, according to Douglas, because their members automatically and unreflectively interpret 'risk' as a marker of prohibition. Douglas argues in her eccentric masterpiece *Purity and Danger* (1966) that all cultures are selectively sensitive to dangers. They concern themselves with some but not other possibilities of future harm. Modern, science-based societies frame their fears in terms of risk. The collective selection of risks, however, is fuelled by cultural contradictions and structural weaknesses. In many modern societies, for example, a disproportionate amount of public attention is given to violent crimes, particularly against children, despite their rarity. Panic is fuelled by wider insecurity about dangerous others. On the other hand, carnage resulting from road accidents is collectively accepted with relative indifference. The former undermines the social order, whilst the latter merely threatens life and limb.

In contrast to Douglas, two other major social scientists, Luhmann and Castel, have drawn a distinction between danger and risk. They have both made an interpretation of the difference between these two terms central to their analysis of risk, but not in the same way. Luhmann (1993) equated risk and danger with the presence and absence of preventability. Risks, he argued, may be avoided, at least probabilistically, as in the case of smoking and lung cancer. In contrast, dangers such as runaway climate change cannot be stopped once the process has started:

> Only in the case of risk, does decision-making (that is to say contingency) play a role.
> One is exposed to danger.

Luhmann acknowledged that many intermediate cases between risk and danger, as he defined them, can be identified. However, he maintained that this distinction between the avoidable and the inevitable does not depend *on the whim of the observer*.

Castel (1991) mapped the distinction between danger and risk to a focus on individuals and populations, respectively. He argued that, since the 19th century, the orientation of health and social services has shifted from the dangerousness of individuals to risk in populations. For instance, Castel argued that, in the 19th century the perceived personal dangerousness of a mentally disordered offender might be managed through a combination of therapy and security measures. In response to the rise of probabilistic reasoning, attention began to move away from dangerous individuals. Instead, epidemiological research was used to identify risk factors in populations. Knowledge of these factors could be used to sift out higher risk sub-populations for preventive attention.

In summary, Douglas regarded risk as a modern variant of danger, i.e. culturally prescribed prohibition. Luhmann and Castel distinguished risk and danger, but in different ways. Luhmann equated this difference with the presence or absence of controllability. Castel distinguished risk from danger in relation to a historical shift of focus from individuals to populations. All three accounts offer informative insights, but seem to have lost touch with the everyday differentiation of risk and danger. Pragmatic analysis investigates the use of language to achieve the speaker's objectives. From this perspective, risks do not differ intrinsically from dangers. Instead, the pragmatic approach homes in on the communication of attitudes towards contingencies. Pragmatically, the speaker selects from a family of related words, usually without conscious reflection, in order to convey a view about how a contingency **should** be managed. Risks, according to the speaker, **may or may not** be taken. Dangers **ought** to be avoided. For example, notices saying '**Danger! Keep Out!**' convey an emphatic prohibition couched in the modern language of health and safety. The underlying message might be articulated more calmly as, 'In your own best interests, you should not take on the unacceptably high risks associated with entry'. In contrast, a notice advising that those who proceed to '**Enter at your own risk!**' is not intended to prevent entry, but to direct legal liability away from the notice writer.

Inevitably, one person's risk may be another's danger. The communication of diverse attitudes towards a contingency is illustrated by the following two quotations (Heyman and Huckle, 1993). The first invokes a prohibition on risk-taking, marked by choice of the term 'dangerous':

> **INTERVIEWER:** Would you ever let [adult relative with learning disabilities] go out on his own?
> **RESPONDENT:** No ... I would worry all the time, wondering what he is doing. It is too dangerous.
> (Research interview with carer of adult with learning disabilities)

In contrast, labelling a contingency as a risk invites consideration of its acceptance, as illustrated below (Heyman and Huckle, 1993):

> **PAID CARER:** *We are all subject to risk, and they will not learn without taking risks.*
> (Research interview with day centre member of staff)

Thus, the same contingency may be labelled as a risk or a danger, depending upon whether the speaker believes that it can be accepted in some circumstances or should be unconditionally rejected.

Uncertainties, probabilities, and risks

The second distinction to be considered as a pragmatic device involves uncertainty *versus* probability. As with the risk/danger distinction, some accounts maintain that the two terms depict different phenomena. For example,

Hacking (1975) argued that uncertainty refers to knowledge limitations, and probability to the unpredictable variability of events. This issue will be discussed in more detail in Chapter 4. The pragmatic approach suggests that the choice of term, again, conveys the speaker's attitude to a contingency. The use of uncertainty language invites a decision-making delay whilst further evidence is collected.

Notoriously, George Bush Jr. justified inaction on climate change by describing the science as 'uncertain' (*New Statesman*, 14 Jun 2007). Similarly, in the clinical practice domain, the language of uncertainty contains an implicit resonance of fools rushing in where angels fear to tread. For instance, Beach and Reading (2005) state that *uncertainty* about whether an event indicates epilepsy leads to frequent misdiagnosis. They recommend recognition of a type of ambiguous case for which reassessment *may prevent a hasty and incorrect diagnosis of epilepsy*. The other side of the same coin is criticism of the invocation of uncertainty as a rationale for inaction. For example, Williams and Sibbald (1999) discuss a *culture of uncertainty* in relation to nurses taking on primary roles traditionally performed by doctors. The authors chose the word 'uncertainty' in order to indicate that this, for them, highly desirable development is being impeded by unwarranted procrastination.

In contrast, the use of both probability and risk language invites decision-making about accepting or attempting to avoid a risk. Middleton and Curnock (1995) found that consultants working in a neonatal intensive care ward used risk discourse, paradoxically, to reduce uncertainty. They thereby legitimated their recommendations by invoking the language of risk. One consultant quoted by these authors asserted, in response to a query from a nurse manager, that there was *no question* that breast-fed babies were *at greater risk* of haemorrhagic diseases unless they were given a vitamin K supplement.

In summary, the term 'risk' belongs to a family of related terms such as danger and uncertainty, all of which can be used to describe contingencies. The social sciences have not as yet developed a coherent analysis of these lexical choices. It has been argued that they can be understood from a pragmatic perspective. Speakers convey a particular attitude to a contingency through their selection of one word rather than another. Describing a possible outcome as a danger conveys a view that it should be avoided. On the other hand, depicting the same outcome as a risk suggests that it may or may not be taken. Referring to uncertainty implies that a decision should be postponed until further information is obtained. In contrast, a reference to probability or risk contains an implicit call for immediate decision-making.

The gulf between 'taking a risk' and 'being at risk'

In this section, a crucial distinction between meaningfully taking a risk and being deemed by an observer to be at risk will be drawn. It is possible to define risk entirely behaviourally, as illustrated by the following quotation (Adams, 1995):

> Everyone is a true risk "expert" ... we have all been trained by practice and experience in the management of risk ... The behaviour of young children, driven by curiosity, yet curbed by their sense of danger, suggests that these junior risk experts are performing a balancing act.

This formulation treats risk-taking as a cultural universal. It also implies, by implication, that non-human animals who appear to balance uncertain costs and benefits should be regarded as taking risks. Whatever term is used to refer to such balancing acts, they need to be distinguished from the conscious calculation of risks, for example about whether to undergo screening. As Luhmann (1993) has argued, consciously calculative risk-taking involves second order observation, in which risk managers imagine themselves acting in alternative ways:

> Anyone who behaves riskily – who, for example, takes risks in traffic or plays with guns – may do so as a first-order observer. But as soon as he considers whether to take a risk, he observes himself from the position of a second-order observer; only then can we really speak of risk communication or risk awareness.

The distinction between first and second order observations can be mapped onto that between 'being at risk' and 'taking a risk'. The latter implies conscious selection from alternatives framed in terms of risk. For example, an individual might decide to avoid fatty foods in order to reduce their risk of coronary heart disease. The virtual character of such risk-taking can be seen at two levels in relation to intentions. Firstly, it exists independently of individual outcomes. For instance, a consumer of saturated fats who decided to ignore the health promotion line can still be said to have taken a risk, even if they never experienced a heart attack. Secondly, the person who opted to continue with a fatty diet could still be said to have taken a risk even if medical science eventually rejected the current view of dietary cholesterol as a risk factor. Status as a risk-taker is not affected by the outcome for the person in question. Nor does it depend on the validity of the beliefs on which risk management decision-making may be based. Instead, it derives from an individual's reasons for making a decision. An individual who continues to eat fatty foods and denies that this diet increases the probability of heart disease does not, in this sense take a risk. They might, however, be deemed, rightly or wrongly, to have placed themselves at risk.

None of the complexities outlined above apply to being 'at risk', a state which does not entail intention. The small linguistic difference between these two widely used phrases conceals the gulf between them. Any structured entity, including all living creatures and organized systems, may be considered to be at risk by an observer who adopts a risk framework. Thousands of species are presently at risk of extinction as a result of global warming without knowing that they face this possible fate. The population of the Roman Empire are now considered to have been at risk of lead poisoning because of the widespread use of this metal in cooking utensils and pipes. But they did not know that low level lead ingestion could harm health (Nriagu, 1983). They did not 'take a risk'.

Risk management encompasses both strategic risk-taking and concern for individuals deemed to be at risk. The latter may be rescued from fates that have never troubled them. Although conceptually distinct, risk-taking and being at risk can become confused in the course of healthcare practice. A health professional who may have grounds to view a service user as at risk, instead considers this person to be taking a risk. By eliding the former into the latter, practitioners inadvertently transfer their own risk perceptions into the minds of clients. This step frequently carries moral force. Even if the person held accountable for an actual or potential disaster did not realize that they were taking a risk, they **ought** to have done so. For example, the legal system quite rightly attributes culpability to a person who drives their car after consuming a large amount of alcohol. This person should have known that they were taking a risk, and placing others at risk, even if they sincerely believed that they could drive safely.

Health professionals who seek to help service users to manage risks occupy this delicate territory. They need to understand the world from the perspective of service users and carers who might not share their perspectives about particular risks, or risk thinking in general. Practitioners cannot understand risk-taking without seeing the world through the eyes of those who might be placing themselves at risk. On the other hand, they share the propensity found commonly in risk-oriented societies to utilize risk thinking as a guide to moral accountability. Examples of the ensuing misunderstandings will be offered in following chapters. They can to some extent be unpicked through the employment of greater definitional rigour.

In summary, it has been argued that taking a risk should be carefully distinguished from being at risk. Risks can only be undertaken, or avoided, by actors who have absorbed risk thinking, and have reflected about a particular risk.

Such reflection may become habitual, and thereby lost to conscious awareness. But it should not be confused with the balancing acts performed by non-verbal animals and pre-linguistic toddlers. The state of being at risk can only be ascribed by observers who have adopted a risk framework. This state can be attributed to actors who might or might not view their situation in terms of risk.

Risk management, managers, and ownership

The discussion so far has attempted to offer a robust definition of risk, to probe the foundations of risk in the visualization of contingency, to locate risk in a wider linguistic context, and to distinguish risk-taking from being at risk. The final section of this definitional chapter will focus on attempts to respond to recognized risks. Perhaps surprisingly, the topic of risk management has been relatively neglected in the academic risk literature, even in books focussing on health and social care. Undue emphasis tends to be placed on risk assessment, which can become an organizational end in itself (Titterton, 2005). Conceptual tools for thinking critically about risk management are not readily available. The present brief discussion seeks only to draw out some implications for management arising from the definition of risk offered above. It will consider the meaning of the related but distinctive concepts of risk management, risk manager, and risk ownership.

Risk management

Risk management is predicated on the assumption that the risk manager can control envisaged contingencies, even if only probabilistically. It entails trying to nudge a contingency so that the probabilities of visualized outcomes are changed in a favourable direction. Hopefully, negatively valued outcomes will become less likely even if they cannot be totally prevented. Attempts at primary prevention aimed at reducing the incidence of disease through trying to persuade people to modify their lifestyles fall into this category.

However, risk management choices tend to produce many effects. Dealing with only a single contingency isolates it from these multiple chains of consequences. Risk managers will usually take more than one contingency into account. But they cannot consider everything. A health professional might, for instance, weigh-up the probability of a frail older person suffering an accident whilst living independently against the chance of mental deterioration if this person was to be institutionalized. For a patient diagnosed with prostate cancer, the odds of dying from the condition have to be balanced against the chances of incontinence and/or impotence. The problem of combining qualitatively different outcomes with varying probabilities is discussed in Chapter 3. The generic definitional point to be taken from the above analysis is that risk managers tend to become enmeshed in multiple contingencies, the implications of which frequently pull them in conflicting directions.

Risk managers

Once a risk has become socially recognized as a problem meriting attention and capable of ameliorative intervention, the question arises of who should manage it. In this section, three different notions of risk manager will be differentiated: firstly that of a formally designated professional who claims expertise in risk management *per se*; secondly, that of a practitioner who views their role through the lens of risk; and, thirdly, that of any person who attempts to manage a risk on behalf of themselves or others. The third, more inclusive, formulation will be recommended, and utilized in the present book.

Power (2005) traced the origin of the formally recognized chief risk officer to the appointment of James Lam at the GE Capital in 1993. He argued that this appointment marked the birth of a new occupational class of *internal regulatory agents or merchants of norms in the competitive field of corporate governance.* The imaginative phrase *merchant of norms* evokes images of renaissance adventurers. At the same time, it suggests that the articles on sale, stripped of their packaging, turn out to be value judgements concealed in claimed risk rationality. Risk manager roles are now firmly established in healthcare systems such as the UK National Health Services (NHS). Corporate risk management, regulation, and the promotion of patient safety in the healthcare sector will be discussed in Chapters 8 and 9. Crucially, the claim to possessing expertise in risk management *per se* depends upon the acceptance of the presupposition that risk knowledge can be decontextualized. It implies that persons who know little about a substantive area such as a form of healthcare can nevertheless supply useful generic risk expertise.

Generic risk managers can be differentiated from practitioners whose roles are now pervaded by risk thinking. They have not developed primary expertise in risk management, but nevertheless find that risk thinking influences everything that they do. As argued in the Introduction, this relatively new interpretive framework shapes clinical practice in particular ways. It has generated novel ways of organizing social and healthcare systems such as clinical governance and population screening.

The broadest formulation of the concept of risk manager includes anyone who deals with risks. This definition encompasses the wider public who fund health and social services which they may need in the future, service users, carers, health professionals, corporate hierarchies, commercial

interests, politicians, and policymakers. Thinking about all of these stakeholders as risk managers avoids the presupposition that experts necessarily know
best (Wynne, 1996).

Risk ownership

Recognition that multiple stakeholders may collaborate or conflict in the
management of a risk raises the question of risk ownership. Risk management
and ownership have been insufficiently differentiated in the social science
literature. Risk owners take on, or are ascribed, accountability for the management of a risk which they may or may not manage directly. In the field of
corporate governance, risk ownership is bestowed on senior figures such as
members of the board of directors. Risk owners are assigned responsibility for
ensuring that identified risks to the organization are managed systematically
and appropriately. The differentiation of risk ownership and management
thus provides a vehicle, not necessarily effective, for centralized organizational
control.

The relationship between risk ownership and management is by no means
clearly articulated in healthcare contexts. Nevertheless, distinguishing the two
concepts provides a useful tool in the analysis of contested risk issues, as illustrated below. The following quotation, taken from a study of a UK forensic
mental health care unit (Shaw *et al.*, 2007), exemplifies the tension which can
arise between risk management and ownership particularly clearly:

> The view from the nurses is that … they have primary responsibility for security and
> risk management. But the experience of the nurses, in our group anyway, is when the
> nurses attend the MDT [multidisciplinary team], that predominance of responsibility
> seems to go to the bottom, in terms of importance and discussion … We also felt that,
> when things went wrong generally, that it would be the nursing staff that would gener-
> ally be criticised.
>
> (Research interview with staff nurse, multidisciplinary workshop, forensic
> mental health service)

The quoted respondent depicted a disjunction between ascribed risk ownership and control. According to this account, nurses are blamed for failures
resulting from risk management decisions which they could not influence.
The question of who owns a risk is sometimes disputed between service
providers and users. The following quotation (Heyman and Huckle, 1993)
illustrates such contention in the context of day care for adults with learning
disabilities:

> Every time I go to the review they keep saying it is time she got a job. But she is epilep-
> tic and could not work in a kitchen. I tell them what she is like. I should know. I made
> her. But the [day] centre don't see this.
>
> (Research interview, mother of adult with learning disabilities)

Previous risk owners may decline to take back possession of a risk which has been subsequently taken on by formal services, as illustrated by the following unpublished data:

> I mean admission into a hospital like this [medium/low secure forensic learning disabilities] can often provide release for the family. They can get on with their lives. They haven't got to be a 24 hour carer, or go down the police station, or the social stigma of every patient, and what they may have offended and done. So you've got other bairns in that period of time, and they don't want to be encroached upon by the child again.
> (Participant in staff group discussion of research findings, forensic learning disabilities hospital.)

Conceptual differentiation of risk ownership and management allows accountability for risk management to be separated out from its mode of production. Risk management can only operate effectively if tensions with risk ownership are carefully addressed.

Conclusion

This wide-ranging chapter has reviewed the definition of risk and its linguistic relatives. Social scientists have exhibited considerable reticence about the meaning of the term 'risk'. Their silence can be defended by arguing that the diversity and ubiquity of its usage has drained the concept of common meaning. However, this line of argument cannot explain why social actors utilize the same term across so many domains. Instead, risk can be understood as a compound concept which draws together four components: categorizing, valuing, uncertain expecting, and time-framing. The perception of each requires active interpretation. Their contingent status gives risks a hypothetical, virtual form. Risks reference what might happen, or might have happened.

The term risk belongs to a wide family of related terms such as danger, vulnerability, safety, and many others. A pragmatic analysis of lexical distinctions emphasizes their use as tools conveying implicit prescriptive views about a contingency. From this perspective, the terms in pairs such as risk/danger and uncertainty/probability do not depict different kinds of entity. Instead they communicate the observer's attitude to a contingency. Speaking about a danger conveys the view that it ought to be avoided, whilst talking about a risk implies that it may or may not be taken. Similarly, choosing the language of uncertainty invites delay, whilst the mention of probability or risk invokes decision-making.

A clinically significant distinction between risk-taking and being at risk can be drawn. Risks can only be taken or avoided by individuals who have consciously recognized a risk and oriented their actions towards it. Toddlers and non-human animals cannot take risks although they can behave riskily. Individuals, social groups, and other organized entities can, in contrast, be deemed to be at risk regardless of their own perceptions. But this judgement can only be made by an observer who is looking through the lens of risk.

The concepts of risk management, manager, and owner appertain to both risk-taking and being viewed as at risk. For instance, health professionals may attempt to help patients to make informed choices about a risk, or to protect individuals who are deemed to be at risk. An inclusive concept of risk manager is required. This definition recognizes all involved stakeholders, including patients, carers, and practitioners, engaged with a particular risk. The requirement for inclusiveness arises from the actively interpretive role of all persons engaged with a risk. Finally, risk management and ownership need to be differentiated. Drawing this distinction allows moral accountability for risks to be considered separately from their day-to-day handling.

The Introduction and the present definitional chapter provide the base for the material which follows. The next four chapters will consider each of the four components identified in the definition of risk in more detail. They will focus, respectively, on the social construction and selection of risks, the role of value judgements in risk thinking, inductive probabilistic reasoning, and the time-framing of risks. Subsequent chapters will locate this analysis in a wider context, considering risk and information, risk representation, risk governance and the patient safety agenda.

Chapter 2

The social construction of health risks

Bob Heyman

Aim

To analyse the social construction of health risks.

Objectives

1. To expose the role of categorization in the creation of health risks
2. To outline the cognitive and social processes which confer a sense of reality on health risks.

Introduction

The next four chapters will each discuss one of the components of risk thinking which were introduced in Chapter 1. There, it was argued that anyone using the lens of risk becomes engaged with the following intertwined mental processes: categorizing, valuing, uncertain expecting, and time-framing. Each has been subjected to intense academic and societal debate spanning many centuries. An introductory text cannot begin to do justice to this material. Nor can busy risk managers, defined broadly as anyone who takes themselves to be dealing with a risk. Typically, their engagement with categorization, values, probability, and time is based on pre-packaged, societally established specifications of particular risks. The attention of practical risk managers is directed outwards towards a risk, rather than inwards towards the nature of risk thinking. The material presented in the following four chapters will merely introduce some of the problematic issues on which risk managers cannot avoid taking a position, usually by making unexamined assumptions. The clinically important implications of this often unwelcome engagement of health care practice with esoteric philosophical issues will be illustrated through examples derived from qualitative research. The analysis of these issues will provide the underpinning for subsequent consideration of practice-related topics, such as the packaging of risk information, media representation of risks, and risk governance.

The first requisite for risk thinking is categorization, the focus of the present chapter. Unless they have been categorized, outcomes cannot be valued, predicted, or located in time. Questions about their management cannot arise. The starting point for the analysis of risk categorization offered below is the recognition of natural variability. All complex material entities, including snowflakes, fingerprints, diseases, and human-beings differ from every other example of any category in which they might be placed. Each case is unique. Inevitably, when individuals are categorized, some of this variability will be selectively disregarded. Categorization establishes an abstract mental representation of individual cases which marks them out as symbolically identical and distinctive from non-cases. These identical conceptual packages can never fully capture the diversity of the physical entities which they represent. The notion that classification can be replaced by direct consideration of the 'actual' (Smith, 2005) must be dismissed as naively romantic. Instead, a creative tension between categorization and acknowledgement of individuality may be anticipated.

It will be argued that the social construction of a risk requires the combination of categorization and consolidation (discussed below). Furthermore, categorization will be considered as a cognitive process requiring two interdependent steps, homogenization and differentiation. Homogenization involves treating cases which meet the criteria for inclusion in a category as identical for practical purposes. Differentiation, the other side of a single mental process, results from separating out cases from non-cases. Thus, categorization brands cases as both similar to each other, ignoring intra-category differences, and distinctive from 'the rest', directing attention away from similarities across categories. A contingency is envisaged when possible futures, or presently unknown, states, are represented through a set of categories defined so that one and only one must occur, as discussed in Chapter 1.

Because contingency refers to what might happen, or might have happened, an indefinite number could potentially become the focus of risk management concern. However, societies could not organize themselves to deal with risks if they attempted to tackle too many contingencies, or if risk managers did not share similar concerns. The second part of the chapter will outline some of the socio-cognitive processes through which health risk categories become socially consolidated. These processes transform a small selected proportion of the infinite number of contingencies which might be managed into 'real' risk virtual objects which demand organized societal attention. Since anything might happen, organized risk management requires a collective narrowing of attention onto some contingencies, but not others. Overall:

Risk social construction = risk categorization (homogenization + differentiation) + consolidation.

Risk homogenization and differentiation

All cultures selectively classify phenomena which matter to them, albeit in widely different ways. Without categorization, abstract thought would not be possible. But categorization comes at a cost. Differences within a category tend to be blurred, whilst dissimilarities between cases and non-cases are exaggerated. Anyone reading the alphabetic series 'A, B, C, D, E, F' followed by the numeric series '11, 12, 13, 14, 15' may note a sequence of letters followed by one of numbers. However, the third number is a copy of the second letter. It is homogenized to the category in which it is located and differentiated from its manifestation in the other series. Similarly, the second component of the two pairs given below will be heard differently, although the two cannot be distinguished acoustically from the other.

I shout, *I scream*
Lollipop, *ice cream*

The conjoint process of homogenization and differentiation would usually occur outside conscious reflective awareness. It only becomes obvious when two categorization contexts are presented side by side.

Rosenhan's famous study *Being Sane in Insane Places* (1973) provides a good health-related example of categorization shaping the views of individual cases via homogenization and differentiation. The study design required field-workers to fake a single symptom, hearing voices, which might be taken to indicate psychosis. They had themselves admitted to a psychiatric hospital, and then began to behave normally. Not one was detected. Examination of clinical notes indicated that everyday behaviour was interpreted as symptomatic of mental disorder. For example, a field worker completing observational notes was seen as exhibiting a writing compulsion. A follow-up study was undertaken at the request of service providers who challenged Rosenhan to send them more pseudo-patients. Several were identified even though none had actually been sent. The two studies illustrate the powerful impact of categorization on clinical judgement. The first study showed that service location can shape diagnosis by providing cues to category membership. Pseudo-patients were seen as having a mental disorder because they were residing in a psychiatric hospital. This sequence reverses the common sense notion that individuals reside in psychiatric hospitals because they are suffering from a mental disorder. The pseudo-patients' everyday actions were homogenized to the categorization of mental disorder, and differentiated from normal conduct. The second study illustrates the power of categorization *per se* to generate the differentiation of cases from non-cases.

Similarly, Parker (Parker and Hickie, 2007) found that 95% of a sample of teachers reported that they were regularly experiencing symptoms which would have produced a diagnosis of depression if they had been drawn to medical attention. Taken to the extreme, it could be concluded that depressed differ from non-depressed teachers only in terms of contact with clinical services. The finding raises doubts about the clarity of the boundary which supposedly differentiates depression cases from non-cases. However, critical consideration of categorization does not imply that they lack any validity, only that they cannot perfectly capture natural variation. Letters and numbers differ, even though classification can shape the perception of ambiguous symbols. The study findings summarized above do not demonstrate that the categories of psychosis and depression lack descriptive validity. But they do illustrate the powerful impact of categorization on perception.

Their nebulous status, together with the philosophical cloudiness of the notion of mental disorder, make psychiatric illnesses particularly susceptible to classification issues. The number of recognized mental disorders has expanded massively over the last century. The *Disease and Statistical Manual of Mental Disorders* (DSM) referred to 108 discrete mental disorders in DSM-1, and 287 in DSM-III-R, published in 1952 and 1987 respectively (Golsworthy, 2004). A naive observer who assumes correspondence between categories and events may conclude that new mental disorders have been discovered, or have recently developed. Alternatively, the main dynamic behind this apparent explosion of diseases can be seen to reside in the expansion of psychiatry. Closer examination of the categorization process reveals its negotiated character (Bowker and Star, 2000). For instance, Manning (2000) traced the history of diagnostic sub-classification for serious personality disorders. He documented the frequent and apparently arbitrary revisions which have taken place, and identified conflict between American and European variants. Manning argued that the international hegemony of the former may reflect the global power structure rather than superior science.

Mental disorders might seem to be particularly nebulous, and therefore susceptible to categorical revision. However, comparable questions can be posed about the classification of apparently more substantial physical disorders. For instance, cancers can be categorized in various ways such as in terms of the bodily parts affected, relevant to surgery, or the genetic processes which fuel them, appropriate for chemotherapy. Gross (2009) has tracked a range of procedures which neuro-oncologists employ in order to fit particular cases to their brain cancer templates. Radiologists may negotiate their reports by 'peeking' at the diagnosis contained in medical notes before writing up their conclusion. Conflicts between contradictory clinical information may be resolved by prioritizing some and discounting others, e.g. by treating imaging as more reliable than patient reports. Sequencing allows inconsistencies to be regarded as signs of deterioration. Discrepancies may be peripheralized by treating them as symptoms of a separate condition. Finally, neuro-oncologists could discount discrepancies as soon as they had concluded that sufficient evidence for a diagnosis had been generated. Diagnostic decisions reduced their sensitivity to further evidence. Such interpretive procedures (Cicourel, 1974) provide a means of assimilating anomalies into disease templates, and thereby affirming their correspondence with specific cases.

As knowledge accumulates, diseases may be reclassified, often through finer sub-classification, with important implications for risk management. During the 1980s a new brain disorder, eventually known as variant Creutzfeldt Jakob disease (vCJD) emerged, with its epicentre in the UK. This disease probably resulted from feeding cows on infected sheep body parts which had been sterilized at an insufficiently high temperature. Cattle became infected by their own new disease, bovine spongiform encephalitis (BSE) which, it turned out, could be transmitted to humans in a fast-acting form affecting younger people (Smith and Charlton, 2000). Before this new risk was recognized, the disease now known as BSE was not differentiated from scrapie, a condition affecting sheep which is relatively uninfectious to human consumers, and develops slowly. Similarly, HIV may be considered as a homogeneous infection or divided into sub-types. The implications for risk management are illustrated by the following contrasting quotations (Davis *et al.*, 2002):

> I know there are different strains out there and I don't want to contemplate too much, because a lot of it is to do with luck … If you get a really bad strain where it knocks you off your perch in two years, well it's just luck.
> (Research interview with HIV-positive gay man)

> I mean if you are positive and your partner is positive … then you're already infected by the virus. Yes, you [risk being] infected by other [sexually transmitted] diseases, but you've already got the main one.
> (Research interview with HIV-positive gay man, present author's additions)

In terms of a distinction presented in Chapter 1, the first respondent 'takes a risk' of being infected by a second strain of HIV, but is prepared to trust to luck. The second respondent might be considered to put himself 'at risk' of a new type of HIV infection. The discrepancy between these two perspectives can be understood in terms of alternative ways of categorizing HIV, either as a homogeneous entity or as distinctive strains. As the example of vCJD illustrates, some ways of dividing and combining the limitless variations of events may work better than others for a particular risk management purpose. Nevertheless, many alternatives will provide a degree of predictive purchase on the future in the fuzzy realm of chance. Crucially, as discussed in Chapter 4, numerical probabilities can be derived from observation for any categorization method. For instance, before the distinction between traditional CJD and vCJD was recognized, the chance of becoming located in this category would have been estimated by observing the combined rate of CJD/vCJD in the population.

Homogenization and differentiation underlie all forms of categorization. They create 'virtual' category members which appear both identical to each other and distinctive from non-members. These simplified mental representations of messily variable material events play a crucial role in risk thinking. They make outcomes countable, thereby enabling their probabilities to be derived from observation. Quantifying a frequency does not make sense unless it is assumed that included cases can be treated as equivalent (O'Malley, 2008). Anyone who counts implicitly makes this assumption. For example, counting the number of apples and oranges on a shelf allows their relative frequency to be calculated, but requires differences within each category to be temporarily ignored. Attention is momentarily directed away from distinctions between large and small, red and green apples, and so on. Reclassification would merely produce different forms of homogenization and differentiation. Although the point illustrated by this example might seem obvious, it is sometimes obscured by the power of categorization. As Lakoff (1987, quoted by Bowker and Star, 2000) put it:

> My guess is that we have a folk theory of categorization itself. It says that things come in well-defined kinds, that the kinds are characterized by shared properties, and that there is one right taxonomy ... It is easier to show what is wrong with a scientific theory than with a folk theory. A folk theory defines common sense itself. When the folk theory and the technical theory converge, it gets even tougher to see where that theory gets in the way – or even that it is a theory at all.

Estimating the probability that women of a certain age will give birth to a baby with Down's syndrome entails treating all children with this condition as equivalent, at least temporarily, for the purpose of probability calculation. At the same time, this particular risk construction draws a line between Down's syndrome and other health problems such as spina bifida. Many different classification schemes might be employed. For instance, children with mild, moderate, and severe disabilities resulting from Down's syndrome might be distinguished. Cases of the selected outcome category must be both homogenized despite their differences, and differentiated from 'the rest' irrespective of any similarities, so that rates of occurrence can be quantified. Service users do not always accept the homogeneity of official risk categories, as illustrated by the following quotations (Heyman and Henriksen, 2001):

> **Pregnant woman:** And it doesn't help, again, people making comments like, what he [acquaintance] just said, 'You could be changing someone's nappy at 21'. I mean, not all Down's syndrome are like that, are they? I have seen them walking around the town. And, apart from their visual looks, they are very intelligent, some of them.
>
> (Research interview with pregnant woman, aged 39, who opted for amniocentesis)

Although risk managers can always opt to query the specification of outcome categories, their descriptive validity tends to be taken for granted. The following statement (Heyman and Henriksen, 2001) illustrates the sense of surprise which can be generated when questions are raised about categorization itself:

> **Interviewer:** Do you talk to them [pregnant women] about Down's syndrome, about what Down's syndrome is?
> **Doctor:** No, I don't actually … interesting. And yet, of course, that is addressed in the film [provided for pregnant women], isn't it? Perhaps I should do.
>
> (Research interview with doctor who advised women about chromosomal testing)

This quotation illustrates the process of 'deletion' (Law, 1996) which obscures the collective mental processes through which categories are created. Deletion does not necessarily result from tyrannical censorship. Instead, it arises from a kind of soft power which directs attention towards events which have been packaged into categories, and away from the categorization process. Focussing on attributes of categories challenges the assumptions which underlie particular forms of healthcare. However, without categorization of some sort, risks cannot exist. High risk status arises from membership of a category in which outcomes viewed as adverse occur sufficiently often to raise collective concern.

Risk consolidation

The second main section of the chapter will consider the processes through which contingencies become established as risks which merit organized societal attention. The important question of **why** individuals, social groups, and societies select some risks rather than others for organized attention will be postponed until the next chapter.

Categorization inevitably involves simplification, achieved through the conjoint mental processes of homogenization and differentiation. The complexity of real life events can be simplified in many ways, generating alternative risk objects, depending upon how outcomes are categorized. However, risk management cannot be effectively co-ordinated unless the categorizations of social actors match up. But this requirement to align contingency visualization constrains perceptions. Bowker and Star (2000) depict the *tyrannies* buried tacitly in any social consensus about how to classify. They note an ambiguity in the much abused notion of 'transparency', which can mean both 'open to inspection' and 'invisible'. The contested 'war on terror' provides a powerful exemplar of the tyranny concealed in categories. The concept lumps together highly diverse phenomena including some but not other lethal attacks on civilians and the possession of nuclear weapons by certain states, but not others. At the same time, this label carries a powerful call to respond forcefully to the risk which it marks out.

A risk will remain no more than an insubstantial will-of-the-wisp unless it becomes organizationally and culturally embedded. Somehow, contingencies, which can only exist in the minds of observers contemplating what might happen, become perceptually transformed into apparently natural entities. They acquire an aura of materiality through the projection of the hypothetical into the external world. The processes through which a risk object may acquire virtual 'weight' have not received systematic social scientific attention. This section of the chapter offers a rudimentary taxonomy of risk consolidation processes, summarized in Box 2.1, below and then briefly explicated.

Box 2.1 Processes involved in the consolidation of risk categories

Risk factor-outcome fusion

Adversity foregrounding

Threshold setting

Risk individualization

Risk-prevention linkage

Institutional embedding

Commercial entrenchment

Iconography accumulation

Risk moralization.

Risk factor-outcome fusion

Risk factor-outcome fusion occurs when an unwanted health outcome becomes culturally bonded with a small number of precursors which are presumed to increase its probability of occurrence. Examples of the simplest binary pairings include smoking-lung cancer, dietary fat-coronary heart disease, sunshine-melanoma and alcohol-liver cirrhosis. Once linked, risk factor and unwanted outcome become parts of a unified virtual object. However, these linkages are always problematic because any number of risk factors related to an unwanted outcome can be specified (Hilgartner, 1992). Unsureness about the causal status of a possible risk factor is conveyed through the notion that individuals 'might be at risk'. This expression communicates a double uncertainty, about the harmfulness of the risk factor itself, and its impact in any individual case. Nevertheless, it carries an action call to those viewing the world through the lens of risk. For example, Hopkins and Williams (1981), writing with critical intent, identified 246 suggested risk factors for coronary heart disease in the medical literature. Potentially, every risk factor can itself be viewed as an outcome to be avoided, and analysis can be extended indefinitely. Thus, those with diets high in saturated fats may be deemed at higher risk of raised cholesterol levels. Poverty might, in turn, be considered as risk factors for a high fat diet, and so on. Big pictures of such chains are rarely presented because individual research studies and reviews tend to focus on small numbers of variables.

Unfortunately, the power of research to disentangle causal spaghetti, distinguishing causation from correlation, is limited. Randomized controlled trials, the gold standard for evaluating medical interventions, cannot be used to assess the long-term impact of environmental and behavioural variables. It is not ethical, for example, to randomly allocate children to receive life-long high or low fat diets in order to determine their impact on health! Experiments with non-human animals also raise ethical concerns. Their usefulness depends on the problematic assumption that findings can be generalized between species. Epidemiologists employ multivariate statistics as the best available alternative to randomized controlled trials. Essentially, the relationship between a selection of variables and a health outcome are assessed conjointly so that the effects of risk factors can be evaluated with allowance for others included in the study. Many thousands of multivariate health risk studies have been carried out, their robustness, apparently demonstrated by the volume of published papers. However, research conclusions are affected by the selection of variables and the ways in which they are measured. For example, a relationship between social class and the risk of ill health has been recognized for over a century, but its explanation still remains unresolved (Link and Phelan, 2004).

In relation to the present analysis, risk factor-outcome linkages can be considered as a sociological phenomenon. Societies become organized to mange some but not other of these linkages. In doing so, they background non-selected risk factors, for instance, genetic rather than lifestyle determinants of obesity (Wardle *et al.*, 2008). In addition, they downplay beneficial consequences of a selected risk factor, e.g. the role of sunlight as a source of vitamin D (Holick, 2004) as well as melanomas. The causal complexity of real life is reduced to simplified forms involving a small number of risk factors.

Adversity foregrounding

Adversity foregrounding directs concern towards those who will experience the unwanted outcome linked to a risk factor, even if they represent a small proportion of those assigned to a high risk category. This way of thinking exacerbates the bad reputation of selected risks. It emphasizes relative risk, the ratio of the rates in the 'high' and 'low' risk groups, over absolute risk, the additional proportion of the potentially affected population who will experience an undesired outcome through exposure to a risk factor.

Adversity foregrounding draws attention to infrequent or even rare events, because high relative risk can be combined with a low absolute level of risk. For example, a probability of 1:1 000 000 is double that of 1:2 000 000, but both are tiny. Notoriously, panic about the increased relative risk of venous thromboembolism drove the contraceptive pill scare of the mid-1990s (Spitzer, 1997). This panic subsided when it was pointed out that the extra absolute health risk was considerably less than that associated with unwanted pregnancy.

The mode of academic production may encourage overemphasis on relative as against absolute risks for two possible reasons. Firstly, researchers have an interest in talking up the importance of their findings so as to enhance their prospects of getting published. Once printed, dramatic findings may be cited with greater frequently in other papers than are those which draw more modest conclusions. The authors thereby earn better scores on bibliometric measures which purport to measure the importance of research by quantifying the number of times a paper is mentioned by others. Secondly, where research is funded by commercial interests such as pharmaceutical companies, emphasis on high relative risk as against low absolute risk may be motivated by the desire to increase sales of products designed to reduce it.

Crucially, adversity foregrounding brings about a metamorphosis of higher **relative** risk into an **absolute** state of perceived high risk. It 'spreads' this stigmatized status to all of those who might be affected, even if nearly all would not experience the risked outcome. It thereby casts a shadow over everyone categorized as at higher risk. It also leads to the selective playing down of the importance of other outcomes. For example, the adversity foregrounding of cannabis use as a risk factor for schizophrenia has directed attention away from other possible consequences, both beneficial and harmful. This issue is briefly discussed in the next section.

Adversity foregrounding is further illustrated below with reference to cannabis-schizophrenia and condomless sex-incurable sexually transmitted disease.

Cannabis use and the risk of schizophrenia

As documented below, only a tiny minority of exposed individuals will experience psychosis because of consuming cannabis. The adversity foregrounding of the cannabis-schizophrenia link can be seen in a UK Government policy statement (HM Government, 2008) which maintained that:

> The MRC [Medical Research Council] already supports basic research on cannabinoid receptors and also a major epidemiological study which will look at how cannabis use is associated with the development of a mental state that is high risk for psychosis.

In 2009, the UK Government, ignoring scientific advice, reclassified cannabis from category 'C' to the more serious category 'B', on the grounds that stronger versions such as skunk, now in use, posed increased risk to mental health. Policies of this sort consolidate the status of a risk factor-outcome linkage, drawing attention away from the vast majority who will not experience the assessed harm.

Epidemiological research can be used to quantify the strength of the relationship between a candidate risk factor and an outcome. However, even the strongest studies are affected by the unavoidable methodological limitations of multivariate analysis, touched on in the previous section on risk factor-outcome fusion. One large-scale, long-term prospective study (Zammit *et al.*, 2002) has assessed the relationship between reported cannabis use and future hospitalisation for schizophrenia. The researchers attempted to control statistically for a range of factors, for example urban residence and prior psychiatric history, which might have increased the probability of both cannabis use and psychosis. It will be assumed for the sake of argument that any identified 'excess' of schizophrenia cases among cannabis users remaining after these factors were controlled for was directly or indirectly caused by its consumption. Similarly, measurement problems such as treating self-reported substance use as an accurate indicator of actual consumption will be ignored so that the issue of adversity foregrounding can be highlighted.

Zammit *et al.* concluded that cannabis consumption is associated with an increased risk of hospitalisation for schizophrenia. They found that individuals who reported using cannabis heavily (>30 times over their lifetime) were

6.3 times more likely to experience this adverse outcome than those who claimed that they had never consumed cannabis. Smaller, 'dose-related' levels of relative risk were found among research participants who reported having used lesser amounts of cannabis. Among heavy users, 3.8% were hospitalized, compared with 0.6% of self-reported non-users. In absolute terms, an extra 3.2% of heavy cannabis users (3.8%–0.6%) appear to have experienced this adverse outcome.

Adversity foregrounding distributes this effect among all of those who behave 'riskily', including, in this case, the 96% who were not known to have been hospitalized for schizophrenia. The above analysis is designed to illustrate adversity foregrounding, not to commend consuming cannabis, or other legal or illegal psychotropic substances. Even a 3% increase in serious mental illness represents a major public health issue, with tragic consequences for affected individuals. Stronger versions of cannabis in current use may be associated with higher levels of relative and absolute risk. However, their long-term impact cannot yet be assessed. (The temporal dimension of risk analysis is discussed in Chapter 5.) Cannabis may have other harmful, but also beneficial, health consequences which selective attention to psychosis risk pushes into the background.

Because of the critical role of adversity foregrounding in conferring a sense of reality on risk virtual objects, a second example, involving the relationship between 'unsafe' sex and the transmission of incurable sexually transmitted diseases, is discussed below.

How risky is condomless heterosexual genital intercourse?

'Unsafe sex' provides another example of foregrounding adverse outcomes which occur infrequently, at least within the majority heterosexual population. The term has become a descriptive synonym for condomless intercourse with possibly infected partners. 'Unsafe' translates into 'dangerous', a term which carries the implicit, unexamined judgement that a risk should not be taken, as discussed in Chapter 1. However, the overall chance of an individual experiencing a serious infection such as HIV or hepatitis C from hetrosexual sex is extremely small in rich countries among the lower risk population. This claim is briefly justified below. The aim is not to recommend unprotected sex with multiple partners which would have disastrous consequences at the population level, but to illustrate the role of adversity foregrounding in the social construction of risks.

The analysis which follows will focus on the risk to an individual of undertaking a single act of genital, condomless, heterosexual intercourse with a new partner. It will be assumed that the individual whose risk is being assessed possesses no further information about the risk status of the other party[1], and is not currently infected with a sexually transmitted disease (STD). Because nothing is known about the partner, she or he might or might not be at higher risk of carrying an STD through having shared needles, engaged in commercial sex, or being a man who has had sex with men. (The relationship between information and probability will be discussed in Chapter 4.) The individual considering sexual intercourse faces risks of a number of sexually transmitted diseases including HIV, hepatitis, chlamydia, gonorrhoea and syphilis. The present analysis will consider only HIV and hepatitis C, the two most serious current sexual health risks at the population level. The following analysis refers only to the UK, and not to other countries such as those with higher infection rates and/or different pathogen sub-strains.

The chance of being infected through a single act of heterosexual genital sex, in the absence of further information, depends upon infection prevalence, the likelihood of infected persons having unprotected intercourse, and the probability of transmission per sexual act. With respect to HIV, roughly 80 000 people in the UK were living with the virus at the end of 2007 (Health Protection Agency, 2008), out of a sexually active population of 48 000 000, a proportion of around 1:600. The overall chance of a new heterosexual partner being HIV-positive is affected by a number of factors. Those who have had more sexual partners are more likely to be infected and will also appear more often as a new partner. This risk-increasing factor is counterbalanced by two others. Firstly, men who only have sex with men, about half of those infected (McGarrigle *et al.*, 2006), will not be available for heterosexual intercourse. Secondly, many of those who know that they are infected, about 70% of UK residents with HIV (Health Protection Agency, 2008), will act in ways which minimise risks to others. Thus, one of these three factors increases the risk that a given partner will be infected, whilst the other two reduce it. Their net effect will be ignored in the following rough calculation. The probability of an HIV infection being passed through unprotected heterosexual genital intercourse has been estimated as 1:2 500 per coital act for female to male transmission, and 1:1 250 for male to female transmission (Boily *et al.*, 2009). Based on these statistics, the chance of infection is 1:1 500 000 for men, 1:(2 500*600), and 1:750 000 for women, 1:(1 250*600). These crude estimates greatly overstate the risks because the findings of Boily *et al.* refer to transmission from a partner who is not

---

[1] This condition of total ignorance will occur only rarely in practice, but provides a baseline against which higher or lower probabilities can be calibrated. The analysis offered does **not** provide a guide to practical decision-making, still less, as discussed below, a commendation for condomless sex with multiple partners!

receiving virus-reducing therapy which cuts infectivity substantially (Wilson *et al.*, 2008).

A higher proportion of the population, including about 0.4% of pregnant women (Sweeting *et al.*, 2008), are infected with hepatitis C. However, even the possibility of transmission via genital heterosexual acts has not been clearly demonstrated. One study of 900 monogamous, sexually active couples with one infected and one uninfected partner ruled out sexual transmission in every case over a 10-year period (Vandelli *et al.*, 2004).

The probabilities presented above are subject to wide margins of error. Nevertheless, it can be concluded that a single act of 'unsafe' heterosexual genital sex in the absence of further information poses considerably less **immediate individual** risk than travelling in an aeroplane. But these statistics will not be found on Government websites. Foregrounding a serious consequence of a risk factor which will directly affect hardly any of those defined as at risk provides a method of attempted behavioural control. Promotion of the 'unsafe', i.e. dangerous, label is intended to reduce the frequency of condomless sex, thereby preventing the spread of sexually transmitted diseases, and the consequent increase in **long-term population** risk. This key issue will be taken up in Chapter 3 in relation to the idea of risk thinking as a form of governmentality. The media representation of risks will be discussed in Chapter 7.

If health professionals uncritically absorb adversity foregrounding, it will then colour their attitudes towards risks affecting patients. For example, mental health service users may be seen as at risk of harming themselves or others even though the vast majority will never do so, as illustrated by the following quotation (Alaszewski *et al.*, 2000):

> I see risk as a very negative thing because most of the risk that I am dealing with is the risk of people [mental health service users] self-harming or committing suicide.
> (Research interview with mental health nurse)

This perspective orients staff towards highly regulated but often infrequent adverse outcomes, discussed in Chapter 9. Adversity foregrounding casts a shadow over all of those categorized as at higher risk, even though most will not experience the adverse outcome being managed. It also leads to the selective playing down of the importance of other outcomes. In this case, the risks to mental health service users from other members of the wider community have received little attention, despite their high prevalence in socially deprived neighbourhoods (Kelly and McKenna, 2004).

Threshold setting

Thresholds provide triggers for preventive options which in practice must either be, or not be, adopted. They define a binary cut-off for the virtual presence of a risk to be registered. Lower risk levels may be treated as non-existent, even if the border between higher and lower risk has to be calibrated arbitrarily. For example, the practicalities of screening systems usually require a sifting process which divides those meriting further diagnostic attention from those who do not. Although recipients may be advised that 'low risk' does not mean 'no risk', and *vice versa*, screening pragmatics lead in the direction of their conflation. Falling below a specified threshold may be equated emotionally with the virtual absence of risk, as illustrated by the following quotation (Heyman and Henriksen, 2001):

> And if I had the serum screening test, that would let me know when it was high risk or a low risk. And if it were low risk, well, I could practically rule out having a Down's baby anyway. So that was brilliant anyway because that gave me peace of mind.
> (Research interview with pregnant woman aged 37 who underwent serum screening for chromosomal anomalies)

Conversely, individuals who screen above a threshold for further investigation may feel overwhelmed by the reality of the risk even if they have merely scraped over an arbitrary boundary. One woman quoted by Heyman *et al.* (2006) had concealed her pregnancy after learning that she faced a 1:249 chance of a fetal chromosomal anomaly such as Down's syndrome. She was offered and accepted diagnostic testing because screening had indicated that the probability of a problem being detected in her case was just above the cut-off (1:250) employed within this particular screening system:

> I'm having problems at work, as to what to wear and things, and hope that nobody notices … And emotionally, from lying to people basically … I think I prefer to do it [conceal the pregnancy], particularly because we have decided that, if the results were very bad [Down's syndrome was to be detected], we would terminate. I don't want to have to tell people that I've had a termination.
> (Research interview with pregnant woman aged 40 who underwent amniocentesis after screening at higher risk for chromosomal anomalies)

On the basis of her age alone, this woman would have been given a probability of about 1:120 of carrying a fetus with a chromosomal anomaly. Despite screening resulting in a substantial lowering of her risk, she experienced intense distress. Such acceptance of the reality of risks generated in relation to an arbitrary cut-off does not occur universally. Some of those who participated in the studies cited above challenged the dividing lines used for differentiating higher and lower risk. Nevertheless, a translation of quantity into quality can be detected. Lower and higher probabilities of an unwanted outcome, distinguished in terms of an arbitrary dividing line, become transformed into its virtual absence or presence. The pragmatic origin of this binary distinction in the requirement to either offer or not offer a preventive intervention tends to be lost sight of.

This transformation of continuous probabilities into the presence or absence of risk underlies intuitively meaningful but logically odd statements of the form 'X might be at risk of Y'. For example, the UK Alzheimer's Society (www.alzheimers.org.uk) opens a fact sheet with the question *Am I at risk of developing dementia?*. The fact sheet continues by noting that, *Many people worry that they may be at risk of developing dementia – particularly if they have a close relative with the condition.* This commonly used phrase implies that risks either do or do not exist. This notion in turn depends upon the assumption that risks possess a material existence, like cancers or infections. However, the question of whether an individual 'may be at risk' can only be answered 'yes' in relation to any contingency which cannot be ruled out as physically impossible. The intuitive meaningfulness of the double uncertainty contained in the widely used phrase 'may be at risk' derives from implicit threshold setting, as well as from uncertainty about the causal status of risk factors, discussed above. Below a certain probability level, risk may be dismissed as absent. This way of thinking gives rise to the questions of how the dividing line between the virtual existence and non-existence of a risk is to be set, and by whom.

Risk individualization

Risk individualization occurs when risk factors established from aggregate statistics are applied to specific cases. Those who are assigned to a higher risk category become transformed into personal 'carriers' of riskiness. The woman quoted below (Heyman *et al.*, 2006) was discussing her feelings after receiving the results of a diagnostic test for chromosomal anomalies which had been recommended as a follow-on to screening at higher risk:

> We kept thinking, 'Well, if it [diagnostic test] is clear … there must, it can't be just that easy. There must be a next stage they're not telling us about'. It can't be, 'Oh yes, the results are clear. You've got a healthy baby'. There must be some other news they were going to break to us.
> (Research interview with pregnant woman aged 36, who accepted chorionic villus sampling for chromosomal anomalies)

Screening located this woman in a category of women among whom 1 in 250 would carry a fetus with a chromosomal anomaly. But she, understandably, transferred this aggregated proportion to her own baby, concluding that it must have some kind of personal problem. Although not universally understood in this way, riskiness readily morphs from an attribute of populations to a characteristic of individuals. This perceptual illusion makes risks seem to possess a tangible physical presence, as if located in the minds or bodies of persons.

Risk-prevention linkage

As risks become culturally and organizationally embedded, they tend to be linked to particular forms of preventive endeavour. Perception of a risk as real does not require that risk-reducing efforts should necessarily be implemented. Risks may be taken. But risk thinking does demand that the implementation of preventive measures should be carefully considered. In consequence, risks become associated, however temporarily, with specific means of attempting to reduce them. Thus, coronary heart disease prevention has become linked to statins, as has weight control to diabetes management and high-security mental health institutions to the containment of persons who have committed 'irrational' crimes. One or more forms or preventive endeavour may become operationally paired with a particular risk, and thereby incorporated into the risk virtual object. Their efficacy then tends to be taken for granted, their disadvantages underplayed, and the potential value of alternatives lost sight of. For example, no clear evidence exists that using statins merely to reduce 'bad' cholesterol levels reduces net mortality risk (Hayward, Hofer, and Vijan, 2006; Hann and Peckham, 2010). The encoding of prescribed preventive packages in healthcare systems will be further discussed in Chapter 6.

Institutional embedding

Risks become institutionally embedded as human services take on board preventive operations which have been incorporated into risk virtual objects. A substantial segment of maternity services are now dedicated to offering prenatal chromosomal screening, for instance. Thirty years ago, such systems did not exist. Neither did medium-secure forensic mental health or genetic counselling services. Prisons provide a major source of employment in some states of the USA. Such risk-oriented organizational forms are not immune to dissolution. Few tuberculosis (TB) sanatoria or leper colonies are to be currently found. Nevertheless, organizational embedding gives further virtual 'weight' to risk objects. A price for their abandonment would be paid by those who directly maintain them and by those who service primary producers. Organizational embedding imparts a certain inertia to risk virtual objects which works against, or at least delays, their dissolution.

As risks become institutionally embedded, the threshold for recognizing the presence of risk may be driven downwards, thereby expanding the requirement for a linked preventive intervention. For example, since the 1980s, the cut-off cholesterol level for offering statins has been progressively reduced, increasing the proportion of the population recommended these drugs (Crinson *et al.*, 2007). Similar historical trends have been noted for glucose intolerance/diabetes (Shaw *et al.*, 2000) and high blood pressure (Amoah, 2003). In contrast, raising the cut-off for detecting risk reduces the demand for a service, at the expense of increasing the probability that opportunities for prevention will be missed. This would happen, for example, if the state responded to any increasing gap between life and healthy life expectancy by focussing risk management on those older people considered to be at highest risk (Tanner, 2003).

Commercial entrenchment

Commercial entrenchment is linked to organizational embedding through the development of markets supporting preventive efforts. The concealed influence of pharmaceutical companies who fund most research can easily be overlooked. It is illustrated in Box 2.2, below. Commercial companies have been accused of constructing medical risks out of everyday problems which they then link to the supposedly risk-reducing drugs which they sell.

Box 2.2 A pharmaceutical example of commercial entrenchment

Double blind randomized controlled trials offer the best available means for assessing treatment efficacy. Patients who agree to participate are randomly allocated to different intervention groups, allowing an innovative drug to be compared with the best currently available treatment. Clinical outcomes are assessed without patients or with those conducting the trial being informed about which drug (or placebo) individual patients have received until their outcome has been recorded.

Despite providing the maximum possible protection against bias, the outcomes of these studies appear to be influenced by commercial interests. Trials funded by pharmaceutical companies are more likely to show that their new drug confers clinical benefits than are those financed by disinterested sources (Yaphe *et al.*, 2001). Publication of medical research in more prestigious journals is associated with drug company sponsorship, a finding which is unlikely to result from this work being of better quality (Jefferson *et al.*, 2009).

Once drugs have been approved, risks from side-effects are less likely to be detected because adverse drug reactions (ADRs) are systematically under-reported. One review of studies covering 12 countries estimated that over 90% of ADRs were not reported, with similar rates observed for more and less serious side-effects (Hazell and Shakir, 2006).

For instance, the diagnosis of child attention/hyperactivity deficit disorder (ADHD) creates a market for drug treatments which bring new risks such as treatment-induced psychosis (Mosholder *et al.*, 2009) and anorexia (Graham and Coghill, 2008). Until ADHD became accepted as a disease entity, the question of its management could not arise. Defenders (e.g. Smalley, 2008) and detractors (e.g. Stolzer, 2005) have become locked in debate about whether a medical category such as ADHD references a real disease or a concoction falsely differentiated from common issues of everyday life. Commercial entrenchment imparts extra virtual 'weight' to risk categorizations through their promotion by powerful, financially motivated organizations.

Iconography accumulation

Iconography accumulation involves the growth of culturally shared, often stigmatizing, imagery and metaphors around a risk. Although such templates may have some statistical justification, they tend to be applied to the entire category judged at risk. For example, the image of a 'gay plague' stuck to HIV infection even though many infected people are not homosexual or bisexual men who practise condomless sex with multiple partners. Kingham (1998) traced the iconography of HIV/AIDS through analysing UK cartoons and public health advertisements and popular jokes. He concluded that the most vivid images, for instance of medieval plague and the grim reaper, were generated during a phase of the pandemic in which the general population were thought to be at risk. During other phases, relatively little imagery was produced. Thus, the most lurid iconography may be produced about risks which generate a collective sense of insecurity. This theme will be picked up in the next chapter in relation to the question of why societies concern themselves with some risks rather than others.

As well as being influenced by prevailing representations, those who interact with a risk may select from a diverse set of available imagery according to their needs. One couple (Heyman and Henriksen, 2001) experienced deep distress after deciding to terminate the woman's pregnancy when Down's syndrome was diagnosed. They used particular images of a child with this condition to support their difficult decision, as illustrated below:

> **Woman who had terminated pregnancy:** I mean you can't get away from the fact that they are ... I mean their eyes come out, they have floppy tongues ... It's just endless.
> (Research interview with woman aged 46 and her husband after pregnancy termination for Down's syndrome)

This way of visualizing the condition helped the above respondent and her husband to come to terms with a decision which left them feeling deeply distressed a year after this interview when a follow-up was undertaken. The couple did appreciate that their images of Down's syndrome were contested by others, as documented below (Heyman and Henriksen, 2001):

> **Woman who had terminated pregnancy:** I read a story. Reading this story has helped me cope with it … I think they [couple depicted in story] are bloody stupid. It's in 'Take a Break' … They look like they are really over the moon because they are having this Down's baby.
> **Husband:** I mean they will have been explained the same as everybody else as to what can happen, or what it is going to be like, and what it means for the future.
> **Woman:** They can have chest infections
> **Husband:** There's any number of things that we know that can happen …
> **Woman:** I mean they are laughed and they are scorned at.
> (Research interview with woman aged 46 and her husband after pregnancy termination for Down's syndrome)

Thus, contested images of a risked outcome may coexist, giving risk managers alternative options for its visualization. Nevertheless, the homogenization process outlined above creates a pressure towards viewing individuals in a risk category as sharing common characteristics. Prevailing iconographies of illicit drug-users, people with mental disorders, the obese, and many other risk categories provide a vector for societal control. However, such images are by no means universally accepted, or immune from historical transformation.

Risk moralization

Finally, iconography accumulation is closely linked to the moralization of risks which individuals are expected to manage responsibly. (The moral component of risk will be further discussed in Chapter 3.) Those assigned to a higher risk category may be considered culpable for placing themselves in a vulnerable position. Moralization transforms a presumed risk factor into an adverse outcome in its own right. It is predicated on the problematic assumption that individuals could have avoided putting themselves at risk. For example, the obese may be blamed for placing themselves voluntarily and visibly into a higher risk category despite the existence of evidence that individuals metabolize food differently, that appetite for food is genetically modulated, and that efforts to reduce weight can cause more health harm than good (O'Hara and Gregg, 2006). Schwartz *et al.* (2003) found that health professionals specializing in obesity were more likely than those who were not to rate an obese person than somebody with a lower body mass index (BMI) as lazy, stupid, and worthless.

Service users quickly detect such negative categorization, often communicated indirectly, as illustrated by the following quotation (Henriksen and Heyman, 1998):

> I gets booked in, you know, and she went, 'And how old are you?' And I went, 'I'm 40'.
> So she writes 40. And then she underlines it in red three times!'
> (Research interview with pregnant woman aged 40)

The 'elderly primigravida' (Aref-Adib, Freeman-Wang, and Ataullah, 2008) may be seen to have voluntarily and culpably put herself into a high risk category by choosing to give birth to her first child at a relatively older age. Moralization, typically unspoken and implicit, ignores circumstances such as fertility problems which might make entry into the high risk category involuntary. In addition, it 'spreads' the problems which will be experienced in a relatively large but often absolutely small number of cases to all category members.

Conclusion

The present chapter has explored the social construction of health risks. This process was considered to result from the combination of risk categorization and consolidation. Risk categorization involves a socio-cognitive process which combines homogenization and differentiation of alternative imagined outcomes. Thinking in terms of contingency, an observer takes the view that one of two or more outcome categories might occur in a particular case. The observer considers some of these outcome categories undesirable, and therefore as risks. Each outcome category must cover a range of possibilities because history never repeats itself precisely. Categorization makes outcomes countable, at the expense of directing attention away from variations present within a category, and from similarities between cases and non-cases. The irreducible diversity of events is replaced by common mental representations.

Outcomes can potentially be categorized in many different ways. Depending upon the view that they take, observers might or might not distinguish sadness from depression, or might subdivide a broad disease category differently, for instance. However, the need for risk management to be socially organized creates pressures to recognize the same risks. A number of consolidation processes give risks virtual 'weight', facilitating shared recognition of their reality. Outcomes may become perceptually linked to a particular risk factor, as with obesity-diabetes and cannabis-schizophrenia. These linkages provide simplified views of the limited, available medical knowledge about health determinants. They may be used to classify large populations as at risk even though many or even most will never experience the outcome of concern. The binary requirement of risk management to either offer or not offer a particular intervention may be transferred to the risk itself, which comes to be seen as existing or not existing, rather than as more or less likely. Particular preventive remedies may become linked to a health risk, as with statins for heart disease. As responses to constructed risks become socially organized, they start to be embedded in institutions, and to be caught up in commercial activities, generating vested interests. Recognized risks accumulate a cultural history and become moral issues. As a result of such processes, risks come to be viewed as natural entities. In consequence, it becomes intuitively meaningful to say that an individual 'might be at risk' even though this double uncertainty is epistemologically empty.

The analysis presented so far gives no account of why a social group or society should focus on some risks rather than others. The issue of risk selection will be addressed in the next chapter, which explores the role of values in risk thinking.

Chapter 3

Values and health risks

Bob Heyman

Aim

To analyse the role of value judgements in health risk management.

Objectives

1. To introduce the concept of valuing
2. To explore the role of value judgements in the attribution of adversity
3. To review the idea of expected value in relation to health risk thinking
4. To consider organized selective attention to health risks.

Introduction

This chapter will examine the role of value judgements in health risk management. It is the second of four chapters, each of which reviews one of the inter-related components of risk thinking, namely constructing, valuing, uncertain expecting, and time-framing. A central argument of Chapter 1 was that the lens of risk offers one variant of a more general human propensity to view the future as contingent.

Risk thinking invariably marks out at least one of the outcomes specified by a contingency as undesirable. However, such value judgements will not necessarily be shared. A frail, elderly person might feel ready to die, or parents might be happy to welcome the birth of a child with disabilities, for example. Moreover, actions generate multiple consequences. The negativity incorporated into risk thinking may be balanced by positive considerations. A risk manager's view of a risk will be shaped by their assessment of the overall picture, which may require numerous values to be combined. Such mixed blessings create a potential for positive risk-taking (Titterton, 2005), but the modern ear will always associate the term 'risk' with the identification of possible unwanted consequences.

The concept of risk has not always carried its present, overwhelmingly negative associations. The term originated from the development of merchant seafaring in the late middle ages. It derives from the Italian word *risicare*, traced to the 16th century, meaning both to venture and to dare. The related French term *aventure* refers to sailing before the wind (Schmid, 2006). Today, the concepts of 'risk' and 'adventure' have become strongly uncoupled. The language of risk now invokes concern about the potential for negatively valued outcomes to occur.

The chapter will, firstly, consider the definition of value and valuing, emphasizing the range of phenomena covered by this culturally universal human response to the world. The second section will discuss the role of value judgements in risk thinking. It will be argued that risk managers may project their values onto events, so that adversity comes to be seen as an intrinsic property of outcomes, rather than being attributed by observers. The third part of the chapter will critically review the idea of expected value, and the associated methodologies for quantifying the value of multiple consequences which might or might not occur. The discussion will highlight limitations of this approach, emphasizing the value judgements which are concealed in numerical models such as that of quality-adjusted life years (QALYs). The final section of the chapter will raise the crucial but sometimes overlooked question of risk selection. The difficult question of why social groups and societies who have adopted risk thinking point the lens of risk in one direction rather another will be raised, if not answered.

Values and valuing

Linguistically, 'value' may take a descriptive adjectival form, depict an action through a verb, or name an abstract entity through a noun. Valuing involves preferring one state of affairs over another. The adjective and noun derive from the verb. Value as an attribute and as an abstract entity both result from the mental act of valuing. Valuing may be grounded in various combinations of economics, taste, aesthetics, lifestyle choices, personal aspirations, and morality. Those who love virtue, are moved by a fine opera production, or enjoy a large steak are all valuing. Every animal demonstrates preferences, a defining characteristic of life. However, behavioural inclination should not be conflated with linguistically mediated choice.

Values may be highly articulated or embedded unreflectively in perception and action. The latter is illustrated in Box 3.1, with respect to the social psychological example of the matched guise paradigm. Consideration of this paradigm demonstrates that individuals may not consciously recognize their own values.

Box 3.1 Unconscious preferencing and the matched guise technique

The matched guise methodology (Lambert, Frankle, and Tucker, 1966) attempts to uncover unconsciously held stereotypes through comparisons of responses to social cues. Essentially, research participants are divided randomly into two or more groups. Members of each group receive the same information concerning a single target person, about whom they are asked to make judgements. As far as possible, the presentations are matched except in one respect which gives clues to the target person's membership of a particular social category. Comparisons of the average judgements made by the different groups provide an indication of the impact of the varied attribute.

Crucially, identification of values does not depend upon asking participants to state their preferences. The values which they express verbally and those implicit in collective responses can be compared. For instance, most people deny being racially prejudiced. But matched guise comparisons might show that judgements about the same performance are influenced by cues indicating the target person's racial identify.

Some work using the matched guise technique to explore health professionals' stereotypes about service users has been undertaken. Brettell (1988) asked health visitor students to make judgements about a client after hearing a recording read by an actor. The same actor read the transcript with a South-East England educated, Birmingham, Yorkshire, or Asian accent. Students, who each heard only one of the tapes, rated the Asian speaker less favourably on average. The operation of this unarticulated stereotype could influence clinical judgement, for instance in potential child protection cases. However, conclusions about unconscious values derived from matched guise studies have not proved to be very consistent, with outcomes depending upon the content of the information presented. In relation to the present focus, the matched guise paradigm provides a useful reminder about the range of phenomena covered by the concept of valuing. In particular, values may be located in actions and perceptions rather than verbally articulated.

The externalization of values

People actively bestow value on phenomena. Those looking at the world through the lens of risk impose negative value on some but not other of the outcome categories envisaged contingently. As Rescher (1983, quoted author's emphasis) puts it, people **ascribe** *values to negativities*. Shakespeare's Hamlet came to the same conclusion when he asserted that *There is nothing either good or bad, but thinking makes it so* (Hamlet, Act II, Scene ii). In consequence, the same outcome may be valued differently (Rosa, 2003). Because the concept of risk has built into it the assumption of adversity, some observers may treat a contingency as a risk whilst others do not. In addition, as discussed further below, people may simply not know how they would feel about a previously unexperienced outcome such as impending mortality.

Some value differences can be explained in terms of personal preference. But culture offers strong guidelines about what should be considered good and bad. For example, those who have internalized Western values may be shocked by female infanticide which, in effect, categorizes the birth of a baby girl as an adverse event. It is much harder to reflect critically on one's own ingrained cultural values, for instance the privileging of achievement over personal enlightenment in materialistic societies. Once the connection between adversity and valuing is recognized, it becomes apparent that risk analysis is always based on presuppositions, usually tacit, about potentially contentious issues. Adversity can appear to be an intrinsic attribute of events rather than a result of valuing only because social groups tend to share certain preferences which they take for granted. Questioning such presuppositions, or even articulating them, raises questions about the existing social order.

Both Rescher, who chose to emphasize the word 'ascribe' and Shakespeare considered that they were challenging prevailing wisdom when they located adversity in acts of judgement rather than outcomes *per se*. The opposite view is embedded in the Royal Society definition of risk (1992, present author's emphasis) as *the probability that a particular **adverse event** occurs*. If it is accepted that value is always ascribed, then adoption of the above definition entails unreflectively projecting acts of judgement onto outcomes. Such externalization corresponds with everyday experience of social consensus. To the extent that observers share similar values they can act as if adversity is intrinsically attached to outcomes rather than invoked by observers. However, when such tacit consensus cannot be correctly assumed, taking it for granted will threaten the coherence of organized risk management.

Externalization mystifies value differences because it transforms judgements into apparently intrinsic properties. In consequence, social actors negotiating the management of a risk may not appreciate that views about the adversity of an outcome differ. They may not realize that they are unreflectively imposing a particular judgement on others who do not share their values. The anti-psychiatry movement of the 1960s has largely lost momentum. Nevertheless, Laing's view of schizophrenia dramatically illustrates the potential for making a different evaluation of an outcome which others consider wholly adverse. He argued that *the cracked mind of the schizophrenic may **let in** light which does not enter the intact mind of many sane people whose minds are closed* (Laing, 1959, quoted author's emphasis). Similarly, some, but not all, deaf people regard this condition as a marker of positive identity which enables them to belong to a linguistic community of sign language users. They reject the categorization of deafness as an infliction to be cured if possible (French, 1994).

Many citizens living in secular Western societies would not wish to develop cancer or become parents to a child with disabilities. But some people, perhaps viewing outcomes from a religious framework, might welcome cancer as a test from God. Parents of children with severe learning disabilities do not necessarily regard the birth of their child as an adverse event, in retrospect at least, as illustrated by the following quotation (Oulton and Heyman, 2009):

> Her every little step she makes is just so phenomenal. And what grace she's got. And, ah, she's just a complete delight all the time.
> (Research interview with mother of daughter with severe learning and physical disabilities)

From this perspective, the achievement of relatively tiny developmental goals became a source of intense pleasure. The parents who participated in the study, by no means a representative sample, all valued their relationship to a severely disabled child highly positively. One mother welcomed the continuing nature of her shared life with a child who would never grow independent. Others framed their experience as a religious or secular challenge to be embraced, as illustrated below. The following powerful quotation portrays caring for a child with severe learning disabilities as offering a rare opportunity to transcend the limitations of Western secular society:

> There aren't many opportunities in twentieth century life in England to be a good person unless you seek it out. And, like a missionary or something, so caring for somebody, and the experience of loving somebody who is different and damaged, and has certain problems, is a very rewarding experience for me personally ... It's a bit like Calvinism. You actually begin to feel as if you're of the elect, and of a very small banded set of special people who are different from everybody else ... It's very dangerous to feel superior to other people. That's why you have to fight it.
> (Research interview with the father of daughter with severe learning and physical disabilities)

By viewing his caring role as offering a *terrific personal journey*, this father inverted the culturally standard interpretation of the birth of a child with severe learning disabilities as a highly adverse event.

If negativity is seen as an intrinsic, measurable property of outcomes, the potential for individuals to value outcomes differently may be overlooked. The presence of such unrealized variations of perspective can fuel overt or concealed conflict. An outcome which counts as a risk for one person will not necessarily do so for another. This dynamic is illustrated by the following extract from a research interview concerning prenatal chromosomal screening (Heyman and Henriksen, 2001):

> **Pregnant woman:** [Hospital doctor] just seemed to think that if I was in that age group I had to have the test [screening for chromosomal anomalies such as Down's syndrome]. And I said, 'Well, what is the point? Even if the test comes back that the baby's Down's, I'm not going to do anything. And, on the other hand, the baby may be healthy, and I may have a miscarriage [from amniocentesis]'. But I couldn't get through to [the doctor]. A just plain headache was turning into a migraine. And [doctor] said, 'Well, I can't just let you go with that. You'll have to talk to the consultant'. And I thought, 'Oh God, I've got to get out of here now'. I said, 'I'll take the blood test then', you know – 'Will that keep [the consultant] happy?' But it's not very, em [accurate]. It's just an indicator whether to take the other test really isn't it?
> **Interviewer:** So it wasn't for you, really, that you had it?
> **Pregnant woman:** It was for [the doctor].
> (Research interview with woman aged 38 who underwent screening for chromosomal anomalies)

This untypical encounter resulted in a patient being pressurized to undergo unwanted screening. Although the procedure requires only a blood test, and does not entail additional direct risk, this woman might have ended up located in the higher risk group for whom diagnostic testing is recommended. If she had declined to undergo amniocentesis she would have been left in a higher-risk limbo throughout the rest of her pregnancy. Service users are not usually subjected to such overt pressure. But they may be more subtly influenced by the organization of services around the prevention of particular risks, as illustrated below (Heyman *et al.*, 2006):

> **Pregnant woman:** Well, I've got a [dating] scan on the 16th of September, and I don't see the midwife until after I've been to the scan. I would only see anybody if I did go for the triple test. That is the only time you see anybody in between …
> **Interviewer:** And how are you feeling about the scan?
> **Pregnant woman:** I can't wait. I will feel better when I go to the scan, because I just can't wait to see something on that screen, because you still don't feel like you are [pregnant].
> (Research interview with woman who declined screening for chromosomal anomalies)

The maternity service provided during the early stages of pregnancy was organized primarily around the prevention of Down's syndrome. Women who chose not to undergo screening were inadvertently excluded during this period. The value judgement that giving birth to a baby with Down's syndrome ought to be avoided is implied by the very provision of a screening service. Although women are given the explicit option of declining to be screened, they have to push against this tacit pressure in order to do so. The quoted respondent appeared to regret the lack of contact which would have helped her to affirm the reality of her pregnancy.

Multiple consequences and expected value

Two ideas can be carried forwards from the last section: firstly, that social actors may ascribe differing values to an outcome which some view as adverse; and, secondly, that these differences tend to be obscured when culturally prevailing values are unreflectively externalized. The analysis will now be progressed by taking into account multiple more or less likely consequences.

The starting point for the analysis of multiple consequences is the observation that any action, including those designed to manage a risk, will generate many effects. For example, prostate surgery might: reduce the long-term risk of dying from cancer; cause more or less pain during a shorter or longer recovery period; create new risks of dying in surgery, and of post-operative impotence and incontinence; and come at a cost to the health service. These consequences will have different probabilities of occurring, take effect over different timescales, and affect different people. Crucially for risk management, causal connections mediated by probability and time draw together qualitatively distinctive consequences. Focussing on merely one risk such as that of dying from prostate cancer with and without surgery excludes other important considerations, providing an inadequate guide to risk management. But the inclusion of multiple consequences raises difficult issues as to how the list of those to be taken into account is to be specified, and how net benefit can be assessed. Despite these difficulties, decisions about the provision and acceptance of health care interventions have to be made. Acknowledgement of this practical necessity should not stand in the way of recognizing the problems which the inevitability of multiple consequences generates.

Cost-benefit analysis (Nord, 1999) provides a quantitative methodology for choosing the best of an available set of options involving multiple consequences. Its claims will be critically scrutinized below. Sassi (2006) provides a useful introduction to the history and mathematical meas ures such as QALYs. The main focus of the present discussion will be critical analysis of the usually implicit assumptions which underpin them.

Box 3.2 The essential steps in cost-benefit analysis

1. List choices in a specified decision-making domain
2. For each choice, list its consequences
3. Work out the expected value (utility) of each consequence by multiplying its positive or negative value by its probability of occurrence
4. Take into account temporal trajectories and time-discounting
5. Add up the expected values associated with each choice in order to measure its overall expected value
6. Select for action the option which turns out to generate the highest overall utility.

The complexity of the mathematics used to calculate QALYs indicators of expected value should not be confused with the clarity of the thinking on which they are based (Carr-Hill, 1989).

Wolff (2007) states that cost-benefit analysis offers a *surprisingly simple* way of deciding, e.g. whether a life saving safety measure should be implemented. However, he goes on to discuss associated complex issues, reviewed in following sections. The simplicity of cost-benefit analysis might be depicted more accurately as 'apparent' than as 'surprising'. Operationally, cost-benefit of any kind can be broken down into the steps outlined in Box 3.2, above.

The rationality of expected value calculations

Eight problems affecting expected value calculations are listed in Table 3.1 below. The difficulties shown in bold will be considered in the present chapter. The others are reviewed elsewhere in the book. In brief summary of the latter, values shape the construction of outcome categories, without which risk

Table 3.1 Difficulties associated with the concept of expected value

1. The influence of values on risk construction (Chapter 2)
2. **Consequence selection**
3. **Value incommensurability and direction**
4. **Value fuzziness and dynamics**
5. **Value/probability combinations**
6. **Personal and moral values**
7. Values and multiple probabilities (Chapter 4)
8. Values and multiple time frames (Chapter 5)

virtual objects could not exist, as discussed in Chapter 2. Values influence the selection of one of the many different probabilities which can be derived from data about the same risk, as explained in Chapter 4. They may influence the setting of temporal boundaries, in the absence of which expected value cannot be calculated, and affect the nature of any time-discounting, both considered in Chapter 5. The other issues listed in Table 3.1 will be reviewed below.

Peterson (2007) concludes from careful consideration of just one of these issues, that of combining qualitatively distinctive values (e.g. pain and reduced mortality risk) in a cost-benefit calculation, that *our present theories of rationality are not sufficiently well-developed.* Unfortunately, cost-benefit calculations are equally undermined by each of the other problems listed above, and, no doubt, by others. However, health risk managers cannot afford the luxury of philosophical despair. They must make recommendations as best they can. Expected value calculations provide a rough and ready guide to risk management decision-making, but require a whole raft of assumptions to be accepted. A critical approach does not call for abandonment of the methods enshrined by the discipline of health economics. Rather it leans towards the adoption of a becomingly modest attitude, so often lacking, towards their potency. Difficulties arise particularly when expected values are expressed in terms of single numbers rather than profiles. The complexities listed in Table 3.1 will now be briefly reviewed.

Consequence selection

Everything which happens is causally connected to everything else, however remotely. In principle at least, the beating of a butterfly wing might trigger a cataclysm at a remote time and place by tipping a finely balanced natural system in one direction rather than another. Health care interventions, like all events, create potentially unlimited chains of causality stretching far into the future, together with feedback loops between them. But risks can only be made calculable by focussing, wilfully, or without conscious awareness, on a small proportion of the indefinitely large number of causal ripples arising from an event. Specification of the consequences to be considered, a necessary preliminary to measuring expected value, entails selection of those which are to be included in the cost-benefit calculation.

In practice, formal risk management usually starts with a metaphorical blank sheet of paper on which contingencies are listed before their probability and value can be assessed. Titterton (2005), advises health and social care professionals to *identify possible outcomes/benefits and disadvantages* for the individual, family and friends, the service, and others. This recipe usefully reminds risk managers that the contingencies associated with an action line potentially affect many different parties. It does not provide any explicit guidance about what criteria should be used to *identify* outcomes, benefits, and disadvantages. The open-ended specification for the category of *others* contained in the above recommendation reflects the indefiniteness of the consequences to be taken into account. Titterton (2005) has argued for a value-based approach to risk analysis. Risk management options cannot be assessed by empirical means alone because criteria for choosing consequences must be drawn upon before observation can start. Peterson (2007) concludes that *there might be more than one way to construct a list of attributes for a given decision problem*. He also asserts that writers who recommend quantification of expected value across qualitatively different consequences *are not aware of the problem*. The sometimes non-transparent processes through which consequences may be unreflectively selected into or excluded from the risk analysis agenda are illustrated in Box 3.3 below.

Box 3.3 The aims of forensic mental health services. An example of implicit consequence selection

The Department of Health (2007a) prescribed three aims for medium-secure forensic mental health services, cited below.

1. Providing ... specialised assessment, treatment, rehabilitation and after-care services for offenders with mental health problems or those at risk of offending, thereby seeking to reduce the distress associated with mental health problems ..., with reduction of risk of harm to others

2. Promoting better services for the client group by teaching, research and development

3. Working closely with other health, local authority social services, non-statutory and criminal justice agencies to reduce and manage the risk posed to others by the client group.

The first aim encompasses two adverse consequences affecting this client group: firstly, that they may experience mental distress; and, secondly, that they may harm others. The third aim, however, focusses solely on reducing the harm *posed to others* after discharge. Carrying forwards the risks posed to others, but not to self, curtails the consequence list. It thereby generates a specific construction of discharged forensic mental health service users as a risk to others which excludes consideration of risks to their own well-being.

Service providers tend to be oriented towards a specific range of consequences, such as medical outcomes, and work-related issues like litigation risk and service overload. Patients and carers who are living with health problems are more likely to consider the personal impact of illness and treatment on their wider lives. The following quotation, drawn from a study of diabetic patients' perspectives (Watson and Heyman, 1998), illustrates concern about a consequence which could not be anticipated in a generic risk analysis:

> Well, with being an insulin dependent diabetic, I can't get my PPL [private pilot's licence], and I think that's probably the hardest thing about it.
> (Research interview with man with diabetes)

The example presented below documents the interpenetration of medical risk and wider concerns in relation to the fitting of a colostomy bag. It is drawn from an unpublished case study[1].

The lady who risked exploding

Julia, a single woman in her 40s, had been diagnosed with early anal cancer, and informed that immediate surgery would offer her a 90% chance of survival. She was told that she would have to rely on a colostomy bag for several months, and that she faced a 50% probability of needing to wear one permanently. Julia was particularly worried about loss of sexual attractiveness, a risk which she raised with her consultant who had not mentioned it:

> **Consultant:** We would expect you to continue with your normal life.
> **Julia:** A fully normal life? ... Apart from having sex and living that kind of normal life ... which I assume I won't be able to do?
> **Consultant:** No, we would – I think once your undercarriage has healed up –
> **Julia:** ... I was looking forward to finding out the name of the whole business.
> **Consultant:** Perineum is the posh word.
> (Transcript of medical consultation at which surgery was discussed)

The (female) consultant's reticence and resorting to euphemisms did not deliver reassurance. Julia communicated worry about loss of attractiveness much more intensely in a subsequent research interview:

> **Julia:** I think it's [colostomy is] the most hideous and revolting thing, and I don't want it.
> **Interviewer:** OK.
> **Julia:** However, I would prefer to live.

---

[1] The author would like to express thanks to Anthony McGrath, currently at the University of Bedfordshire, and to the patient whose case is discussed for giving permission to utilize this data.

Interviewer: OK.

Julia: I'm not so sure you know. I don't know if I would prefer to live with no sex life. And I don't know if I would ever be able to persuade a man to fuck me, excuse my language, with a stoma. Would you [male interviewer?] [Long pause]

Julia: I really don't know because it's really bad news.

Interviewer: Right, apart from the sexual aspects, is there anything else?

(Research interview with patient shortly before surgery)

The male interviewer, an experienced colorectal nurse, displayed as much reticence as the female consultant quoted above about addressing this issue. The patient, perhaps responding to this double experience of non-communication, dealt with her personal risk concern in a way which put herself at considerable clinical risk:

Julia: So I just left the hospital the day after the operation and came home ... and had sex with my boyfriend ... I'd absconded from the hospital without telling anybody, and [thereby] really upsetting them.

(Research interview with patient following surgery and recovery)

The nurse interviewer commented that the patient's insides might have 'exploded' as a result of her having sex so soon after an operation. This case study illustrates, admittedly in a stark form containing an element of black comedy, the main theme of this section. Gaps between the narrow reach of any risk analysis and the unending chain of consequences which it segments cannot be avoided. A specific cost-benefit calculation can shed only limited illumination on the indefinitely large range which might be taken into account. Some concerns which matter to patients may be firmly but unreflectively excluded from the risk assessment agenda.

The first step in expected value calculation, the identification of consequences for risk analysis, raises problematic issues. The following sections will consider the additional difficulties associated with adding up the components of expected value, given that the list of consequences to be considered has somehow been specified.

Value incommensurability and direction

Risk managers have to weigh-up qualitatively different consequences which are connected by their certain or probabilistic association to a possible action. The net gain or loss in expected value resulting from interventions with multiple consequences can only be calculated by deciding on the relative value of each. The relative value of a miscarriage and giving birth to a child with Down's syndrome, or of death from prostate cancer and impotence, for instance, cannot be objectively determined. The terms of trade between consequences need to be calibrated with reference to the values of those who are affected.

Consequences may differ not only in their specific content and probability, but also in their 'direction'. In other words, the same action can have different consequences for a variety of social actors. For example, the immunization of children reduces not only their own probability of being infected by diseases such as measles, but also that of others. At the same time, immunization is associated with a very small risk of brain damage to the recipient. Hence, risk managers have to weigh-up costs/benefits to the child and to others (Wroe et al., 2005). Similarly, patients with TB may stay healthy after terminating treatment prematurely, but at the expense of stimulating the evolution of drug-resistant strains which affect others (Ormerod, 2005).

Value fuzziness and dynamics

Because values are ascribed by people, rather than residing intrinsically in outcomes, consequences can only be calibrated by measuring subjectivity. A range of methods for attempting to measure subjective value have been developed. Only one, the standard gamble, will be outlined for illustrative purposes. Other measures include direct questions, expert judgements, and indirect inference from observation of the money which individuals or societies actually spend in order to reduce a risk. In standard gambles (Nord, 1999), survey participants are asked to indicate the probability of an outcome such as immediate death, which they would accept in order to remove a health problem, for example pain. Acceptance of higher probabilities is taken to indicate that removal of the health problem has greater value for an informant.

In the same way, pregnant women considering screening for Down's syndrome can be asked what probability of a miscarriage they would accept in order to be certain that their fetus did not have this condition. One study using a related approach concluded that Chinese women living in Hong Kong considered the birth of a child with Down's syndrome 2.75 times worse than losing a fetus through invasive diagnostic testing (Chan et al., 2006). Taking this finding at face value for the moment, it would follow that, for example, a 1:100 probability of losing the fetus due to amniocentesis would equate, for these women, to a 1:275 chance of giving birth to a baby with Down's syndrome. As it happens, these relative values correspond roughly to those embedded in current prenatal screening systems. The probability of diagnostic testing causing a spontaneous abortion is considered to be about 1% (Alfirevic, Sundberg, and Brigham, 2003). Diagnostic testing is usually recommended for women whose chance of a chromosomal anomaly is estimated as greater than 1:250–1:300, depending on screening system design.

Health economists use techniques such as the standard gamble to calculate average 'exchange rates' between qualitatively different consequences. As with any other average, they do not depict the characteristics of individuals who may ascribe adversity differently. Even more seriously, the meaningfulness of hypothetical questions about imagined but never experienced health states must be questioned. Individuals may simply not know their personal trade-offs between qualitatively different values (Peterson, 2007). Perhaps for this reason, survey results concerning public attitudes to healthcare interventions are strongly affected by minor changes in question wording (Ubel, 1999). Respondents who have not experienced a health problem can value interventions behind *a veil of ignorance* (Nord, 1999). But their responses to hypothetical circumstances will be more or less meaningless. On the other hand, those who have encountered a health issue may become lobbyists for pumping resources into its management. They cannot know how they would have valued prevention before they were affected.

As well as being often fuzzy and ill-defined, values are not fixed and may change in response to encounters with health problems. Experiencing disability or the diagnosis of a terminal illness inevitably changes attitudes. Nobody can know with certainty how they would feel in presently hypothetical circumstances. For instance, Menzel *et al.* (2002) cite evidence suggesting that patients rate a long-term condition as less severe than do members of the general public, perhaps because patients learn to make the best of their circumstances. The incorporation of such adaptations into expected value calculations would perversely reduce the utility of risk-reducing interventions.

Service user perspectives should be treated respectfully. Nevertheless, their limits need to be considered. For example, patients who have not experienced aggressive surgery cannot know with any certainty how unwell they would feel afterwards. Papagrigoriadis and Heyman (2004) found to their surprise that patients with later stage colorectal cancer expressed an overall preference for receiving radical surgical intervention aimed at cure even if they were advised that their chance of survival would be increased only slightly. The potential for regret needs to be acknowledged, undermining the credibility of measuring value through patient testimony about the future. In this case, patients who die soon after painful surgery may come to wish that they had used their final span of life differently.

Value/probability combinations

Outcomes may vary both in their value and in their anticipated likelihood of occurrence. The validity of value assessments, critically discussed in the last section, will temporarily be taken for granted, along with the selection of consequences, so that the issue of combining value and expectation can be scrutinized. In general, a more likely desired result will be preferred over a less likely one and *vice versa*. However, all is rarely equal. Risk managers may be faced with weighing up consequences which differ in both probability and value.

Quantitative procedures for tackling this problem such as the estimation of QALYs rely on multiplying values by probabilities. This multiplicative step is illustrated by the following simple examples:

Expected value 1 (death) = $-1000 \times 0.01 = -10$

Expected value 2 (pain relief) = $+20 \times 0.5 = +10$

The above formulae might apply to surgery which carries a 1% (0.01) risk of mortality with a subjective value of -1000 and a 50% (0.5) chance of relieving chronic pain, with a value of $+20$. They indicate that a particular or average patient rates death in surgery 50 times worse than continuing to experience pain. Multiplication of probability by value gives the same expected value, negative and positive respectively, for these two consequences. In this case, the costs and benefits of undergoing surgery balance out exactly. In the jargon of decision theory, the above expected value calculation indicates that whoever made this judgement is 'indifferent' to the two options of undergoing or declining surgery.

But like is not being compared with like. The whole calculation process relies on the assumption that patients will equate a lower probability of a highly adverse outcome with a higher probability of a less severe one. Unless this presupposition is made, the calculation of expected value becomes extremely complicated, if not impossible. Its acceptance is not justified by evidence, but driven by the requirements for calculability. For example, some risk managers may view low probability catastrophic events as worse than more likely but less severe ones (Renn, 2008). On the other hand, very low probability outcomes may be dismissed as virtually non-existent, leading to the conclusion that individuals are not at risk, as noted in Chapter 2 in relation to the commonplace notion that somebody 'might be at risk'. These complications have received little research attention, perhaps because they throw a spanner in the extensive works of health economics, subverting faith in 'metrics'[2].

Risk and moral values

The multi-attribute approach to expected value takes an implicitly 'consequentialist' approach to decision-making (Cranor, 2007). This approach assumes that the value of a choice derives entirely from the results of its implementation. According to Piaget (1965), very young children also adopt a consequentialist

---

[2] In 2009, NICE relaxed its cost-benefit requirement for end of life drugs, thereby recognizing the greater value of time for those with little remaining. This shift, a response to public pressure, adds yet another complication to simple multiplicative utilitarian models.

view of morality. For instance they consider it naughtier to accidentally cause a lot of damage than to deliberately cause a smaller amount. Older children will differentiate between intentions and results. The UK National Institute for Health and Clinical Excellence (NICE) and the huge army of health economists who seek to evaluate health care interventions by quantifying their consequences are not reverting to early childhood! Their investigations are confined to a specific context in which resource limitations dictate that healthcare priorities must be set. Nevertheless, an exclusive focus on 'what works' can obscure the role of moral judgements in risk management. Nord (1999) attempts to banish morality from QALY judgements as follows:

> Broadly speaking, the utility of a health state is the same as the "goodness" of it to the individuals who are in it. By goodness I thus mean the well-being or quality of life associated with the state. (Note that goodness in an ethical sense is not implied).

The above description excludes a key ingredient of valuing, its penetration by moral judgement (Erikson and Doyle, 2003). Taken to its logical conclusion, the consequentialist approach generates conclusions about healthcare which most people would intuitively reject. For example, medical researchers might be able to save millions of QALYs for arthritis sufferers by performing experiments on 1000 babies, each of whom would face a 1% chance of dying as a result of their participation in the research. Despite, the prospect of a huge net health gain at the cost of a mere 10 deaths, this proposal seems immediately and obviously unacceptable. Moral intuition conflicts with utilitarian calculation. It can be argued that this moral intuition is simply mistaken. Alternatively, it can be maintained that such reductions to absurdity demonstrate the limitations of the simple forms of utilitarian reasoning built into expected value formulae. Such proposals do not have to be dismissed because they will not be envisaged. However, the obviousness of their unacceptability derives from a taken-for-granted 'common sense' which requires analysis. Closer inspection suggests that an outrageous proposal to sacrifice babies and current medical practice cannot be sharply separated.

Reviled totalitarian regimes such as Nazi Germany sanctioned experiments in which Jewish and other victims were sacrificed in the cause of scientific progress. Democracies have also risked lives in the cause of knowledge, for example when military personnel were deliberately exposed to fall-out from nuclear explosions. The practice of randomized controlled trials provides a more subtle and currently plausible example of moral tension between the rights of individual patients and the collective benefits derived from extending medical knowledge. Because patients have only one life, they may well opt for a new treatment of a terminal illness if they think that it might improve their survival chances. However, healthcare systems which adopt new treatments too readily will end up investing in large numbers of useless or even harmful interventions.

A collective, long-term interest in ensuring that medicine is firmly evidence-based conflicts with the immediate needs of patients who might be offered promising treatments. But the underlying value judgement about the balance between individual and collective benefit remains undebated because it is concealed behind the myth of 'equipoise' (Fries and Krishnan, 2004). Official accounts maintain that the expected values of treatment alternatives assessed in a randomized controlled trial should be roughly equal. This condition would hold true if, for example, an innovative drug treatment for a terminal illness might do as much harm as good. However, it is difficult to see how equipoise could apply when the possibility of cure, or at least a long period of remission, is balanced against inevitable rapid death.

Following through on a strictly consequentialist perspective would imply that health resources should be concentrated on groups with greater life expectancy, including the young, women, and the middle classes. For instance, women living in developed societies experience a longer average life expectancy than men. All else being equal, curative interventions such as expensive cancer treatments should, therefore, generate more added QALYs for these groups than for men. If the worthiness of interventions was assessed solely in terms of their net consequences, it would follow that more healthcare resources should be directed to women than to men. This logic applies both to the approval of publicly funded treatments and to decisions about providing them in individual cases. Such a proposal seems almost as intuitively absurd as the baby sacrifice example outlined above. Its rejection illustrates the unspoken mental work over and above the calculation of expected value which goes into health economic assessment. Bodies such as NICE do not make such recommendations, and indeed would not dare to do so. Their judgements take into account unspoken moral assumptions.

The influential 'fair innings' argument (Williams, 1997) provides a rights-based alternative perspective to the brutal but only partly practised logic of consequentialism. Every individual is considered to be entitled to enjoy a minimum number of QALYs. Society cannot guarantee this distributive outcome, but can do its best to achieve it. One QALY advocate (Nord, 1999) has attempted to incorporate distributive justice into the quantification of expected value. The 'fair innings' position generates its own contested implications. For instance, it could be argued that men should receive a greater amount of healthcare investment than women in order to compensate them for their lower life expectancy. More plausibly, but still controversially, a case could be made for investing more in saving or improving the lives of younger people on the grounds that the elderly have had their turn (Nord, 2005). Even if a societal consensus of this sort could be reached, it would pose new questions for the calculation of expected value. An additional set of conversion factors between absolute health gains and equity would have to be established.

Furthermore, the moral dimension of value judgements cannot be reduced to the single, possibly quantifiable, issue of distributive justice. Valuing in practice combines numerous utilitarian and ethical considerations. The specification of the latter is inevitably mediated by historically evolving cultural processes. For instance, the murder of a child in the UK and similar countries triggers major media attention, whilst the death each week on the roads of several children is calmly accepted as a fact of life. Further moral complications arise from the intersection of voluntariness and consequence direction (Breakwell, 2007). Risk-taking viewed as optional may be considered more acceptable if judged to affect only the risk-taker. But these judgements are riddled with problems. For example, some risks, such as those which motorists cause to pedestrians forced to inhale exhaust fumes, do not attract societal censure.

Consequentialism as expressed in health economic models obscures ethical debates about rights and desserts. Such considerations demonstrate that the *surprisingly simple* appearance of cost-benefit analysis mentioned by Wolff (2007) conceals extraordinary complexity. Maintaining the façade of simplicity preserves a sense that health risks are quantifiable, transforming their evaluation into matters of science. It removes resource allocation from the arena of political debate, allowing a fragile consensus to be maintained. But it also obscures necessary critical discussion.

Risk selection

The second main section of this chapter will consider the influence of values on the selection of risks as objects of organized concern. Societies and social groups do not give equal attention to all the risks which might trouble them, appearing strangely indifferent to some whilst seeming to worry disproportionately about others (Douglas, 1966; Van Loon, 2002; Hacking, 2003). Risks are not usually selected via conscious decision-making. Rather, their existence as virtual objects emerges out of societal processes which result in 'successful' risks becoming institutionally embedded. Others are simply ignored or neglected until, perhaps, the flow of history brings them into greater prominence. Health risks such as the so-called modern epidemics of depression, autism, and childhood hyperactivity present themselves as 'problems' to which health care systems become geared to respond.

Given that risk selection itself tends to be taken for granted, the question of why societies and social groups concern themselves with some risks rather than others can easily be overlooked. Risk managers become immersed in dealing with particular risks which appear to present themselves as material entities. The phenomenon of societal risk selection, a central concern for the student of risk, may seem rather obvious once it is thought about. However, the concept needs to be carefully unpacked.

Identifying organized risk selection bias

The idea of organized risk selection must be qualified to take into account perceived differences in expected value. All else being equal, more serious risks should attract greater societal resources. The charge of risk selection hints at discrepancies between expected value gains and quantities of preventive endeavour. For instance, it might be anticipated, not necessarily correctly, that more money would be spent on preventing global pandemics than on avoiding middle-aged hair loss. By implication, a society or social group accused of risk selection is seen as giving more or less attention to certain risks than their severity and preventability merit. Such judgements can only be made comparatively. On the one hand are the gains in expected value anticipated from available management strategies for two or more risks. On the other hand are measures of the effort put into prevention in each case. Discrepancies between these two series provide a marker of risk selection bias.

For example, campaigner Georgina Brown won a high court ruling (later reversed) requiring the UK Government to give more attention to the risks posed by pesticide residues to people living in the countryside (*The Guardian* newspaper, 15th Nov 2008). Instructively in relation to the present theme of risk selection, the court based its ruling on the detection of incongruity between the protection afforded to bee-keepers and rural residents. This state of affairs is more accurately depicted as risk selection bias. Its detection requires differences in expected value gains to be filtered out from comparisons of responses to different risks. However, the difficulties inherent in the assessment of expected value, discussed above, make the detection of health risk selection bias problematic and open to contention. Furthermore, because expected values can be calibrated differently, its assessment can itself be regarded as biased. Notoriously, for instance, drug manufacturers attempt to downplay risks allegedly posed by their products.

Little empirical work into health risk selection bias has been undertaken, perhaps because researchers have mainly focussed on particular risks. Such research explores specific risks singly, but does not address the question of why certain risks and not others are being addressed. One exception to the more general neglect of risk selection bias, a paper evaluating the legal classification of psychotropic substances (Nutt *et al.*, 2007), is outlined below.

The risk severity of psychotropic substances

Most countries attempt to restrict the consumption of certain 'drugs' which are considered to place their consumers at risk of physical and/or mental harm, although the specifics vary from country to country. The very term 'drug' raises categorical issues as it implicitly excludes substances such as alcohol which are legally used to change mood. The same word is used to depict pharmaceuticals, often similar to banned substances, which are prescribed by doctors. The UK and other countries classify illegal drugs into three categories, A, B, and C, in terms of the physical, mental, and social harm which they supposedly cause, with 'A' the most serious. Categorization of substances affects both the legal penalties for consumption, and the amount of societal effort invested in prevention.

The ground-breaking study undertaken by Nutt *et al.* (2007) attempted to assess the overall harm caused by a range of 20 banned and legal substances. Three types of harm, physical, mental, and social, were considered. Each was divided into three sub-categories: physical into acute, chronic, and intravenous; mental into 'intensity of pleasure', and mental and physical addiction; and social into intoxications, and social and health care costs. Two panels of experts rated each substance on these nine types of harm, with the ratings summed to give an overall score. Obvious difficulties with this methodology, mostly unavoidable and acknowledged by the authors, can be identified. Reliance on expert opinion implicitly locates adversity in events rather than in individuals' variable value judgements. Overall harm was quantified by simply adding up scores for these qualitatively distinct outcomes. Potential benefits were not considered, tacitly excluded from the risk analysis agenda. Ironically, 'intensity of pleasure' was considered as harmful. Consequences intrinsic to substance use and arising from societal responses were not distinguished. Thus, widespread availability of needle exchange systems would reduce, at least, the risk of infection from this source. A substantial proportion of the damage caused to self and others from illegal substance consumption arises from criminalization. For instance, it has been estimated that 750 000 arrests were made for cannabis possession in the USA during 2006 (Coghlan, 2009).

Having measured harmfulness as best they could, Nutt *et al.* identified major discrepancies between it and substance legal classification, although the category A drugs heroin and cocaine were ranked first and second on both counts. Barbiturates, which are prescribed by doctors, were closely followed in fifth position by alcohol. Cannabis, currently a category B drug in the UK following its upgrading from category C in 2009, at 11th place, was rated less damaging than smoking, which came ninth. Defenders of this upgrading can argue that stronger varieties of cannabis such as skunk do far more harm than traditional ones. Whatever view is taken, the work summarized above illustrates both the complexity of the reasoning on which judgements of risk selection bias must be based and the resulting uncertainties[3].

Explaining organized risk selection bias

It was argued in the last section that the identification of risk selection bias is by no means straightforward. Differences in value gains expected from alternative risk management interventions have to be taken into account. Greater organized attention may be given to a risk simply because the belief prevails that it can be tackled particularly cost-effectively. Unfortunately, for the reasons outlined above, the assessment of expected value raises a number of difficult, if not intractable, issues. The analysis will now be taken forward through consideration of why risks may be given more or less attention than warranted by the utilitarian considerations built into risk thinking. Doubts about the measurement of expected value will be temporarily set aside so that this issue can be addressed.

Even if incongruence between expected value gains and risk management attention can be demonstrated, it does not follow that the observed discrepancy results from deep-seated psychological, societal, or cultural processes. Policy-makers and opinion formers such as the mass media may have simply failed to take on board the evidence about a particular risk. In this case, they may be expected to forcefully respond as soon as scientific conclusions are drawn to their attention. Official reactions, in developed countries at least, to research documenting the risks arising from smoking perhaps falls into this category.

Differences in societal risk attention may result from particular historical processes which become difficult to reverse once established. Hacking (2003) makes this point, noting the contrast between France which has embraced nuclear power and Germany which has not. A self-sustaining process in which research leading to the development of therapies results in the expansion of service provision, and encourages more research, can bring a particular risk to increasing prominence, as has happened with breast cancer (Booth *et al.*, 2007).

---

[3] In October 2009, Professor Nutt was sacked as chairman of the UK Advisory Council on the Misuse of Drugs for criticizing current drug classification. In the ensuing heated debate about the proper relationship between science and government policy, the fragility of the former was grossly underestimated.

Effective lobbying by groups championing patients with a particular condition may kick-start this cumulative process. On the other hand, deeper forces, in this case linked to gender, might be involved.

Risk management priorities may be set by administrative fiat, particularly in hierarchical bureaucracies such as the UK National Health Service. However, top-down attempts to drive organizational change often fail to take root. For instance, regulatory pressure to reduce UK accident and emergency waiting times, through the use of a star rating system, transferred delays to elective surgery (Bevan and Hood, 2006) and even ambulance waits. This system has subsequently been modified. Nevertheless, its dysfunctionality illustrates the power of regulation backed by incentives to shape risk selection, all too often with unintended consequences. Risk and regulation will be further discussed in Chapter 8.

Risk selection in social scientific theories

The identification of more deep-seated reasons for organized risk selection bias implies the presence of powerful inclinations to recognize or ignore certain kinds of risk. Such biases tend to be detected and accounted for retrospectively rather than predicted. Notoriously, events which have already happened can be explained in many different ways. The whole range of social scientific theories, not just those which specifically address risk, can be called upon. For example, a Marxist would explain risk selection in terms of the implications for the means of production. The manufacture of new conditions which require expensive pharmaceutical interventions provides an obvious example. In contrast, a classical psychoanalyst would relate risk selection to unconscious inner conflicts and anxieties. The attention given to individually horrific but statistically rare cases of serious child abuse could be explained in this way. Douglas (1966) offers an account which similarly emphasizes emotional factors, but in relation to weak points of particular cultures, rather than to psychodynamics. She argued that the small-scale 'primitive' cultures studied by classical anthropologists use powerful beliefs about pollution and taboo in order to shore up fault lines in their fragile social order. Such devices are mostly not needed in larger, more complex societies. But images of pollution may be invoked even in modern societies in response to marginal individuals such as discharged prisoners and mental health patients who cannot be readily fitted into prevailing social structures (Douglas, 1966).

Risk theories provide a variety of explanations for deep-seated organized risk selection bias. The positions of three such theories are briefly outlined below, for illustrative purposes only, rather than to offer comprehensive coverage.

Beck's risk society thesis has stimulated considerable controversy in relation to the issue of ecological determinism. However, the powerful image of

science-based societies collapsing under the weight of unintended consequences remains compelling even if it lacks sociological correctness. Beck
(1992, quoted author's emphasis) anticipates that *in its mere continuity industrial society **exits the stage of world history on the tip-toes of normality, via the
back stairs of side-effects.*** This analysis sees side-effects of valued technologies
ignored until too late. Their damaging consequences, magnified through
unpredictable interactions, eventually force themselves to societal attention.
In a healthcare context, the accumulation of resistance to antibiotics provides
an illustrative example. Their widespread use in intensive farming and over-
prescription to humans may eventually be paid for through accelerating a
catastrophic collapse in the recently won power to control bacterial diseases.

The governmentality approach derives from the work of Foucault (1991). It
focusses on the negotiation of social power, analysing the historical evolution
of the *diverse ways in which we may govern the conduct of others **and** ourselves*
(O'Malley, 2008, quoted author's emphasis). Written with hyphenation,
'govern-mentality' fuses the notions of sovereignty and interpretive framework. Social power is understood, transmitted, and legitimated within systems
of ideas. According to governmentality theorists, social power is always located
in multiple sources which interact dynamically.

Risk thinking has provided the foundation for a new technique of governmentality which fuses a focus on the relatively new idea of population with a
call for self-governance. Statistical analysis of population data provides the
grounds for 'responsible' personal self-management guided by epidemiological findings. This mentality directs societal attention towards risk factors such
as diet and exercise which individuals can supposedly control for themselves;
and away from larger-scale issues such as poverty, inequality, and pollution.
Neo-liberal emphasis on the responsible individual is balanced by light touch
regulation of organizations (Power, 2007). For example, the Healthcare
Commission for England and Wales, which existed from 2004 to 2009, was set
up on the principle that it should be *risk-based to make it more effective and to
reduce unnecessary burdens on business* (Commission for Healthcare Audit and
Inspection, 2009). The light touch approach reduced the amount of attention
bestowed on risks caused by healthcare organizations themselves. (Following
the global financial meltdown, and also recurrent UK tragedies involving systemic child protection failures, the attitude expressed in the above quotation
might seem to belong to a bygone era.)

Risk systems theory (Luhmann 1993; Japp and Kusche, 2008) will be discussed in greater detail as it provides particularly useful insights into risk selection in healthcare systems. This approach focusses on the ever increasing
differentiation of roles in modern societies. For example, a modern hospital

depends upon the collaboration of literally hundreds of occupational groups, including doctors, nurses, radiologists, physiotherapists, laboratory technicians, information scientists, administrators, accountants, catering and security staff, cleaners, and many others. Greater role differentiation enables an organization or society to maintain a wider range of specialist expertise, thereby overcoming the limitations of individual learning capacity. This type of social evolution is required if the constantly accumulating stock of expert knowledge is to be maintained and developed.

Increased role differentiation produces two unintended consequences. Firstly, it complicates the task of co-ordinating the growing number of roles, as discussed below. Secondly, it weakens central authority because each sub-system organized around a specialism becomes more and more dependent on a greater number of others. According to systems theorists, modern societal preoccupation with risk itself derives from the uncertainty arising from this weakening of central authority. (Pessimistically, it could be argued that increasing complexity dooms societies to eventual self-destruction as co-ordination problems expand exponentially out of control. The near collapse of the global financial systems in 2007 perhaps provides a harbinger of this fate. In the same way, looming climate change confirms the prescience of the version of the risk society thesis summarized above. Unfortunately, these two types of failure, one derived from the evolution of human societies and the other from the limitations of nature, are now combining. Their interactions appear set to reinforce each other in the near future, creating massive, unmanageable risks to human health.)

Risk systems theorists argue that members of sub-systems employ different interpretive frameworks which generate distinctive risk virtual objects. In consequence, interactions between sub-systems are characterized by endemic misunderstandings because each is oriented to differently constructed risks. Anyone who has worked in a multi-professional environment such as a hospital or a university may recognize this predicament. It is illustrated by the following quotation from a study of multidisciplinary communication in a forensic mental health service (Shaw *et al.*, 2007):

> I think it's always been too medically centred, you know. The medical profession, they are the ones that make the decisions. If you are lucky, they'll ask your opinion. I mean, obviously, there are variations across consultants, but, you know, there is a constant battle. And it's not just consultants. I mean the registrars and the senior house officers will come in and make decisions that are, you think, 'Hold on. You've known someone for six minutes. We have been working with them for a year. We might have a different idea'.
>
> (Research interview with psychologist working in a forensic mental health service)

The quoted respondent felt that doctors viewed patients from a solely medical perspective, and were therefore blind to other frameworks for understanding their problems. The quotation illustrates the disorder which can arise from the selection of parallel but distinctive risk objects in sub-systems within the same organization. Cross-institutional collaboration poses even more severe problems.

Critics of Luhmann's system theory have argued that it's portrayal of barriers to risk communication are overstated (Van Loon, 2002). However, systems theory proponents do not argue that co-ordination across specialities cannot be achieved, only that it tends to break down. This approach offers an important insight into risk selection bias. Self-organized groups may, without realizing it, orient themselves to different risks, each generated by a specialized role. Moreover, risks which cut across the foci of service sub-systems tend to be under-detected. For example, some drugs used to treat heart disease can trigger dermatological conditions such as psoriasis (Mrowietz, Elder, and Barker, 2006). This risk may not be recognized by health professionals who specialize in coronary medicine. Such trans-system risks remain largely unexamined because most research is confined within disciplinary boundaries.

Comparing theoretical explanations of organised risk selection bias
Comparison of theoretical perspectives such as the three outlined above can generate new insights into risk selection bias. In brief, the cited strand of Beck's risk society thesis emphasises the overlooked build-up of side-effects into catastrophes which can no longer be ignored. Luhmann's system theory explains risk selection bias in terms of historically increasing societal role differentiation. Each sub-system selects a distinctive set of risks, thereby impeding overall functional co-ordination. According to the governmentality perspective, societal risk selection provides a means of attempting to achieve social control. However, governmentality theory, like the risk society and systems approaches, also points to disorganising processes which disrupt prevailing risk selections. Prevailing forms of governmentality are weakened and eventually brought down through combinations of historical social change and their own internal contradictions. For example, as discussed at length in chapter 4, risk thinking as a form of governmentality is undermined by tensions between the individual and the aggregate.

Reflection on possible causes of societal risk selection bias yields important insights for health care practice even though a multiplicity of processes can be speculatively proposed. Risk selection is bound up not only with the evidence-based estimation of expected value, but also with deeper, ill-understood social forces which periodically convulse the apparently stable tectonic plates of organised risk selection. Healthcare practitioners need to appreciate the concealed fragility of the risk ground on which they tread.

Conclusion

Thinking about a contingency in terms of risk inevitably points to some kind of undesired outcome. The adversities which the lens of risk highlights do not reside intrinsically in events themselves, but in the value judgements which individuals make about them. However, risk thinking does not deal solely with negativity. Actions designed to manage risks, like any other, bring about multiple consequences. Assessing them will usually require consideration of numerous qualitatively distinctive consequences, valued positively and negatively. Their probability of occurring and temporal significance will also vary, and must be taken into account. The task of validly summing overall expected value can only be performed with difficulty, if at all. It requires the conversion of qualitatively distinctive outcomes into the terms of a common virtual currency.

The social science of risk highlights the organized selection of risks. Since contingency, whether or not viewed through the lens of risk, refers to what might happen, there is no limit to the number of possibilities which could be considered. Some but not others become locked into place as social groups organize themselves to deal with those which they have collectively chosen to recognize and respond to.

Challenges to the prevailing societal prioritization of risks rest on a conviction, warranted or unwarranted, that risk management efforts and potential expected value gains do not match up. For example, those who believe that alcohol causes more harm than cannabis may seek to explain why the latter but not the former is illegal. Discrepancies between expected value gains and risk management effort do not necessarily arise from organized bias. Risk managers may have simply lacked knowledge of available evidence. Particular risks may be currently emphasized or ignored for historical reasons which become difficult to reverse. On the other hand, risk selection bias may result from more deep-seated causes. Unfortunately, any number of psychological, sociological, and anthropological explanations for such bias can be put forwards retrospectively.

Healthcare professionals attempting to help service users to manage risks cannot resolve all these issues. But they can question the allocation of resources to the management of particular risks. In addition, they can appreciate that risk prioritization is influenced by organizational processes as well as by evidence-based appraisal of expected value.

Chapter 4

Health risks and probabilistic reasoning

Bob Heyman

Aim

To critically analyse the use of probabilistic reasoning in health care contexts.

Objectives

1. To differentiate uncertainty from randomness
2. To distinguish predictive from causal risk analysis
3. To uncover the heuristic (rule of thumb) foundations of probabilistic reasoning
4. To draw out some implications of the probability heuristic for health risk management.

Introduction

This chapter will explore the role of probabilistic reasoning in health risk management. It is the third of four chapters, each of which reviews one of the interrelated components of risk thinking identified in Chapter 1, namely constructing, valuing, uncertain expecting, and time-framing. Probabilistic reasoning provides the crucial ingredient which differentiates risk thinking from older ways of attempting to manage future contingencies, such as consulting oracles, or fatalistically accepting divine will.

The present chapter will raise questions about the nature of probabilistic reasoning, and discuss the implications for health risk management. The chapter is divided into two main parts. Firstly, the concept of probability will be explored in relation to the associated ideas of chance, uncertainty, complexity, and expectation. The starting point for the analysis to be developed will be a challenge to the distinction between probability and uncertainty. It will be argued that probabilities represent projections of uncertain expectations onto the external world. One source of such expectations, inductive probabilistic reasoning will then be discussed in more detail because of its key role in healthcare risk management. This method of developing expectations depends upon assigning outcomes to two or more categories, and then observing their rates of occurrence. Two limitations of this procedure will be documented: its reliance on the past as a guide to the future; and its assignment of probability statistics derived from categories to their individual members. The status of inductive probabilistic reasoning will be demoted to that of a useful heuristic (simplifying rule of thumb). The heuristics used by members of the public in an attempt to grapple with probabilities will then be further demoted to the status of heuristics about heuristics.

The next part of the chapter will draw out three non-obvious implications of this analysis for health risk management. Firstly, it will be shown that many probabilities of the same outcome can reasonably be derived from evidence. Individuals can choose from these alternatives, exercising some control over chance simply by managing their receipt of information. Unfortunately, they cannot determine their personal outcome in this way, although they can influence their healthcare options. Secondly, it will be demonstrated that inductive probabilistic reasoning encompasses entire categories of people, such as those with a higher body mass index (BMI), or those who consume cannabis. All the members of a high risk category become sucked into risk management endeavours even if most would not have been personally affected if left well alone. Thirdly, it will be argued that preventive efforts based on inductive probabilistic reasoning can themselves weaken the evidence base for risk management. Individuals, social groups, and societies who have put in place risk-reducing measures can only reassess what would happen without these measures by taking the now new risk of at least partly abandoning them.

The nature of probabilistic reasoning

The Royal Society (1992) definition of risk as *the probability that a particular event occurs during a stated time period, or results from a particular challenge* has been cited several times as its terms are recast into matters of interpretation. The text elaborates the notion of probability as follows: *As a probability in the sense of statistical theory risk obeys all the formal laws of combining probabilities.* The linguistic clumsiness of this sentence in a generally well-written document perhaps reflects unconscious unease about its clarity. The quotation conveys an aura of scientific precision by invoking 'laws', and, by implication, abstruse mathematics. But it glosses over the question of what 'probability' actually means. Hájek (2008, quoted author's emphasis) related the following anecdote in illustration of the same point:

> Once upon a time I was an undergraduate majoring in mathematics and statistics.
> I attended many lectures on probability theory, and my lecturers taught me many nice

theorems involving probability ... One day I approached them after a lecture and asked him ... '**What is probability?**' He looked at me like I needed medication, and he told me to go to the philosophy department.

Debate about the nature of probability has continued since the 17th century (Hacking, 1975). Ironically, an aura of mathematical rigour has been attached to a concept which is used to encode imprecision. Exactly predictable outcomes, such as the timing of sunrise, do not need to be thought about probabilistically. Instead, probability is applied to outcomes which cannot be accurately foretold at the individual level, e.g. in relation to survival after major surgery or the presence of a condition flagged up through screening. Patients may be told that 'they' face a 10% chance of dying during surgery or of giving birth to a baby with Down's syndrome. What they and health professionals would really like to know is whether an adverse outcome will occur in their particular case. Unfortunately, medicine, like other disciplines applied outside the laboratory, rarely offers this degree of precision. As discussed below, probabilistic reasoning sheds some light on the future. But a price has to be paid for the illumination gained in terms of inescapable acceptance of simplifying assumptions. However, the perspective provided by probabilistic reasoning can easily be projected outwards. In consequence, individuals included in a high or low risk category may seem to 'carry' this riskiness as a personal attribute.

Chance and uncertainty

The quintessential exemplar of probability involves games of chance, with which the concept has strong iconic associations. For example, if a fair die is thrown, its probability of landing with the number six uppermost is $1:6 = 16.5\%$. But what does this mean? In everyday terms, it might be said that the six specified possible outcomes occur randomly. Their relative chance of happening can be determined empirically by throwing a die many times, observing the outcomes and calculating the proportion of each. This 'evidence-based' statistic would closely approximate to the long-run probability providing that a sufficiently large number of observations were made. It would show that the die was a fair one, or perhaps that it was biased towards certain numbers.

The following example provides a slightly less obvious, apparently contrasting, example of probabilistic reasoning. A driver who is totally lost in the middle of a strange city approaches a large roundabout containing six exits. Completely uncertain which way to go, the driver takes the first exit which turns out to be the right one. It makes good sense to say that the driver made a random choice. Its correctness can be put down to luck. Although involving the same odds of 1:6, these two examples seem intuitively different. Hacking (1975) in his widely cited and excellent history of probability maintained that probabilities can take two forms, illustrated by the examples outlined above. 'Aleatory' probabilities describe outcome rates which remain constant even though their sequence varies irregularly. 'Epistemic' probabilities express strength of belief. A popular science book about chance (Casti, 1992) goes further, equating irregularity with randomness:

> Roughly speaking, we can identify two main sources of the uncertainty we want to banish from our everyday lives: randomness and imprecision.

However, imaginatively removing the limitations of standard human observers shows that the distinction between randomness and imprecision is more apparent than real. A super-powered robot could, in principle, anticipate the results of dice throws with perfect accuracy. Concealed roulette computers with sensors allow punters to predict outcomes sufficiently accurately to make a profit over a casino, or so it has been claimed (www.selmckenzie.com/roulettecomputer.htm):

> Using a range of sensors, a roulette computer measures the speed and deceleration of the wheel and ball to predict where the ball is most likely to land. If the roulette computer has been designed correctly, they enable predictions that are clearly accurate enough to overcome the house edge. This means the user can consistently beat roulette.

The quoted website does not claim perfect accuracy, merely to tilt the odds in favour of the punter. Whether or not this claim is justified, it illustrates the illusory nature of the distinction between aleatory and epistemic probability. For mere humans, the results of spinning roulette wheels and other outcomes of complex physical processes can only be predicted by applying the laws of chance. However, enhancing predictive power transforms the same phenomenon into an epistemic one. In principle a robot might predict roulette wheel outcomes with perfect accuracy, banishing chance. What changes is not the behaviour of the roulette wheel itself, but the observer's knowledge about it's motion. The only difference between the lost driver and fair die examples given above is their relationship to 'normal' predictive power. The driver could have navigated correctly if he had possessed sufficient information, whereas an ordinary observer could not have predicted the outcome of a fair die throw. Above the level of quantum particles[1] at least, the attribution of randomness entails no more than the projection of uncertainty onto the external world. As Bedford and Cooke (2001) conclude, drawing on the idea of Winkler (1996), *the distinction between these* [aleatory and epistemic] *uncertainties is of a more practical than a theoretical significance.*

---

[1] Risk analysis offers no more than a cookbook approach to the future behaviour of large, complex objects. Notions of randomness drawn from quantum theories can only be applied loosely and metaphorically within the realm of risk thinking.

Historically, advances in scientific knowledge narrow the scope of 'chance', as the uncertain becomes more predictable. For example, proponents of personalized medicine seek to remove randomness from the prediction of drug reactions. Its advocates hope that genetic markers can be used to indicate which patients will benefit or suffer side-effects. The full achievement of this feat would transform 'random' outcomes into 'determined' ones. Even its partial accomplishment would narrow the domain of chance, confining it to variations which could not be predicted in terms of identified genetic factors.

This reframing of chance as the projection of uncertainty can be seen most clearly with respect to unknown outcomes which have already happened. For instance, a pregnant woman who has undergone non-invasive but inaccurate screening tests might be told that her 'personal' probability of carrying a fetus with chromosomal anomalies such as Down's syndrome is 1:100. But the chromosomal status of the fetus was determined at conception. Despite its existence as a historical fact, the outcome of the binary contingency 'chromosomal anomaly/no chromosomal anomaly' can be thought of as a matter of chance. However, its 'random' status is merely metaphorical. This transformation of uncertainty into chance, the central feature of risk thinking, is imposed by the lens of risk. Its implications for health risk management will be explored below.

Bayesians, taking their cue from the famous 18th century mathematician Thomas Bayes, view probabilities as expectations justified by evidence (Suppes, 1994; Heyman, Henriksen, and Maughan, 1998). The conceptualization of probability as the projection of uncertainty onto the world put forwards in Chapter 1 reflects a firm commitment to the Bayesian view. The notion of projection is intended to convey the additional idea that, in risk-oriented societies, expectations about the future based on counting past outcomes tend to be perceptually transferred to events. Hence, the lens of risk morphs uncertainty into randomness. From a critical perspective, framing probability as uncertain expectation refocuses attention on risk analysts' knowledge and beliefs about outcomes. Similarly, risk thinking projects categories (Chapter 2), values (Chapter 3), and time frames (Chapter 5) onto external events. Through the lens of risk, these categories are experienced as intrinsic attributes of unknown outcomes rather than of the risk manager's relationship to them.

Randomness and independence

Everyday outcomes are not determined randomly. Instead, they result from interactions of forces which preclude accurate prediction on account of their complexity. Despite their non-randomness, outcomes may occur more or less independently of each other. For instance, a fair die does not 'remember' its previous behaviour. The result of the next toss is not affected by its predecessors. Providing that the assumption of independence holds true, probabilities can be combined using the 'laws' referred to in the Royal Society document quoted above. The rule of addition allows probabilities of alternative outcomes to be summed. Thus, the chance of a fair die throw producing a 5 or 6 is given by adding their individual probabilities (1/6 + 1/6 = 1/3). The rule of conjunction enables the combined chance of independent outcomes to be calculated through multiplication. Hence, the probability of obtaining two sixes with a pair of fair dice equals 1/36 (1/6 × 1/6).

The uncoupling of randomness from event independence draws attention to the crucial role of the latter. The laws of chance will not provide a useful approximation for complexity unless it is true that knowledge of one outcome does not allow the occurrence of another to be predicted more accurately. The lens of risk tends to blur this issue because it leads metaphorical wearers to view separate events as inherently random, and therefore automatically independent. The clinically significant problems which may arise from uncritically assuming the independence of health outcomes are illustrated by the case, discussed below, of Sally Clark who was falsely imprisoned for murdering two of her babies as a result of flawed statistical reasoning.

Does the occurrence of two unexplained cot deaths imply murder?

Sally Clark died tragically in March 2007, possibly through suicide. After spending several years in prison, she was released when her conviction for murdering two of her children was quashed by the Court of Appeal. Her trial was heavily influenced by the testimony of Professor Sir Roy Meadows who had advised the court that the probability of a second, unexplained natural cot death in a family was about 73 000 000:1. A review of the case estimated that this probability was actually 200:1. Meadows calculated the probability of two cot deaths occurring by chance by squaring the probability of one such death, estimated to be 1:8 600. (Similarly, the chance of throwing two sixes with fair dice is given, in this case correctly, by $6^2 = 36$, as noted above.)

The enormous discrepancy between 1:200 and 1:73 000 000 can be explained in terms of the combined impact of two separate errors in probabilistic reasoning, involving confusion about time-framing and statistical independence. The former will be considered in Chapter 5. In brief, a crucial distinction must be drawn between the probability of **two** and of a **second** unrelated event. Given that one unexplained death is known to have occurred, the chance of a second one is only 1:8 600. At the time when the second death is observed, the first one has already been observed, and is not a matter of chance. Similarly, the chance of getting two sixes from a dice throw is 1:36, but only 1:6 after the first 6 has become history.

Secondly, if the probabilities of two events are positively associated, then the conjunction (multiplication) rule does not work because the outcomes are not independent. Knowledge about the first outcome should change the expectation about the second. Linkages of this sort will occur if cot deaths are caused by factors such as unknown inherited genetic problems which remain constant across births to the same parents. If families who have suffered one cot death from unexplained natural causes are 43 times more likely to experience a second one, then 1:200 (8 600/43) families who have suffered one such death would experience another one. Meadows referred to the chance of two unexplained cot deaths. This formulation would exclude known causes such as identified genetic problems, but not unknown ones. Chance operates in just this zone of knowledge limitations.

Meadows was struck off the medical register for unprofessional conduct. He was reinstated after appealing on the grounds that his expert testimony, although flawed, was given in good faith (Samanta, 2006). He was considered to have erred by straying from medical to statistical matters about which he lacked expertise. However, the mistakes which he made relate to the philosophy of probability rather than to the technicalities of statistics. Furthermore, medical and statistical knowledge cannot be disentangled as medicine engages increasingly with risk. Health professionals cannot afford to take the meaning of probability for granted. This issue is considered further in the next section.

Inductive probabilistic reasoning

The belief that an outcome is more or less likely to occur can be grounded in expectations derived from a diverse range of sources, including detailed knowledge about a single case and introspection about one's own intentions. For instance, a woman's belief that she is at risk of domestic violence might be based on personal knowledge about her partner. A student's anticipation that she will 'probably' work on her assignment this evening does not derive from statistical analysis, but from an assessment of her level of determination. Such expectations may incorporate quantification of degree of certainty. For example, a social worker might feel '90% certain' that a child is being abused by a family member. An alternative explanation is not ruled out, but would be surprising. Probability quantifications do not necessarily depict the results of exhaustive statistical analysis. They may communicate an approximate degree of uncertainty. However, the central case in the health care domain involves inference from observed frequencies, discussed below.

As noted in the introductory chapter, the complexity of the human organism mostly precludes health outcome prediction for individuals. On the other hand, the existence of large quantities of humans allows the past occurrence of all but the rarest outcomes to be reliably counted. Expectations can be grounded in previous experience on a large scale. For example, the probability of dying before a certain age such as 70 could be estimated by counting the proportion of these deaths occurring within a large sample. Individuals might be told that 'their' risk of experiencing this fate is the same as the observed proportion. The epidemiological estimation of risk is based on this form of thinking. Although practically useful, it is predicated on two fundamental fallacies. The fallacy of inductive reasoning is committed when it is assumed that because a type of outcome has occurred in the past, it will therefore happen in the future. The ecological fallacy is committed when a property of a category is attributed to its individual members.

Logically, it is not true that outcomes will necessarily recur. Historical observation will provide a good guide to the future, providing that relevant background conditions have not changed. All swans were considered white until Australia was discovered. In the case of mortality, the assumption that the future reproduces the past can easily be challenged. Death rates for people aged less than 70, for instance, cannot be observed for people who are presently younger than that age. Applying the rate derived from the recent past to younger people entails assuming that death rates found in an older generation also apply to them. Acceptance of this assumption enables life expectancy statistics to be calculated for young people, but is obviously problematic.[2]

Inductive probabilistic reasoning requires acceptance of the ecological fallacy as well as the fallacy of induction. A contingency is first constructed by developing a set of outcome categories defined so that every case must fall into one and only one of those specified. A human-being might die before their 70th birthday or still be alive on that date, for instance, as already discussed. The specification of the contingency channels the possible futures of an individual younger than this age in two directions. Their probabilities of travelling down one or the other of these paths can be estimated by observing their past relative frequency. Even if the *ceteris paribus* (all else being equal) assumption necessary for inductive reasoning holds true, the further problem associated with the ecological fallacy would remain. The quantification of probability requires the assumption to be made that individuals 'carry' the rate observed in the category to which they belong. Each person will die after living for a fixed span of time which can be measured precisely in retrospect. Risk thinking projects multiple possible futures which coalesce into an actual outcome only after the event is observed. But this projection of a collective distribution of fates onto individuals remains virtual, as argued by Luhmann (1993):

> Probabilistic calculation has frequently been used in an effort to provide the present with a consensual basis on which decisions can be made. However, such calculations

---

[2] The current yawning financial pension shortfall has arisen, in part at least, because actuaries did not take sufficient account of historic increases in average life expectancy.

fail precisely in this function ... Even if one knows that one suffers a fatal accident driving on the motorway every twelve million kilometres, death could still be waiting round the next bend ... In social evaluations, the calculus leaves all eventualities open for the individual case.

The accident statistic conjectured in the above quotation conflates all drivers including young men racing sports cars, drunks and families proceeding at a leisurely pace. Although more differentiated and accurate statistics could be generated, they would merely aggregate at a finer level. In theory, this process would finish when the occurrence of individual accidents could be precisely predicted. In that case, probability and therefore risk would then have been replaced by certainty. Probabilistic analysis is utilized only because correct forecasting in individual cases remains out of reach. Hunt (2003) notes *a constant moving back and forth between individualizing and totalizing logics* in risk analysis. Aggregated alternative futures coexist with singular, individual, past outcomes.

Luhmann perhaps judges inductive probabilistic reasoning too harshly when he asserts that it 'fails'. Analyses based on acceptance of the inductive and ecological fallacies provide practically useful pointers for the direction of organized risk management. But its limitations must be acknowledged, a form of modesty sometimes sadly lacking in the medical literature. The implications for clinical risk management of accepting the inductive and ecological fallacies are discussed and illustrated in the second part of this chapter.

Conditional probabilities

In the simplest form of inductive probabilistic reasoning, considered above, rates observed in an entire population are applied to new individuals. But it is known that probabilities of a particular health outcome are linked to many risk factors. For example, men, smokers, and poorer people are more likely to die young. Bringing risk factors into consideration allows conditional probabilities to be calculated. These statistics provide estimates of an individual's chance of experiencing a particular outcome **if** specified conditions apply. Risk factors may be considered to possess causal or merely predictive significance. Causal factors can, if possible, be controlled in order to directly reduce the chance of an adverse outcome occurring. Knowledge of predictive factors can be used to identify cases at higher risk of an adverse outcome, thereby guiding healthcare attention towards those in most need.

The most basic type of conditional probabilistic reasoning can be displayed in a two-by-two contingency table, as illustrated in Table 4.1a. A number of probability statistics can be derived from a table such as this. These statistics are summarized in Table 4.1b, and explained below.

Table 4.1a First trimester screening for chromosomal anomalies such as Down's syndrome. (Bindra *et al.*, 2002)

		Fetus has chromosomal anomaly	Fetus does not have chromosomal anomaly	TOTAL
		1	2	3
A	Screened at higher risk (≥1:300)	129	967	1096
B	Screened at lower risk (<1:300)	14	13 273	13 287
C	TOTAL	143	14 240	14 383

Table 4.1b First trimester screening for chromosomal anomalies such as Down's syndrome: Summary screening statistics. (Bindra *et al.*, 2002)

Statistic	Calculation[1]	Probability	95% Confidence intervals
Base rate	C1/C3	1%	0.8–1.2%
Sensitivity	A1/C1	90%	85–95%
Selectivity	B2/C2	93%	92.5–93.5%
'False positive' rate	A2/A3	88%	86–90%
'False negative' rate	B1/B3	0.1%	0.05–0.15%
Positive predictive value	A1/A3	12%	10–14%
Negative predictive value	B2/B3	99.9%	99.8–100%
Attributable positive gain	A1/C3	1%	0.8–1.2%

[1]The cells of Table 4.1a which need to be divided in order to calculate the displayed probability

Confidence intervals are required because probabilities are estimated from observations derived from samples of cases. If sample members are selected in an unbiased fashion, statistics obtained from them will not necessarily match the underlying rate in the population from which they are drawn. On average, larger samples will generate more accurate results providing they are not systematically biased. In the same way, a fair coin may not land on heads 50% of the time for a given number of tosses. However, it will on average approximate more closely to this rate if thrown a larger number of times.

Confidence intervals give a rough indication of the range in which the true values are likely to fall. By convention, 95% confidence intervals are usually calculated. These statistics indicate the range in which the true underlying probability would occur 95% of the time if an unbiased sample had been selected. In this case, the size of the sample ensures that the calculated probabilities are only modestly susceptible to sampling error. However, the sensitivity measure, discussed below, has relatively wide confidence intervals of 85–95%. This statistic indicates the probability of a true case being identified through screening. Because chromosomal anomalies such as Down's syndrome occur relatively rarely, this statistic includes a small number of cases, only 143 in this data set (see cell C1 in Table 4.1). It therefore has relatively wide confidence intervals.

The base rate refers to the overall probability, estimated by inductive reasoning, of the outcome in question. In this case, 143/14 240, or about 1:100, fetuses were observed to have chromosomal anomalies. The relatively high probability (1%) observed by Bindra *et al.* reflects the older average age of the women included in their study, 47% of whom were aged 35 or older. The overall population rate is itself rising on account of a historical increase in average maternal age in many developed countries (Luke and Brown, 2007).

The base rate given in Table 4.1 covers all chromosomal anomalies. It includes 82 fetuses with trisomy 21 (three instead of two 21st chromosomes) which causes Down's syndrome, and 41 fetuses with other anomalies such as trisomy 18 which brings about Edward's syndrome. Different probabilities will be generated depending upon whether conditions are analysed separately or merged into the same category. The likelihood of Down's syndrome is often considered separately because children with this condition have a good chance of surviving into adulthood, whilst babies with other chromosomal anomalies have a very short life expectancy. Implicit in this way of categorizing outcomes is the assumption that the main aim of screening is to avoid the presumed burden of caring for children and adults with disabilities. If the aim of screening is to prevent **live** births of children with Down's syndrome, it will overestimate the risk because a substantial proportion of fetuses with this condition are aborted spontaneously. Diagnostic tests would indicate that these women were carrying a fetus with chromosomal anomalies, but they would not give birth to a living baby. As discussed in Chapter 5, the size of a probability depends upon the time frame over which it is considered.

The sensitivity of a screening system measures its ability to detect true cases. The value of about 90% (129/143) is obtained by dividing the number of fetuses with chromosomal anomalies who were categorized as being at higher risk by the total of true cases. This probability indicates that only 10% of true cases would be missed, i.e. classified as lower risk and therefore not considered for further investigation. These women would continue to carry an undetected fetus with chromosomal anomalies despite having been screened.

The selectivity of a screening system assesses its capacity to filter out non-cases. The value of 93% (13 273/14 240) is estimated by dividing the number of cases marked as being at lower risk by the true number of non-cases.

The so-called false positive rate of 88% (967/1 096) gives the probability of cases identified as higher risk not being true cases. The often-used term 'false positive' is misleading. Case identification merely indicates a relatively greater probability of the outcome in question being present. In this and many other screening systems, **most** cases marked as higher risk will not turn out to have the condition screened for. Nevertheless, these patients will be invited to undergo invasive diagnostic tests which carry additional risks, and have to manage uncertainty during the waiting period for further test results. Screening systems for relatively unusual conditions often suffer from high 'false positive' rates, for reasons explained in the next paragraph.

The positive predictive value of 12% (129/1 096) indicates the probability of cases identified as at higher risk being true cases. This statistic provides the inverse of the false positive rate (88% + 12% = 100%). Thus, only about a 10th of women informed that they are at higher risk and invited to consider invasive diagnostic testing will turn out to have the condition screened for. Positive predictive values and false positive rates tend to give a less flattering picture of the predictive power of a screening system than do the more frequently cited sensitivity and selectivity statistics (90% and 93%, respectively, for this system).

Most screening systems are designed to prioritize prevention over false detection. They tend to be set up with the intention of minimizing the chance of true cases being overlooked. This is done by setting the dividing line for 'higher' risk at a relatively low level, usually 1:250–1:300 for prenatal chromosomal screening. A price of additional cases for whom further investigation is recommended has to be paid for reducing the chance of overlooking true cases. This policy results in screening systems suffering from low positive predictive values. Bindra *et al.* (2002) estimated that increasing the cut-off for higher risk to 1:9 would increase the positive predictive value of their system from 12% to 65%, but would result in only 60% of true cases being detected. Fewer women would undertake diagnostic tests, but more fetuses with Down's syndrome would slip through the net[3].

It was argued in Chapter 2 that in risk management practice, higher and lower risk tend to be elided into the presence and absence of risk which comes to be viewed as either existing or not existing. But the necessary dividing line between them has to be set by compromising between sensitivity and selectivity.

----

[3] Receiver operator characteristic graphs can be plotted for different probability cut-offs between 'positive' and 'negative' cases. More predictively accurate screening systems will offer greater sensitivity at different levels of specificity and vice versa.

The so-called 'false negative rate' of 0.1% (14/13 287) gives the probability of cases marked as at lower risk being true cases. As with the false positive rate, the term is strictly inaccurate since low risk does not equate to no risk. Nevertheless, the 'tuning' of screening systems towards sensitivity ensures that only a tiny proportion of true cases will be overlooked.

The negative predictive value of 99.9% (13 273/13 287) quantifies the chance of cases marked as at lower risk not having the condition tested for. This screening system, like many others, is far more likely to generate 'false positives' than 'false negatives', as already pointed out.

The term **attributable positive predictive gain** refers to the probability of an individual who has not yet been screened being eventually diagnosed with the condition being investigated. To the author's knowledge, no standard term for this rarely discussed statistic exists, perhaps because it reveals the smallness of the health gains generated by present screening technologies (Gigerenzer, 2002). The chance of a woman taking a screening pathway in which chromosomal anomalies will be eventually diagnosed through a follow-up test such as chorionic villus sampling is about 1:1 000 (129/14 383) in the system under consideration.

In addition, as already noted, some fetuses with Down's syndrome would not make it to live birth. Bindra *et al.* (2002) suggest that about 30% of fetuses with Down's syndrome are lost between 12 weeks, when first trimester screening is undertaken, and the end of pregnancy. These women would end up with the same pregnancy outcome as those who decide to terminate their pregnancy after Down's syndrome is diagnosed. The remaining 70%, only 90 women out of 14 383, gained extra leverage over their future by being able to choose whether or not to abort a fetus who would otherwise have developed into a living child with Down's syndrome.

Heuristics about heuristics

Social scientists, particularly psychologists, have expressed scathing views about the probabilistic reasoning abilities of non-experts. Even Douglas, an anthropologist trying to understand the world from diverse cultural perspectives, has criticized the public in this respect. She considered that *the ordinary lay person, the man in the street, is weak on probabilistic thinking* (Douglas, 1992). The gloomy litany of failings emerging from psychological laboratory research (Breakwell, 2007) is worth quoting at length:

> Humans appear to fail miserably when it comes to rational decision-making ...
> They ignore base rates when estimating probabilities; commit the 'sunk cost fallacy' (continuing to invest in failure because they have done so before), are naively optimistic, take undue credit for their achievements and do not recognise self-inflicted

failures. In addition, they underestimate the number of others who share their beliefs, demonstrate 'hindsight bias', have limited understanding of chance, perceive illusory relationships between non-contingent events and overestimate their own ability to impose control. The list could be extended: they are overconfident in their judgements; they engage in spurious hyperprecision when making predictions; they ignore the limits of the data available to them, and so on.

Probabilistic reasoning gives rise to endemic confusion, at least in psychology laboratories, and perhaps also in clinical settings (Lloyd, 2001). However, it was argued above that probabilistic reasoning itself requires pragmatic acceptance of crude but useful rules of thumb. It follows that its further simplification in everyday life involves the use of a double heuristic. The implicit contrast between the lofty precision of science and the weak thinking of the person in the street does not apply in the fuzzy realm of probability. Non-experts who misunderstand probability merely simplify a simplification.

For the present purpose of introducing the idea of the double probability heuristic, a brief outline of one way of simplifying probabilistic reasoning will suffice. An individual who is using the availability heuristic, arguably the most important in relation to the simplification of probabilistic reasoning, will assess the chance of an adverse outcome occurring on the basis of exposure to specific incidents. For instance, research participants overestimate their risk of being murdered, and underestimate their chance of dying from a stroke (Slovic, 2000). They are heavily exposed to murder cases through obsessive media coverage. Strokes, at the other end of the availability scale, receive virtually no media attention despite their much higher incidence. In general, awareness of specific occurrences provides some information about probability since more common outcomes are more likely to be encountered. But conclusions derived in this way should not be relied on, for two reasons. Firstly, underlying rates cannot be reliably estimated from small numbers of cases, any more than the fairness of a coin can be assessed by tossing it 2 or 3 times. Secondly, socially organized processes draw some outcomes to popular attention more than others. For example, following publicity about the death at the hands of relatives of Baby 'P' in 2007, the number of child protection referrals in London increased by 30% (*The Guardian* newspaper, 26th Jan 2009). The child abuse rate had not changed, but instead had acquired a higher profile. A specific example illustrating these issues is discussed below.

An example of probabilistic reasoning about health outcomes (Heyman and Henriksen, 2001)

A woman who had declined prenatal screening for Down's syndrome expressed scepticism about the view that older women like herself faced a higher probability of giving birth to babies with this condition. She justified her doubt as follows:

> **Pregnant woman:** My husband knows someone who was only in his early 40s now, and he's got a Down's syndrome boy, and he's in his 20s. And both him and his wife were in their early 20s when they had him. And I think, well, it can happen at that age, it can happen any time.
>
> (Research interview with woman aged 38 who declined screening for chromosomal anomalies)

The research participant quoted above stated correctly that outcomes which scientists characterize as unlikely can still occur. However, she used her observation of one such case to support her decision not to undergo screening.

Three issues can be raised about this frequently used way of thinking, in which conclusions are drawn from observation of a single case. Firstly, individual examples provide no information about likelihood, as already noted. Secondly, mothers of children with Down's syndrome are actually more likely to be younger than older even though older women are more likely to give birth to such children. This apparent anomaly arises because the majority of pregnant women are younger. More formally, the probability of A given B should not be confused with that of B given A. **Given that** an expectant mother is younger, she is **less** likely to deliver a baby with Down's syndrome, as women are informed when screening is discussed with them. On the other hand, **given that** a child has Down's syndrome, its mother is **more** likely to have been younger rather than older at the time of the birth simply because of the age distribution of pregnant women. A third issue with drawing probabilistic conclusions from observation of cases is that it ignores the impact of screening. The implementation of effective preventive interventions selectively lowers the probability of an adverse outcome occurring in the targeted higher risk group. At the time when the research under consideration was undertaken, screening for chromosomal anomalies was only offered routinely in the research catchment area to women older than 35-years. Although screening for Down's syndrome is now mostly offered to all pregnant women in the UK and other rich countries, selective effects have not been eliminated. The systems in use offer higher detection rates to older women, at the expense of a greater proportion of 'false positives' (Spencer, 2001), a trade-off considered above. Moreover, older women are more likely to accept the offer of screening (Dormandy et al., 2005), probably because they see themselves as being at higher risk. This 'prevention paradox' is further discussed below.

Implications of using the probability heuristic

The heuristic status of official probabilistic reasoning gives rise to some counter-intuitive paradoxes. These paradoxes illustrate the limitations of risk thinking which projects uncertainty, metamorphosed into randomness, onto external events. They also impact significantly on health risk management. Three such paradoxes will be outlined below: the paradox of multiple probabilities; the ecological prevention paradox; and the inductive prevention paradox.

The paradox of multiple probabilities

The operation of inductive probabilistic reasoning entails attributing rates observed in outcome categories to their members. It follows that many probabilities of the same outcome can be generated, depending upon how cases are categorized. Furthermore, individuals can control 'their' probability of experiencing an adverse outcome by choosing whether to obtain more information about such factors.

Children of a parent with Huntingdon's disease face a 50% probability of developing this inherited fatal condition. Because Huntingdon's disease does not cause symptoms until well into adult life, children may 'stick' with this probability for a considerable proportion of their lives. Alternatively, they may decide to undergo diagnostic DNA tests, available only since the 1980s, which will determine with certainty whether or not they will develop the disease. Hence, presymptomatic individuals can choose one of two options. Firstly, they can leave 'their' odds at 0.5. Secondly, they can accept further information which will change this probability to either 1 or 0. They know with certainty that their chance of developing the disease will change to one of these values. But they cannot know in advance which one will hold true. This choice has implications not only for themselves but for the genetic health of any offspring. Some individuals decide that they could not cope with this knowledge (Goizet, Lesca, and Dürr 2002), or do not wish to weigh down existing children with this burden (Binedell, Soldan, and Harper 1998).

A related opening for the 'management' of probabilities arises within established systems which allow progressively finer partitioning of risk categories. The overall rate of Down's syndrome for women using a particular hospital offers one undifferentiated probability, as illustrated by the following quotation (Heyman and Henriksen, 2001):

> **Pregnant woman:** That sort of, like, cheers me up, when [the doctor] said I was one in 4 200, I think, or 4 500 or something ..., and only five of them were Down's Syndrome.
>
> (Research interview with woman aged 39 who opted to undergo amniocentesis without prior screening)

This woman opted for an invasive diagnostic test, having been advised that her age took her over the higher risk threshold. Nevertheless, she took comfort from attributing the hospital base rate to herself. This much lower rate of about 1:4 000 reflected the predominance of younger women in the population of maternity service users. At the same time, she appreciated that her age-related probability was 1:120, although, understandably, she felt some uncertainty about these multiple statistics.

Women were told their age-related probability of giving birth to a baby with chromosomal anomalies when they attended the consultation at which screening was discussed. They could not 'unknow' this statistic. They could further manage 'their' probability by selecting a route through this system, as illustrated below (Heyman and Henriksen, 2001):

> **Pregnant midwife:** I didn't want to have the, em, I could have had the amnio, because I didn't want to be placed in a position of having to decide about a termination, because I knew I wouldn't want one. But I thought, once you know for a fact that you have a Down's syndrome child, would that change you? Would you then want to have a termination because you would feel pressure … from other people?
> (Research interview with woman aged 36 who declined to be screened or tested for chromosomal anomalies)

In effect, the respondent quoted above opted to keep 'her' probability at its age-related level rather than proceed to acquire further knowledge. Testing would have increased or decreased her chance of carrying a fetus with a chromosomal anomaly. But she could not know in advance which of these two outcomes would occur. In either case, the resulting change would have affected the prediction, not the actual chromosomal status of the fetus. Although not mysterious when carefully considered, this argument can seem counter-intuitive at first sight. It appears to imply that the fetus itself is changed through screening. Instead, screening merely locates the fetus in a different predictive category.

This limited power to control the chance of a future or otherwise unknown event is inherent in the nature of inductive probabilistic reasoning. Even if outcomes themselves cannot be modified, expectations based on induction from observed frequencies can be managed in this one respect. Individuals who can choose whether to receive further information can opt to leave 'their' probability at its existing level, or to investigate further. Additional inquiry will either decrease or increase this prior probability. But which of these outcomes will turn out to occur cannot be known in advance. Once prognostic information has been received, it cannot be 'unknown'.

The ecological prevention paradox

Inductive probabilistic reasoning works by attributing rates observed in categories to individuals who meet the criteria for membership. Patients who are informed that they face a certain probability of an adverse event may wonder whether they will be one of the unlucky ones. The impossibility of providing personal probabilities opens up a gap between this fundamental limitation of risk analysis and the informational needs of service users who wish to know what is going to happen to in their particular case.

Attribution of higher risk status to individuals located in a category makes them all targets for preventive endeavours. It is entirely possible for an average health gain to be achieved through a health-promoting activity such as dieting which confers no benefits on most of those who undertake it (Davison, Davey Smith, and Frankel, 1992). Ecological prevention paradoxes can be identified in relation to health promotional message which recommend limiting pleasurable activities such as eating fatty or sugary foods, sun-bathing, and alcohol consumption. Weight loss, discussed below, provides a good illustrative example.

High body mass index as a health risk factor

The risks arising from being overweight or obese have been widely publicized. Globally, the prevalence of these two 'conditions' has increased substantially over recent years (Caballero, 2007). In the UK and elsewhere, numerous governmental campaigns promoting diets considered healthy and exercise have been launched. However, food companies remain more or less free to market products high in fat, sugar, and salt to adults and children.

Traditionally, the states of being overweight and obese have been assessed through measuring body mass index (BMI), defined as a person's weight in kilograms divided by their height in metres squared. An individual with a BMI between about 27 and 30 is considered overweight, and someone with a BMI of 30 or more is classified as obese. Although internationally accepted, these boundaries have an arbitrary character which affects individuals at the margins between categories. At the aggregate level, people with higher BMIs are more likely to experience a range of health problems, including pregnancy complications (Galtier-Dereure, Boegner, and Bringer, 2000), diabetes (Jung, 1997), heart disease (Willett *et al.*, 1995), strokes (Rexrode *et al.*, 1997), prostate cancer (Gronberg, Damber, and Damber, 1998) and post-menopausal breast cancer (Huang *et al.*, 1997). A higher BMI marks out individuals as having high risk status, creating personal and social pressure for them to extricate themselves from this position. Blame tends to be attributed even though genetic factors can explain some or all of the additional body weight in many cases, as discussed in Chapter 2.

Crucially for the present argument, higher risk status derives from categorizing persons with increased BMIs. An aggregate statistic is applied to all the individuals whom it encompasses. However, a higher BMI does not directly cause health problems such as those mentioned above. The category of obesity, defined in terms of BMI, captures both individuals who will suffer and those who will not. It merely marks out a set of individuals who will collectively experience greater rates of risked conditions, thereby 'spreading' higher risk status across all category members. In consequence, higher risk status becomes a virtual feature of all individuals in the marked category. But, as noted in Chapter 2 in the discussion of adversity foregrounding, many or even most of those defined as at higher risk will turn out, with the benefit of hindsight, to have been unaffected.

More recent research has suggested that waist circumference may provide a better predictor of health outcomes than BMI (Janssen, Katzmarzyk, and Ross, 2004; Yusuf *et al.*, 2005). According to this new risk construction, individuals with slim waists but high BMIs would be wrongly flagged up as being at higher health risk. However, even if waist circumference offers a better predictor, BMI would still provide some predictive purchase. The higher BMI category would contain more individuals with large waists than the lower BMI group. The former would therefore also include a larger proportion of individuals with health problems. It would lump together individuals with big waists and heavy people with slim waists, all of whom would acquire higher risk status.

Any gains in predictive power arising from an improved specification of risk factors can be identified through research after it has been proposed. In this case it has been shown, in effect, that the category of individuals with slim waists but higher BMIs does not face an increase in health risk. They could be discharged from higher risk status. Unfortunately, such prognostic refinements can only be tested for risk factors which have been considered. Those remaining will continue to retain higher risk status. This tentative state of affairs can only be resolved by perfect prediction about individual outcomes. In that case, neither risk thinking nor acceptance of the ecological fallacy would be required.

The inductive prevention paradox

To the extent that preventive efforts are believed to reduce the probability of an adverse outcome occurring, their implementation weakens the evidence base for detecting risk. Once a medical intervention has been implemented, it becomes difficult or impossible to know what would have happened if it had not been employed. Conversely, if a patient is not treated, the outcome of the intervention which might have been carried out becomes unknowable.

This little discussed consequence of attempted prevention applies to risk categories, considered below, as well as to individuals. In relation to the latter, a frail older person who has suffered a distressing fall outside the home might decide that the risk of going out is too great to accept. By remaining at home, this person will remove the flow of information from which the chance of another fall might have been estimated. Having opted for risk avoidance, she cannot know whether she might have been able to go out in the future without experiencing harm.

Patients with inflammatory bowel disease (IBD) may be able to control their condition by taking non-steroidal anti-inflammatory drugs. Although cleared for long-term use, these drugs carry their own iatrogenic risks. Patients who have consumed them for a long duration without experiencing major IBD symptoms face a difficult decision. If they stop taking these drugs they might experience a further flare-up which, through a process of positive feedback, might make future events more likely. On the other hand, if they continue to take anti-inflammatory drugs, they increase their risk of suffering unwanted side-effects, perhaps unnecessarily. But they cannot find out what would happen without risking their present flare-up-free status. Restarting to take the drug if flare-ups recur might not take them back to their previous state. Thus, the inductive prevention paradox places risk managers in a trap which fuels the 'reality' of the virtual object that they are attempting to control, as discussed in Chapter 2.

The evidence base for risk management is weakened whenever a risk is managed through attempted prevention. For instance, forensic mental health patients may live in secure environments designed to protect the public. They will be discharged when their risk of reoffending is assessed to be acceptably low. But the hospital environment removes direct evidence of patients risk predisposition through the very measures taken to stop them from committing further offences. Risk assessment must therefore rely on assessment of how patients might behave in the very different environment external to the secure unit.

Staff faced with this risk management conundrum may seek to test patients through drawing inferences from their limited exposure to environments in which offending becomes possible. This testing out process is illustrated by the following quotation (Heyman et al., 2004):

> **Nurse:** I personally think, when he goes out [on parole], that's a big test for him, because he goes out on a Saturday to [large town], and [large town] is quite far, and anything can happen then … If something really pushed him, he would do something.
> (Research interview with nurse, forensic mental health unit)

Staff called this individual the *star patient* on account of his pleasant manner and apparent lack of personal problems. They viewed him with suspicion because of his offending history. Their 'suck it and see' approach to risk management can be compared to that traditionally adopted for testing the safety of novel foods by eating progressively larger amounts. It tends to be adopted in the absence of a better alternative when an inductive evidence base is lacking. Its limitations can easily be identified. Patients who intend to reoffend may be able to conceal their inclinations until they are discharged. Others may be able to avoid reoffending for a short period only. Staff may resort to such an approach because nothing better is available. However, those conducting formal inquiries into cases where a patient seriously reoffended enjoy the benefit of hindsight. The following quotation is taken from an inquiry into the release of John Barrett who murdered a member of the public, Dennis Finnegan, shortly after his release from a medium-secure unit:

> Too much confidence was placed in clinical judgements unsupported by evidence and rigorous analysis.
> (South West London Strategic Health Authority, 2006)

Such accounts place excessive faith in the potential for 'rigorous' analysis. They overlook the limitations to predictive power which arise from prevention itself. On the one hand, risk managers are obliged to take the possibility of adverse outcomes seriously, and may be blamed when they occur. On the other hand, the implementation of preventive measures itself removes the evidential grounds for assessing risk.

At the collective level, the war on drugs is continued despite its evident failure for fear that its abandonment would trigger an irreversible expansion of addict numbers (Califano, 2007). However the impact of decriminalization could only be observed if the present legal regime was suspended. Similarly, the now widespread use of cervical cancer screening in combination with vaccination clouds the picture of their separate efficacy (Kiviat, Hawes, and Feng, 2008). The extent to which vaccination might reduce the need for screening cannot be easily assessed as long as they are both being provided. But the withdrawal of screening can hardly be contemplated, just because it might still play an important preventive role.

Conclusion

This chapter reviewed the logic of inductive probabilistic reasoning, considered as merely one approach to developing expectations. Essentially, cases are located in outcome categories and their relative frequencies are observed.

These rates are then applied to new cases, so that an individual's probability of experiencing alternative outcomes is derived from the proportion observed in past cases. Although inductive probabilistic reasoning proceeds by treating outcomes as if they occur randomly, this way of thinking is merely metaphorical. The randomness which might rule at the level of quantum particles does not apply to probabilistic reasoning about the everyday large-scale world.

Inductive probabilistic reasoning involves no more than the application of a simple, practically useful, but potentially misleading, rule of thumb. Individuals are treated as if they 'carry' the risk detected previously in a category of cases. This way of thinking allows a risk to be managed by motivating preventive action within the higher risk group. However, it generates some esoteric and even counterintuitive consequences.

Firstly, many probabilities of the same outcome can be derived from evidence, depending upon how cases are categorized and what information is obtained in individual cases. Patients can 'manage' their probability of experiencing an outcome by deciding whether or not to obtain further information. They cannot, unfortunately, control the presence of disease so easily. But they can influence their risk status together with any associated moral pressures or new risks arising from preventive measures. Secondly, inductive probabilistic reasoning lumps together all of the individuals who are assigned to particular levels of risk, e.g. those with large bodies, older mothers, or those consuming illegal drugs. They are all tarred with the same higher risk brush even though a proportion, or even a large majority, are not expected to be affected. Thirdly, preventive efforts are designed to change the causal conditions producing higher risk. They thereby cloud the view of risk factors which could be seen before prevention was implemented. Individuals and societies can find themselves trapped in self-sustaining, virtual risk 'bubbles' because they do not dare to find out what would happen if measures adopted to reduce risk were abandoned.

The potential for multiple probabilities, the ecological prevention paradox and the inductive prevention paradox jointly imbue risk analysis with an inescapable fragility. Individuals can exercise a degree of control over 'their' probability of an adverse outcome. Those who are assigned to a higher risk category might lose this status if cases were grouped differently. And individuals who are apparently protected by preventive measures might learn that they were not needed if their abandonment could be risked. Accurate prediction in individual cases offers the only way out of these paradoxes. But risk analysis and management are resorted to just because science cannot deliver such precision.

Chapter 5

Time and health risks

Bob Heyman

Aim

To explore the role of time and its interpretation in health risk thinking.

Objectives

1. To consider the setting of time frames for health risk management
2. To introduce the concept of time-discounting
3. To analyse retrospective views about health risks.

Introduction

The previous three chapters have offered a reinterpretation of the Royal Society (1992) definition of a risk, which they described as:

> the probability that a particular adverse event occurs during a stated time period, or results from a particular challenge.

The discussions of risk events, adversity, and probability have recast these elements of the risk compound as categorizing, valuing, and uncertain expecting, respectively. The final chapter in this set of four will attempt to perform the same task for *the stated time period*, reconstituted as the active interpretive process of time-framing. The second idea of a *particular challenge* mentioned in the Royal Society definition does not offer an alternative to time-framing. Instead, it suggests that a risk may be considered over the full span of time in which it continues to have adverse effects. Risks cannot be analysed, assessed, or managed unless a time period for consideration is specified. In addition, the expected timing of adverse outcomes within the selected time frame affects their valuation, most commonly through time-discounting. Delaying a currently unavoidable outcome such as the progression of incurable cancer will usually be welcomed. Hence, the interpretation of time influences risk management in relation to both the period which is covered and event timing inside the chosen temporal horizons. However, as argued below, the value of such gains to individuals will depend upon their specific meaning for their wider lives.

Despite its critical importance, the temporal dimension of risk management has received relatively little attention in the social science literature, although Luhmann (1993) does offer a whole chapter on this topic. The puzzling nature of time makes analysis of its role in risk thinking particularly difficult. Neither the past nor the future manifests itself directly to the senses. The present remains tantalizingly intangible, poised fleetingly between the remembered past and the imagined future, neither of which exists materially (Luhmann, 1993). How time is experienced is equally unclear. Time sense derives from conscious memory, but understanding that memories reference the past requires a prior intuitive grasp of time. Without a sense of travelling through time, individuals could not maintain their personal identities. Despite its problematic relationship to experience and the material world, time appears more irreducibly physical than the other three risk ingredients discussed previously. Categorizing, valuing, and uncertain expecting do not belong directly to nature, but to its interpretation by sentient beings. In contrast, time remains stubbornly unstoppable. The arrow of time moves in one direction only, towards increasing entropy, i.e. a less ordered universe, regardless of whether its progression noticed or not. Yet, one of the few points of agreement in the vast literature speculating about the nature of time concerns its thoroughly social nature (Adam, 1990). Time consciousness is culturally mediated, as exemplified, for example, by the emerging dominance of clock time associated with the industrial revolution, and by the current anxious focus on climate change over the next century.

Risk managers, being people of business, cannot be expected to take on board the entire philosophy, science, and social science of time. Giddens' (1991a) much quoted idea of attempted *colonization of the future* provides a good starting point for analysing the key role of temporal considerations in risk thinking. The discussion which follows is divided into two main sections. The first will examine risks from a prospective perspective, considering the related issues of time-framing, time-discounting within a selected time frame, and management of future intentions. The second main section will be concerned with retrospective views of risks, at a vantage point from which one of the possible outcomes envisaged in a contingency has actually occurred.

Prospective views of risks

Time-framing in health risk management

Time-framing establishes boundaries within which risks can be qualitatively or quantitatively assessed. The expected value calculations discussed in Chapter 3 require the consequences of a choice to be categorized, valued, and multiplied by their probabilities, so that their total net utility can be measured. Time-framing must be added to this list of issues because utility simply cannot be assessed unless temporal horizons have been set. Utilitarian calculations cannot be performed over an infinite time period. This point might seem fanciful. However, with respect to major environmental risks to health, such as soil erosion, radioactive waste, and climate change, the outcome of cost-benefit analyses will depend upon how far into the future the calculations are projected. The nuclear industry has mostly assessed the health impact of storing radioactive waste over a 500-year period. More favourable risk assessments will be generated if appraisal is confined within this time horizon than if effects over tens, or even hundreds, of thousands of years are taken into account (Atherton and French, 1999). In general, the theoretically unlimited length of consequence chains, stretching to the end of history, stands in contrast to the requirements of risk analysis which must segment causal sequences somewhere in order to make expected values calculable.

Prospective time-framing will be discussed below from two points of view: firstly, as a socially organized phenomenon; and, secondly, with respect to the varying personal time horizons which individuals may adopt when they manage health risks. The co-ordination of risk management will tend to break down unless those dealing with a risk adopt a similar time frame, or at least recognize their differences. But the meaning of time derives from personal lives, and therefore varies considerably, as will be illustrated in the second part of this discussion. A tension can be identified between the need to standardize the temporal span of a risk in order to facilitate the organization of its management and the variability of its meaning to individuals.

Collective time-framing

The temporal management of health risks is shaped by the human condition, as well as influenced by broad societal trends and the requirements of organized risk management. The limits of the human lifespan impose a boundary on consequences which might, at first sight, appear to offer a simple solution to the question of temporal boundary-setting in the health domain. Individuals may reasonably feel untroubled about risks to their health which are unlikely to translate into adverse consequences during their expected lifespan. For example, terminally ill patients do not need to concern themselves about the long-term effects of taking morphine. Given that some prostate cancers develop so slowly, many individuals would die of other causes totally unaware of its presence in the absence of medical investigation (Harris and Lohr, 2002). Unfortunately, the speed with which prostate cancer grows cannot as yet be predicted. On the other hand, longer life expectancy requires time horizons to be extended. For instance, children cannot rely on steroids for more than a brief period because of the side-effects resulting from long-term use.

Some health risks span generations, and might therefore be considered across more than one lifetime. In this case, risk managers would attempt to colonize far-distant health futures. Such cross-generational risks include genetic transmission, the ongoing effects of environmental hazards, and enduring social patterns. Parents are enjoined to manage the genetic health of their offspring by accepting prenatal screening and selective reproduction (Beck-Gernsheim, 1996). The health implications of transmitting genetic problems may span many lifetimes. Epigenetic processes can transmit environmental signals across more than one generation by controlling which genes are switched on in the developing embryo (Godfrey *et al.*, 2007). For example, inadequate maternal diet increases risks for the unborn child in later life, particularly of obesity and diabetes (Hazani and Shasha, 2008). Social processes influence children across generations. For instance, the child rearing practices of grandmothers towards mothers have been linked to the personal development of grandchildren (Brook, Whiteman, and Brook,1999). It is well-established that abused children are more likely to become abusive adults (Dixon, Browne, and Hamilton-Giachritsis, 2004). In all these cases, health risks have been tracked across time frames which extend well beyond the life-span of one individual.

On the other hand, the time span within which a risk is considered may be confined to a period considerably shorter than that in which it might still be affecting health. Taking into account a longer period causes too many practical problems. One reason for such foreshortening is to limit accountability. For instance, UK confidential inquiries into the suicides of discharged mental health service users usually employ a 1-year time frame. Incidents are subjected to an inquiry if a patient had been in contact with relevant services within 12-months of taking their own life (Robinson and Bickley, 2004). Services cannot be held to account for suicides which take place decades after contact terminated. However, cut-offs for appraising responsibility can only be set arbitrarily. Thus, a 6-month time horizon would generate fewer enquiry cases than one of 12-months. But the processes which put patients at increased risk do not suddenly cease to affect them after a set period. Specifying an accountability time horizon creates an artificial boundary which causality is deemed not to cross. In turn, the presence of such boundaries will affect service provision. Service providers are likely to give more attention to risks for which they expect to be held accountable if adverse events occur.

Temporal horizons for considering risks associated with medical interventions also tend to be narrowed for pragmatic reasons. For example, prospects after treatment for a life-threatening condition such as cancer are usually assessed in terms of 5-year survival. This time frame speeds up research by limiting the period over which outcomes have to be considered, and reduces its cost. Sharing the same time span also helps to makes research findings comparable. But the risk of recurrence beyond the period covered by data collection becomes obscured. Lengthier time periods are not systematically investigated, resulting in research blindness about possible longer-term risks. For instance, an annual recurrence rate of 1–2% after 10-years has been found for one form of testicular cancer (Dearnaley, Huddart, and Horwich, 2001). Research confined to 5-year survival would not detect such effects, and might not identify the best overall treatment.

Online searching yields a feast of literature discussing 5-year survival for life-threatening conditions, and calling for longer-term follow-up, but a famine of studies which actually do so. For example, Williams *et al.* (2005) note that the time frame for intensive care survival studies has ranged from 16-months to 13-years, and calls for studies covering longer periods. The conclusion, nevertheless, offers an estimated 5-year survival rate of around 50%. This collective clinical myopia is not necessarily shared by patients. For instance, women recovering from breast cancer treatment interviewed 10-months after intervention expressed concern about the risks of eventual recurrence and treatment side-effects (Gil *et al.*, 2004). Not surprisingly, their personal time horizons stretched much further than the conventional 5-years. With respect to interventions aimed at morbidity rather than survival, even shorter time horizons may be adopted, possibly resulting in a distorted view of treatment effectiveness. One study of a minimally invasive surgical procedure for relieving chronic pancreatic pain (Súilleabháin *et al.*, 2002) concluded that the proportion needing opiates, 96% pre-operatively, was only 22% 6-months after surgery, but rose to 39% after 1-year, and 54% after 2-years. The clinical picture 6-months after surgery provided a misleading view of its longer-term benefit.

The apparent cost-effectiveness of any procedure depends upon the time frame which is selected. The use of a drastically foreshortened time frame to create an impression of successful risk reduction is illustrated in Box 5.1, below, which discusses the UK smoking cessation programme.

Shortening the time frame flatters therapeutic interventions such as smoking cessation programmes which are undermined by longer-term relapse. Conversely, lead-time bias may generate a misleadingly positive impression of the efficacy of screening for conditions such as prostate cancer which progress at variable rates (Brawley, 2001). Lead-time bias occurs because screening will detect cases before symptoms have been noticed, thereby bringing forward and lengthening the time frame in which mortality and morbidity are considered.

Box 5.1 The time-framing of the UK smoking cessation programme

The NHS publishes data on the outcomes of its smoking cessation programme. Success is measured in terms of the number of people intending to quit, and the proportion of this group who are not smoking 1-month after they have joined a programme. According to the official statistics for April–December 2007, (The NHS Information Centre, 2008):

> 462 690 people set a quit date through NHS Stop Smoking Services, an increase of 23% over the same period in 2006/07 and 17% over the same period in 2005/06. At the 4 week follow-up 234 060 people had successfully quit (based on self-report), 51% of those setting a quit date. This compares with 192 527 successful quitters in the same period in 2006/07 (an increase of 22%), and 208 878 successful quitters in 2005/06 (12% increase).

The document equates being a successful quitter with reported abstinence over a 1-month period. A footnote to the table states that: *A client is counted as having successfully quit smoking at the 4 week follow-up if he/she has not smoked at all since two weeks after the quit date*, reducing the effective time frame to 2-weeks. The obvious limitation with this construction of the risk virtual object is that it does not take into account cumulative relapsing over subsequent months. Research findings demonstrate consistently that abstinence rates decline over time. One unusually lengthy study concluded that about half of those who had stopped smoking after 1-year relapsed over an 8-year period (Yudkin *et al.*, 2003). Cynics might conclude that the 1-month time frame utilized in the official statistics was chosen in order to present the campaign against smoking as favourably as possible.

Even if earlier intervention such as surgery and radiotherapy provide no net clinical benefit whatsoever, screened patients would appear to survive longer on average simply because their condition was identified earlier. (They would also seem to live longer on average because the screened, but not the unscreened, population would include people with pseudo-disease. These individuals would not have noticed their condition, and would have died of other causes, if they had not been screened. However, once they have been given treatment it becomes impossible to know in individual cases whether the intervention might have been unnecessary. This example provides another illustration of the inductive prevention paradox, discussed in Chapter 4.)

Doubts about the benefits of screening can be resolved through randomized controlled trials in which older men who consent to participate are randomly allocated to be offered or not offered screening. Conclusive evidence has not as yet been generated (Dragan *et al.*, 2007). Currently, prostate cancer screening is offered widely in North America, but not in Europe. This difference illustrates the impact of cultural and organizational factors on risk management policy in circumstances of evidential uncertainty.

Time-framing can affect the establishment of the evidence base for treatment efficacy. For instance, early US trials of zidovudine as an HIV treatment were stopped prematurely because clear clinical benefits were identified. But subsequent research showed that these gains did not last, and that multi-drug interventions were needed (Kinloch, de Loës, and Perneger, 1997). The issue of premature clinical trial termination is further considered below.

Terminating clinical trials earlier than planned. Who benefits?
In both the EU and the USA, randomized controlled trials may be stopped before the planned number of research participants has been recruited. Premature termination is permitted if the non-complete data demonstrate that the intervention is clearly benefiting or harming patients. In April 2008, the large US JUPITER trial of statins as a risk reducer for cardiovascular disease was terminated prematurely on the grounds that it had generated definite evidence of reduced morbidity and mortality. A trend for an increasing number of trials to be stopped prematurely in this way has been documented in both the USA (Montori *et al.*, 2005) and the EU (Trotta *et al.*, 2008). The title of the latter review, *Stopping a trial early in oncology: For patients or for industry?* raises the suspicion that early trial termination may benefit pharmaceutical companies rather than patients.

The widespread introduction of this practice can lead to treatment benefits being exaggerated, as explained below. In many cases, trials are funded by pharmaceutical companies who have a financial interest in maximizing the apparent benefits of an intervention. Their behaviour can be compared to that of football supporters who urge the referee to finish a match when their side is winning. Proponents of a particular set of medical interventions can similarly stack the cards in their overall favour. Although trial managers are enjoined to also stop trials prematurely if adverse reactions are identified, they can bend the evidence in their favour simply by detecting health gains more readily than adverse events. In the same way, football supporters will hope that the referee delays blowing the final whistle when their side is losing.

The methodology of randomized controlled trials was adopted in order to protect researchers from their own wishful thinking. But flexibility about time-framing allows bias to reassert itself. Once an intervention has been approved, challenges become less likely because of the expense associated with mounting further randomized controlled trials. In consequence, the evidence base may become temporarily or permanently locked even though, in some cases, clinical benefits have been exaggerated. On the other hand, it is unethical to continue with a demonstrably inferior treatment for research purposes. Policy-makers and agencies conducting trials face a difficult temporal risk management dilemma.

Personal time-framing

The above discussion focussed on official risk time-framing. Individual risk managers, including service users, carers, and practitioners, will themselves adopt time frames which may correspond more or less to those adopted by other participants in health care transactions. Such variations in time horizon may underlie conflicts and misunderstandings which arise from differences in unexamined presuppositions about the length of time to be taken into account. Personal management of the temporal dimension of risks has been little considered in the research literature. But the construction of a time frame impacts significantly on the form of the risk virtual object.

For instance, pregnant women thinking about prenatal chromosomal screening for genetic anomalies such as Down's syndrome adopt varying time frames. Some women respond to being offered screening options by focussing on the time span of the pregnancy itself, as illustrated below (Heyman and Henriksen, 2001):

> **Pregnant woman:** Well I thought, if I had the blood test, four out of five, there is one out of five high risk or something. And I thought, well, if I'm at high risk, then you are waiting. You go and have the amniocentesis, and you are waiting three weeks for that. And then they could say there is something wrong, but, at the end of the day, there might not be. So you've got all those months of chewing and preparing yourself, and then you have a normal baby. So why not have a 9-month happy pregnancy, and then worry at the end of the day?
>
> (Research interview with woman aged 36 who declined genetic tests)

The respondent quoted above interpreted the probability of receiving a higher-risk test result as one in five rather than one in 20, the correct statistic. This misunderstanding supported her preferred risk management decision which was driven mainly by the time frame she had adopted. Her time horizon encompassed the remaining 6-months of her pregnancy, excluding the birth and the consequences of giving birth to a baby with Down's syndrome. (This specific time management issue is avoided if more modern, 'one stop' screening and testing technology is adopted (Bindra *et al.*, 2002). But the point of the present discussion is to illustrate the impact of personal time-framing.) Another woman had made the opposite decision in relation to the same time frame, of the pregnancy period itself:

> **Interviewer:** Why did you want the amnio?
> **Pregnant woman:** The reason I wanted it is, because I don't think I could have gone, 'til, until the baby's birth and not knowing if there's anything wrong with the baby.
> (Research interview with woman aged 40 who underwent amniocentesis)

Her main concern was to reduce the period of anxious uncertainty during which the risk of a chromosomal anomaly would continue to exist. In contrast, the respondent cited below looked much further into the future, beyond the time when she would be able to parent a child with Down's syndrome:

> **Pregnant woman:** I would have got rid of the baby ... I felt that I've got three kids ... It shouldn't be their responsibility to look after their younger brother or sister if they were Down's syndrome or whatever ... But I think I've got my kids into such a way. They are very compassionate, they are caring kids. You know that they would feel the way I would feel, that, if anything would happen to mum and dad, I would look after. And I wouldn't want that for them, to have that responsibility.
> (Research interview with woman aged 37 who underwent amniocentesis)

This woman's time frame was *embodied* (Lippman, 1999), i.e. located in a specific social context of family relationships, since she was concerned that the compassion with which she had imbued her children would cause them to take on caring obligations long after she had died.

It is tempting to consider a longer time frame more rational than a shorter one. At the very least, clinicians who seek to communicate effectively with service users and carers need to appreciate the variety of temporal perspectives which may be adopted, and the implications of such differences for risk management. Western culture tacitly encourages individuals to privilege the biographical future over the present, but individuals will not necessarily adopt this attitude to time in their own lives. Moreover, chains of causation, as against thinking about them, can never be confined within any time horizon. Worrying about the future can itself become a risk factor, a consideration which persuaded the woman quoted below to avoid thinking ahead about her diabetes (Watson and Heyman, 1998):

> **Woman with diabetes:** I just try to take things as they come. I think if you worry about things sometimes, it just makes it more of a problem. Worrying about it won't help anyway. I think if you are aware of the problems, you've just got to take it as it comes.
> (Research interview with woman aged 47)

Similarly, the pregnant woman cited below feared that worrying about the presence of Down's syndrome would itself harm her unborn child (Heyman and Henriksen, 2001):

> **Pregnant woman:** Oh it was awful. The result, waiting. It was just, it was, em, I was just crying and everything again, like I did when I found out I was pregnant. 'Cos I was saying, 'Ee, this baby will come out miserable little' ... I mean, when you read the books and that, you think, 'Oh well, you know, three, four weeks'. But, like, you're wishing your life away, and it's awful, you know.
>
> (Research interview with pregnant woman aged 40 who underwent amniocentesis)

The woman quoted above had opted for amniocentesis, thereby enduring a month of intense anxiety whilst she waited for the result. She worried that the ensuing temporary stress might itself generate long-term adverse consequences through its impact on the development of the fetus. This concern is supported by a large body of research evidence that maternal stress is a risk factor for mammalian fetal development (e.g. Wright, 2007).

As this example illustrates, time frames can only be cut out of the tangled spaghetti of causation by accepting simplified selective models which exclude consideration of some potential causal pathways.

Temporal accounting in health risk management

The discussion so far has been concerned with the setting of time horizons which confine risk analysis within a potentially variable time frame. Temporal accounting involves calibrating outcome values in terms of their position within an established time frame. Usually, but by no means always, temporal accounting involves progressively discounting the future. Most people would prefer to be affected by a serious condition later rather than sooner in their life. Cost-benefit analysis methods such as the calculation of quality-adjusted life years (QALYs), discussed in Chapter 3, discount time at a standard rate. This is usually done through using the 'real' (inflation-adjusted) rate of return in financial markets to reduce the estimated value of future benefits (Viscusi, 1992).

Setting the discount rate for declining health in this way requires a conceptual leap from money markets to human life. Moreover, the meaningfulness of any fixed discount rate for health risks is questionable. The valuing of healthy and survival time cannot be separated from personal life projects. For instance, top national athletes might prefer to endure the consequences of injury well before the next Olympic Games. Scientists engaged in projects such as space missions which are implemented over decades might strongly desire to live long enough to see them through. On a much shorter timescale, epidemiological evidence suggests that the terminally ill may postpone their deaths for short periods in order to enjoy valued festivals such as Christmas and Chanukah (Skala and Freedland, 2004). In all such cases, time is not valued only for its own sake, but as a means towards the end of attaining life goals.

Patients with life-threatening conditions may be offered risk management choices which require them to confront stark questions about the personal value of time. For example, patients with lung cancer have been found to prefer to avoid surgery which would increase their overall 5-year survival chances at the price of an immediate increased risk of death resulting from the operation (McNeil, Weichselbaum, and Pauker, 1978). Overall, on average, they perhaps preferred to maximize their chances of immediate survival. Each person will discount time differently, and much will depend upon how choices are framed in particular health care contexts.

Risk and the management of future intentions

When ongoing or staged risk management is required, future intentions become part of the uncertain future. The goal of the selected strategy requires a particular line of action to be adhered to. Anyone who has attempted to sustain their own or others' motivation during the completion of a long-lasting arduous task will know how difficult it is to predict motivation along the way. Novelty wears off and fatigue sets in. In addition, partial completion of a project may itself alter both circumstances and attitudes. Such internal dynamics threaten the coherence of temporally structured actions. The weary voyager may come to regret having started their journey as travel fatigue sets in, but unfortunately now finds turning back as difficult as carrying on. Beginning the voyage, in retrospect, no longer seems sensible. Faith in their future self has turned out to have been ill-founded.

From a future-oriented perspective, willingness and ability to see the project through become matters of risk management concern. For example, some patients with tuberculosis will stop taking prescribed drugs when they start to feel better, despite pledging to complete the full treatment. Their sincerity at the start of this process does not provide a guide to their motivation after symptoms disappear. Unfortunately, non-completion provides the ideal environment for drug-resistant strains to develop. Risk management must address the sustainability of compliance. Regimes such as direct observation of treatment appear to have little impact in both developing (Walley et al., 2001) and developed countries (MacIntyre et al., 2003).

Individuals progressing through health screening systems typically face a two stage process in which higher risk cases are first identified through non-invasive, but less than accurate, testing. This sub-population is then offered precise but invasive diagnostic tests. For instance, older people screened for colorectal cancers will first take a fecal occult blood test (FOBt). Those who screen at higher risk will then be invited to undergo colonoscopy. This unpleasant procedure carries an approximately 1:800 risk of colon perforation which can in turn cause potentially fatal complications such as peritonitis (Bowles *et al.*, 2004). About half of those flagged as higher risk from FOBt are found to have either colorectal cancer (8%), or potentially pre-cancerous polyps (38%) (The UK CRC Screening Pilot Evaluation Team, 2003). Around 20% of patients categorized as at higher risk do not complete colonoscopy in England, and this proportion rises to 25% among ethnic minority groups (The UK CRC Screening Pilot Evaluation Team, 2003). Patients who do not proceed to colonoscopy are not necessarily acting inconsistently. They may have decided from the outset to keep an open mind about how to respond to a higher risk screening outcome. Nevertheless, they cannot return to the state of affairs which existed before they decided to be screened. They cannot 'unknow' their acquired higher risk status. Nor can they exit from this status into certainty, one way or the other, without undertaking diagnostic steps. They become trapped in a higher risk no-man's-land.

Risk retrospection

The first part of the chapter focussed on thinking about the future. Risk managers need to select temporal horizons, and to decide how to account for time within the boundaries they have set. These interpretive steps are forward-looking. In addition, risks may be viewed retrospectively after actual outcomes become known. From this backward-looking vantage point, it can be seen that a possible adverse outcome actually did or did not occur. Past risk management tends to look different when viewed through the 'retroscope', as happened when the global banking collapse of 2007 spectacularly exposed the failings of financial risk regulation. On the other hand, the non-appearance of the much feared millennium computer bug on 1st Jan 2000 generated accusations of computer security company hype. In both cases, a risk looked different with hindsight.

Risk retrospection involves looking back at risk management after an adverse event has or has not detectably occurred. The notion of detectable occurrence must be fitted into a time frame, as argued above. For instance, longer-term risks arising from medical interventions may not be noticed because they happen outside the temporal span of clinical trials. In retrospect, a patient may realize that symptoms which they or health professionals dismissed as trivial should have been regarded as early warning signs of major disease. In the light of present knowledge, a patient may regret not having taken preventive action, or may feel angry with the healthcare system for not having identified a serious risk. The intervention which could have been provided might not have bene-fitted the patient, but at least an attempt to deal with the risk would have been made. On the other hand, as noted in Chapter 4 in relation to the discussion of the inductive prevention paradox, the individual efficacy of an intervention cannot be known retrospectively. The patient who was treated might have prospered even if left well alone.

Hindsight bias occurs when knowledge of an actual outcome influences judgements about the risk management process which was previously fol-lowed. Perceptions of the farther past are coloured by knowledge of the more immediate past which could not have been available at the time when risk-management decisions were made. Psychological research suggests that hind-sight bias powerfully affects human judgement, and that the strength of its influence tends to be underestimated. It is simply too difficult to reconstruct how one would have viewed risk management at the time when the outcome was still uncertain. By definition, risk managers cannot know what will actu-ally turn out to happen at the time when they take a decision. The difference between their informational state and that of later observers looking back at an outcome can be easily overlooked. For example, Mitchell and Kalb (1981) asked nurses to adopt the role of a supervisor who was required to evaluate a subordinate's performance. Research participants who were told that the nurse's failure to replace a bed rail had resulted in injury to a patient rated this outcome as more likely than those who had not. Individuals given hindsight about an adverse outcome also saw the subordinate as more responsible for the behaviour than did those who were not told about the accident.

Underestimation of the hindsight effect's power appears to arise from a striving to maintain a consistent view of the world rather than merely from faulty memory (Stahlberg and Maass, 1998). When research participants are provided with records of their previous views, they preserve coherence by recalling a greater degree of uncertainty about their past belief (Bradfield and Wells, 2005). Crucially in relation to one of the main ideas put forwards in the present book, research participants are more likely to exhibit hindsight bias if it reinforces their own values. Holzl and Kirchler (2005) found that supporters of the Euro currency showed more hindsight bias in relation to beneficial consequences of its adoption than to damaging ones, and *vice versa*. This find-ing suggests that hindsight bias can be considered as an example of a broader process in which the interpretation of evidence is shaped by values.

Official inquiries create a fertile environment in which 'expert' hindsight bias can flourish. An adverse event such as a murder committed by a released mental health patient, or a death which might have been prevented through timely medical intervention, triggers the investigation. In these circumstances, the potential influence of hindsight can never be ruled out. Unlike the inquiry team, the professionals held accountable could not know that their risk management choices would be associated with a subsequent adverse event. Inquiry teams have an inherent vested interest in discounting hindsight bias which would raise doubts about the value of their conclusions. Their societally derived authority may embolden these teams to assume an omniscience which underestimates the cloudiness of prospective uncertainty. The official report into the death of abused child Jasmine Beckford expressed the view *that hindsight is of assistance to us in our task, being no more than reasonable foresight, with the additional benefit of knowledge of what has actually occurred* (London Borough of Brent, 1985).The panel's faith in their ability to avoid the trap of hindsight bias may not be entirely justified.

In addition to drawing attention away from the fundamental difficulties arising from prospective risk management, insensitivity to the power of hindsight bias can stimulate an excessively cautions approach. The inexorable rise of the Caesarean section is considered below from a temporal perspective.

The inexorable rise of the Caesarean section

Temporal risk management dynamics may go some way towards explaining the remorseless increase of the Caesarean section rate in many developed societies, and in emerging economies such as Brazil. The appropriateness of opting for this approach to managing the risks arising from the birth process is decided through clinical judgement in individual cases. However, continually rising aggregate rates, well above WHO guidelines (Johanson, Newburn, and Macfarlane, 2002), provide evidence that Caesarean sections are being increasingly overused.

The informational disjunction between prospective and retrospective perspectives may partly drive this trend. Low probability adverse outcomes such as serious pregnancy complications in rich countries will sometimes occur. Doctors and other paid health risk managers will appreciate their vulnerability to hindsight bias in such cases, and to its associated personal risks, including litigation and damage to professional status. Undertaking a Caesarean section erases knowledge about what would have happened if the procedure had not been actioned. If the patient declines to accept the recommended treatment, health professional vulnerability to hindsight bias is removed because risk ownership reverts to the patient who declined to follow advice.

If implementation leads to an adverse event, as when a Caesarean section goes wrong, health professionals can argue that new risks had to be incurred in order to deal with the initial risk. The inductive prevention paradox obscures retrospection. What might have happened if a less intense procedure had been adopted can never be known. Doctors can also be challenged for undertaking clearly unnecessary procedures which failed, but are far more likely to be sued for not intervening (Bassett, Lyer, and Kazanjian, 2000). A large grey area exists in which intervention can be unverifiably justified. The combination of the inductive prevention paradox with hindsight bias drives intervention intensity upwards, creating unnecessary iatrogenic risks. Health professionals do not, on the whole, deliberately set out to over-treat. Nevertheless, a certain *realpolitik* pushes them in that direction.

Conclusion

This chapter has analysed the role of temporal considerations in risk thinking. The lens of risk generates a resolutely forward-looking orientation towards uncertain health outcomes. Risk thinkers focus on contingencies, imagined alternative possible futures which either have not yet happened, or are presently unknown. Expectations about health outcomes can only be considered within a specific time frame which has to be set. Time-framing sets up temporal horizons beyond which risk managers do not take outcomes into account. Although the lifespan provides a natural boundary for health risk considerations, it is by no means the only one which can be applied. The sheer difficulty of obtaining data over long time periods may lead to considerably shorter time frames being set in practice. On the other hand, many health effects, including genetic and epigenetic abnormalities and risk factors for the mental health of children, may be considered across generations.

Temporal selection can itself become an active ingredient in risk management. Shortening the future period under consideration may flatter healthcare interventions such as smoking cessation, or stack the odds in favour of new pharmaceuticals. Official time frames such as 5-year survival do not necessarily match those of directly affected individuals. Patients have no reason to carve their lives up to suit clinical or research convenience. Personal time scales can only be understood in relation to individual lives and particular responses to risks. For example, pregnant women think about chromosomal screening over periods which vary between the end of pregnancy and the lives of their existing children. Individuals may discount time within the temporal horizons they have set, often valuing delays to risked outcomes actually occurring. However, time-discounting, like time-framing, can only be understood in relation to wider personal aspirations, e.g. to support a much loved child until their adulthood.

The forward-looking focus of risk thinking can be contrasted with the retrospective view which appears after it becomes known that a risked outcome has or has not occurred. Through the retroscope, previous risk management may take on a different meaning. It becomes apparent that an actual adverse event might have been prevented if only prophylactic measures had been adopted in good time. Those conducting official inquiries, perhaps enboldened by their authoritative position, can underestimate the power of hindsight bias over their own perceptions.

Chapter 6

Information about health risks

Andy Alaszewski

Aim

To examine the ways in which information is used in the context of uncertainty about health risks.

Objectives

1. To identify increasing awareness in late modern society about the limitations of current scientific knowledge

2. To consider alternative strategies for managing health risks and uncertainties

3. To critically review current approaches to increasing public confidence in health care systems through the development and application of encoded knowledge.

Knowledge in late modern society

Modern science has created a sophisticated body of knowledge about the causes and most effective ways of treating diseases. For example, research programmes such as the human genome programme have deciphered the human genetic code, facilitating the identification of genetic errors associated with breast and cervical cancer (Human Genome Project Information, n.d.). The development of disease-specific research networks (Department of Health, 2006a) means that new treatment regimes can be rapidly tested, enhancing treatment outcomes. Such developments have had clear measurable benefits. In 1970, approximately 50% of women diagnosed with breast cancer survived for at least 5-years. Currently, 80% survive (Lyall, 2006). (Time-framing of mortality risks is discussed in Chapter 5.)

However, such objective population-wide improvement in health and well-being is not reflected in individual subjective assessments of health and security. Indeed, anxiety appears to have increased in contemporary societies, creating the paradox of anxious or timid prosperity (Taylor-Gooby, 2000):

> Material levels of security in the western world are higher than ever before ... However, the sources of uncertainty and the mechanisms available to most people to deal with

them have changed, leading to the paradox of timid prosperity – growing uncertainty amid rising affluence.

Anxiety and uncertainty are especially associated with illness and disease, whether this is the threat of pandemic disease such as swine flu or the more personal experience of chronic illness. Locker noted that uncertainty arising from many long-term conditions often starts *when the individual first notices that something is wrong and may continue throughout the entire course of the illness* (Locker, 2003).

Science may be seen as a source of knowledge which can reduce uncertainty. But, paradoxically, it may also increase uncertainty in a number of ways. While science, and the professions that applied science to practical issues such as medicine, commanded considerable public support in the early 20th century, more recent events have tended to undermine this authority. For example, Moran (2003) notes the ways in which in, the UK, the BSE disaster and subsequent Inquiry exposed the limitations of scientific knowledge, and was part of a larger crisis of confidence in the food safety regime that produced periodic 'food scares'. The Inquiry report (Phillips, Bridgeman, and Ferguson-Smith, 2000) noted that the Ministry of Agriculture, Food and Fisheries relied heavily on experts. The Inquiry concluded that, although the Government had not sought to deliberately mislead, its misplaced attempts to reassure the public backfired, undermining public confidence:

> The Government was preoccupied with preventing an alarmist over-reaction to BSE because it believed that the risk was remote. It is now clear that this campaign of reassurance was a mistake. When on 20 March 1996 the Government announced that BSE had probably been transmitted to humans, the public felt that they had been betrayed. Confidence in government pronouncements about risk was a further casualty of BSE.

While disasters such as BSE can emphasize the limitations of current knowledge, undermining public confidence, there are other more fundamental problems in applying and using knowledge in contemporary societies. In pre-modern societies, knowledge systems used to explain and manage threats to collective and individual's well-being such as illness tend to incorporate religious and supernatural systems. Such systems provide both an explanation of past events, e.g. why a particular individual died, and a means of managing the future. For example, Evans-Pritchard (1976), in his classic study of a traditional society in Southern Sudan, demonstrated the ways in which the Azande could explain all misfortune. They often combined empirical evidence, for instance termites eating through the wood support of granary, with religious ideas such as witchcraft to explain why a particular individual was sitting under a granary when it collapsed. They used the same knowledge to predict the future. Evans-Pritchard acknowledged that if he had not demonstrated that he accepted Azande knowledge and practices he would not have been able to participate in their everyday life (Miller, 1978). For example, his Azande hosts would not have accompanied him on a journey unless he provided 'evidence' that it would be safe.

Such systems explain everything (and therefore, to modern minds, nothing). They have no space for uncertainty. In contrast, the scientific theories and knowledge that have partly replaced such belief systems in developed societies make more limited claims. As Ilkka notes *good scientific theories typically are false but nevertheless close to the truth* (Ilkka, 2002). The limitations of a theory become evident when it is replaced by a new one. For example, the limitations of the 'humour' theory of the body which underpinned medical practice until the 17th century were exposed when the body was reconceptualized as a system of interconnected organs. However, at any particular time, it is difficult to be sure how 'close to the truth' accepted theories are. Scientific knowledge is always provisional and uncertain. For Beck (1998), this uncertainty underpins contemporary concerns with risk:

> Risk society begins where tradition ends, when, in all spheres of life, we can no longer take traditional certainties for granted. The less we rely on traditional securities, the more risks we have to negotiate. The more risks, the more decisions and choices we have to make.

While science has considerably enhanced knowledge of the natural world, it does not necessarily provide the type of information which individuals can use to manage their lives. Epidemiology which is based on a mapping of the incidence of diseases in defined circumstances, e.g. time and space, provides information on the factors associated with the development of disease. For example, since the publication of the first findings in 1950 that smoking was linked to lung cancer (Doll and Hill, 1950; Wynder and Graham, 1950), the consensus is that about half of regular cigarette smokers will be killed by the habit (Peto, 1994). However, an individual smoker cannot know for sure which group they are in, as discussed in relation to inductive probabilistic reasoning in Chapter 4. This uncertainty opens up a gap which the individual can exploit to disregard information that would suggest an undesired change in behaviour, whether this is stopping smoking (Sutton, 1999) or changing diet to reduce the risk of heart disease (Ruston and Clayton, 2002).

The growth and increasing fragmentation of scientific knowledge into specialist disciplines creates an additional area of uncertainty. As experts become increasingly knowledgeable and specialized, so the gap between their knowledge and that of non-experts increases. Thus, while consultations between Azande experts and their clients are underpinned by the assumption that they share the same knowledge and beliefs, equivalent consultations in contemporary society are based on the premise that the parties do not share the same knowledge. A crucial part of the interaction is 'communicating', i.e. translating between different bodies of information. Morgan (2003) suggested that experts such as doctors can either seek to impose their knowledge by focussing *on objective descriptions of symptoms ... within a reductionist biomedical model* or strive to translate these accounts, adjusting to *patients' own illness framework*. These alternative sources of knowledge can also be exploited to reject advice that individuals do not find acceptable. For instance, Carrier, LaPlante, and Bruneau (2005) noted the ways in which the limits of professional knowledge, e.g. an inability to explain why a person who had tested positive for hepatitis C subsequently tested negative, created uncertainty and *space for competing discourses about body and disease, for example, that life is animated by a spirit that science could never grasp.*

The growth of science has created social benefits, at least in the present historical period for developed societies. A healthier population is living longer, but such knowledge does not reduce uncertainty. Indeed for a variety of reasons, it actually increases it. The management of such uncertainty will be considered in the next section.

Responses to uncertainty and risk in contemporary society

One way in which an individual can manage risk and uncertainty is to rely on agents, with appropriate knowledge, who make decisions on their behalf. This approach reduces *the potentially high costs associated with the actual process of decision-making and those associated with making the wrong decision (i.e. anxiety costs)* (McGuire, Henderson, and Mooney,1988). This is the 'officially' sanctioned approach in state health care systems, such as the UK's NHS, and insurance systems in Europe and the USA, with expert professionals acting as agents for their patients. However, such an approach can only work effectively when there is trust, i.e. the individual believes that the agent will act in good faith and that their claims to knowledge are valid. Boon and Holmes note that trust can be defined as the *confident expectations about another's motives with respect to oneself in situations entailing risk* (Boon and Holmes, 1991). Therefore, trust is an important resource and mechanism for dealing with ignorance and uncertainty (Giddens, 1991b).

The rationale for the UK's NHS which was established in 1948 centred on the doctor-patient relationship. The Government entrusted the profession with the provision of comprehensive medical care and treatment (Webster, 1988), and expected the population to trust their doctors. While the doctor-patient relationship, and the agency structure which underpins it, remain central to the delivery of healthcare, it has changed substantially. Trust has become problematized. Current governmental efforts are directed at maintaining and restoring trust. These developments will be reviewed in the next section.

Trust, informed consent, and clinical governance

The development of informed consent is a relatively recent phenomenon in medicine. Percival, in a text on medical ethics first published in 1803 (Leake, 1927), argued that it would be *gross and unfeeling wrong to reveal the truth* to a patient if such truth was harmful. His friend the Rev. Thomas Gisborne expressed a different view, arguing in 1794 that the *physician … is invariably bound never to represent uncertainty or danger as less than he actually believes it to be.* Percival's arguments prevailed until well into the 20th century. As the Ethics Committee of the American College of Obstetricians and Gynecologists noted, until the 1970s medical practice was grounded in paternalism. Doctors decided how much information to give their patients, using *the medical well-being of the patient* to justify their decisions (The American College of Obstetricians and Gynecologists, 2004). In some areas of medical care, there was a consensus that fully revealing the diagnosis and prognosis would harm the patient either by undermining their confidence or by exposing them to stigma. For example, Holland (2002) pointed out that before the 1970s most patients with cancer were *not* informed of their diagnosis. In the 1970s, there was a 'paradigm shift' (The American College of Obstetricians and Gynecologists, 2004) from a 'protective' approach to one in which the patient is deemed to have the right to receive enough information to make an informed decisions. The doctor is now expected to effectively communicate all relevant knowledge, including the risks and uncertainties associated with available treatment options. The above body stated that the patient should be *given adequate information about her diagnosis, prognosis, and alternative treatment choices, including the option of no treatment.*

The development of informed consent involves a major shift in medical practice. The doctor can no longer make decisions on behalf of the patient, but becomes an adviser who provides information about both the benefits and risks of treatment, so that the patient can make an informed choice. Thus, the doctor has a duty to effectively communicate information on risks. This change in medical roles resulted from a combination of factors, including the increased involvement of the law in medical cases, a decline in deference, the rise of consumerism in post-industrial democracies, and responses to medical scandals.

Dissatisfied patients have long had recourse to the law. For example, in the 18th century, an English patient sued two doctors who had rebroken and reset his fractured leg without his consent (Slater v Baker and Stapleton, K.B. 1767). In the 20th century, informed consent became a well-established issue affecting legal judgements. Justice Cardozo presided over a US case in which a woman had consented to an abdominal examination but not an operation under anaesthetic. During the operation, the doctor had found and removed a tumour. In a landmark decision, the Judge found in the patient's favour ruling *that an individual had the right of bodily self-determination* (Schoendorff v Society of New York Hospital, N.Y. 1914).

A decline in deference in post-industrial societies appears to be a long-term trend which sociologists and social historians have detected in a variety of areas. For example, Neville (1996) noted, on the basis of a study of changing attitudes in Canada, the USA, and Europe during the 1980s, a decline in deference evidenced by *declining confidence in both governmental and non-governmental institutions and the emergence of non-traditional forms of political participation*. The authors of the NHS Plan (Department of Health, 2000a) also observed this change in the healthcare arena. They argued that, in 1948, an attitude of unconditional trust prevailed, as deference and hierarchy defined the relationship between citizens and services. But changes in public attitudes meant that the NHS now had to earn the trust of citizens. There is some empirical evidence supporting the hypothesis that public and patient deference have declined. Blaxter and Paterson (1982) studied the attitudes of three generations of working class women living in a town in Scotland to health and healthcare. They found that women born after the formation of the NHS were less deferential, were less willing to tolerate the symptoms of illness, and had higher expectations of healthcare.

With the decline of deference, users of healthcare are increasingly seen as active consumers rather than passive patients. In the UK and elsewhere, the development of the consumer movement in the 1970s provided a stimulus for this shift. The Consumer Association and its publication *Which?* initially focussed on providing the public with information on commercial services and goods, but expanded to include public services, especially healthcare which now forms one of the 10 key topic areas on its campaign website, www.which.co.uk/portals/p/campaigns/index.jsp/. The Government endorsed this consumerist approach with the publication, in 1991, of the Patient's Charter. The Charter outlined patients' rights and the standards of service which they could expect to receive. Although the Government formally abolished the Charter in 2001, it still endorses its underlying principles.

Subsequent to the year 2001, the consumerist impulse underpinning the Patient's Charter found expression in a number of new policy initiatives. The Department of Health directed that, as of 2006, all patients should have the choice of four or more providers when they are referred for a planned admission. Central to the new system is the provision of information about hospitals. Localities produce local information booklets in up to 18 languages and a range of formats. The Department has created a website which, it claims, *gives people the opportunity to directly share their experiences and generate user ratings of the services they have received* (Department of Health, 2006b). Currently the website is very basic, and highly reliant on official information. But it should evolve as and when patients add their own views (Patient Opinion, 2006).

The Expert Patient programme is a service user led self-management project in which patients with chronic illness are taught to be effective users and consumers of healthcare. They are trained in five core self-management skills: problem solving; decision-making, resource utilization; developing effective partnerships with healthcare providers; and taking action (Department of Health, Chief Medical Officer, 2006). The use of the term 'expert' in the title of the programme indicates that it is designed to restructure the relationship between users and providers of healthcare, challenging the assumption that expertise belongs exclusively to health professionals. Only patients and carers can understand what it means to live with ill health and risk. As argued in the first part of the present book, all risk knowledge must be based on presuppositions, e.g. about values and time frames, which cannot be established objectively. Expertise about these issues, for instance about the meaning of giving birth to a child with disabilities, can only be derived from those directly affected.

A key factor in changing perceptions about the nature of medicine, especially medical research and knowledge, has been medical scandals. In 1946, 23 Nazi doctors and administrators were brought before the Nuremberg War Tribunal for undertaking medical experiments which led to extreme suffering and death of inmates in concentration and prisoner of war camps. The basic principles used by the tribunal to judge these cases were documented in the 1947 Nuremberg Code which affirmed the right to informed voluntary consent and the obligation to minimize risk and harm to participants (Yeide and Lifton, 1987). More recently, medical scandals in the UK have contributed to changing conceptions of doctor-patient relationship, providing a justification for the Government to increase the regulation of medical practice. In 1999, the Government established a public inquiry into the treatment of dead children's bodies at Alder Hey Hospital. The Inquiry found a *long-standing widespread practice of organ retention without consent* (Redfern, Keeling, and Powell, 2001). The Inquiry concluded that these practices were unacceptable, reflecting an outdated approach to medical ethics and practice:

> Their [the medical profession's] approach has been paternalistic in the belief that parents or relatives would not wish to know about the retention of organs and the use to which they were put ... In the current climate of frankness and openness it should no longer be possible for organs to be retained without the knowledge or consent of the parents.

The policy response focussed mainly on the regulation of medical and other health research through the development of research ethics and governance frameworks (see Chapter 8).

The Bristol Royal Infirmary Inquiry (2001) examined the services provided by the paediatric cardiac surgical team at Bristol Royal Infirmary between 1984 and 1995. The Inquiry found that the service was so poor that it exposed children under the age of one to an unacceptable level of risk. The Inquiry concluded that, between 1991 and 1995, about 30 children died who would not have done so if the quality of services at Bristol had been comparable to that achieved in other regional centres. As at Alder Hey, problems with informed consent were identified. At Bristol, parents were not aware of the risks to which their children were being exposed. The Inquiry found that a club culture had developed at the hospital in which a core group of managers disregarded information, withholding it not only from parents but also from other professionals, managers, and the public:

> Bristol was awash with data. There was enough information from the late 1980s onwards to cause questions about mortality rates to be raised both in Bristol and elsewhere had the mindset to do so existed. Little, if any, of this information was available to the parents or to the public. Such information as was given to parents was often partial, confusing and unclear. For the future, there must be openness about clinical performance. Patients should be able to gain access to information about the relative performance of a hospital, or a particular service or consultant unit.

The Inquiry drew on and stimulated contemporary government thinking linking enhanced medical regulation and clinical governance (see Chapter 8). These changes were designed to improve public confidence in healthcare through a process of quality assurance which linked openness to professional self and external regulation (NHS Executive, 1999, present author's emphasis):

> Clinical governance will be the process by which each part of the NHS quality-assures its clinical decisions ... Professional self-regulation provides clinicians with the opportunity to help set standards. **People need to be confident** that the regulatory

bodies will exercise rigorous self-regulation over the standard and conduct of health professionals and will act promptly and openly when things go wrong.

This new approach to regulation was based on a critique of the ways in which knowledge has been used in the NHS. It was designed to replace local knowledge derived either from group custom and practice or personal intuition with evidence-based, scientifically grounded practice. In the 'new' NHS, national systems for encoding knowledge in guidelines and national frameworks are supposed to provide the basis for the regulation and scrutiny of healthcare provision.

While the NHS and related research programmes are designed to provide the knowledge base for healthcare practice, a variety of institutions which are supported by the Department of Health, such as the Cochrane Collaboration and the National Institute for Health and Clinical Excellence (NICE), summarize and codify this evidence. The Cochrane Collaboration (2009) sees itself as *a reliable source of evidence in health care* while the National Institute for Health and Clinical Excellence (2009) emphasizes its role as:

> an independent organisation responsible for providing national guidance on promoting good health and preventing and treating ill health … [including] guidance on the appropriate treatment and care of people with specific diseases and conditions within the NHS.

This codified knowledge is now supposed to provide the grounds for clinical decision-making. Doctors are expected to base their practice on it, and managers are expected to check that it is being used. The main source of evidence for compliance with national standards is measurement of clinical practice outcomes. The 1997 White Paper asserted that the NHS *will place greater emphasis on the outcomes of treatment and care. It will focus on things that really matter* (Department of Health, 1997). Centralized regulatory and information systems were designed to ensure that high risks such as those arising from organizational failures would be rapidly identified, and that normal practice would be soundly evidence-based. The reforms were predicated on the assumption which was challenged in the first part of the present book that risks exist as objective measurable entities. The social science of risk emphasizes the negotiated but normally unspoken interpretive processes which underpin the perception of risks. The final section of this chapter will consider whether the centralized approach to healthcare risk management is likely to succeed.

New relations between the NHS and patients: rhetoric or reality?

The UK Government has attempted to increase its control over the production and use of health knowledge. But this approach may not increase public confidence in the healthcare system. The shift may be seen as one of rhetoric rather than reality. There are also some fundamental flaws in the strategy. Knowledge encoded in generalized clinical guidelines by itself is not an adequate basis for clinical decision-making in particular cases. The policy conflates confidence in the NHS, a relatively abstract concept, with trust in the doctors and nurses delivering the service, which is based on concrete face-to-face relationships and experiences. In seeking to restore confidence, policy-makers have modelled patients as rational actors, and thereby neglected the emotional components of trust.

There has been a major shift in the rhetoric of healthcare from paternalistic compliance with treatment to that of partnership based on concordance over treatment (Marinker *et al.*, 1997). The concordance model is based on communication and exchange of knowledge between expert and patient. According to this model, the expert provides knowledge on prognosis and the risk and benefits of treatment, whilst the patient is provided with an opportunity to articulate their beliefs about, and priorities for, treatment. Concordance emphasizes the importance of patient knowledge and belief (Marinker and Shaw, 2003):

> Patients have their own beliefs about their medicines and medicines in general. They have their own priorities and their own rational discourses in relation to health and care, and risk and benefit.

When expert knowledge and patient belief are irreconcilable, then precedence should not be given to the expert's knowledge, as in the paternalistic compliance approach but to the patient's view (Marinker and Shaw, 2003). This approach to healthcare decision-making has been widely endorsed. For example, the World Health Organization sees concordance as a key step in supporting patients with tuberculosis through the process of treatment (Maher *et al.*, 2003). In England, the Department of Health endorsed the principle in 2002 and established the Medicines Partnership to promote the concept of concordance, or shared decision-making, as an approach to help patients to get the most from their medicines (Medicines Partnership, 2006).

The issue of concordance exposes the tension in health policy between building an efficient health service based on the codification and application of best available evidence and developing a health service which gives precedence to patients' beliefs and priorities (Marinker and Shaw, 2003). In practice, precedence still tends to be given to codified knowledge. This 'knowledge' carries with it unspoken presuppositions, such as implicit preferences about the value of outcomes and their timing, analysed in the first part of the present book. The conflict between the rhetorics of choice and evidence-based care can be seen in areas in which Government has evidence of risky and harmful behaviour which it wants to change in order to improve public health. For instance, Lee (2007) has undertaken a study focussing on the experience of mothers who have bottle-fed their babies. Lee found that official information emphasized the benefits of breast-feeding and the risks of bottle-feeding. Lee notes that, in the USA, the scientific adviser to the Department of Health and Human Sciences had equated the risk of bottle-feeding with those of smoking in pregnancy. Similarly, in the UK, the provision of information on bottle-feeding has been restricted. Group demonstrations of bottle-feeding are no longer sanctioned, and mothers who chose to bottle-feed are informed of the risks. Lee found no evidence of concordance between health professionals and bottle-feeding mothers, some of whom felt such pressure to comply that they concealed the fact that they were bottle-feeding.

A similar trend is evident in the treatment of coronary heart disease. Crinson *et al.* (2007) noted that Government policy as expressed in the National Service Framework (Department of Health, 2000b) identified two interacting causes of coronary heart disease: broader socioeconomic factors such as poverty; and individual risk factors like raised blood pressure and cholesterol levels. The Government has chosen to concentrate on the individual risk factors. Its guidelines for general practitioners (GPs) advise them to identify high-risk patients, and to use drugs to reduce blood pressure and cholesterol levels. These guidelines are now backed up with financial incentives for GPs. Effectively, this system is designed to *ensure* compliance of high risk individuals with recommended drug therapies by appealing to their essential 'rationality' (Crinson *et al.*, 2007). Crinson *et al.* noted that this emphasis on compliance served to limit patient choice over the management of their condition, and marginalized their treatment preferences. In particular, changes which patients did not understand, such as reductions in officially acceptable level of cholesterol, and regular changes of prescriptions to achieve the maximum effect, had the effect of reducing patient confidence in expert advice.

Thus, where there is a conflict between evidence-based practice and a patient-centred, choice based system, policy-makers tend to favour the former. They have, after all, invested heavily in developing the evidence base, and believe that it will deliver more effective and safer health care. However, pressuring patients into compliance is likely to undermine their confidence in the system, conflicting with the rhetoric of patient choice. Furthermore, this approach does not acknowledge limitations to the knowledge base on which healthcare prescriptions are grounded. But patients may not be so uncritical, particularly when recommendations change, are inconsistent, seem arbitrary, or ignore the personal costs of compliance.

The limits of encoded knowledge

The encoding of knowledge about health risks is designed to structure and control professional decision-making. Attempted implementation creates an unexamined tension with the rhetoric of patient-centred care, discussed above. In addition, encoded knowledge is incomplete. It needs to be interpreted and appropriately applied, and therefore requires other forms of knowledge. For example, Prior *et al.* (2002) examined the ways in which clinicians used Cyrillic, a computer-based programme, to estimate patients' risk of cancer. Cyrillic made risk 'visible' by using inputted data on relatives to draw a family tree of cancer and provide a numerical estimate of personal risk. However, clinicians had to make 'sense' of results and images, which involved craftwork, especially in the laboratory. Such craftwork meant that professional decision-making required inputs of additional 'tacit' knowledge.

Even where there is a major shift to the use of encoded knowledge, research has found that such knowledge does not provide an adequate or sufficient basis for decision-making. In an analysis of two projects designed to promote patient safety by reducing drug errors and preventing falls, Procter (2002) found that, in practice, technical developments grounded in the use of encoded knowledge were combined with recognition of the broader social context. Successful application of encoded knowledge depended upon engaging patients, carers, and professionals, which in turn required recognition of their experiential knowledge. Similar findings have come from research on NHS Direct, a telephone advice service in which nurses use knowledge encoded within computerized decision support software to advise callers about self-care and use of other services. In an observational study, Ruston (2006) found that, following an initial conversation with a caller, nurses often made a judgement on the best course of action. They then checked their own view against that prescribed by the computer algorithm, overriding the algorithm if there was disagreement.

Rationality and trust

The development of a health care system based on the application of encoded knowledge is designed not only to improve outcomes and reduce dangerous practice, but also to increase public and patient confidence in the NHS, creating a 'high trust' organization (Department of Health, 2000b). In the UK, the publication of league tables, star ratings, and surgery outcome indicators is intended to guide rational patient choice, drive up clinical standards, and improve patient trust in the quality of health services. Leaving aside the practical problems involved in developing this system, i.e. whether it really works in terms of providing patient choice and controlling professional decision-making, there is a serious flaw in the logic. It emphasizes the instrumental rationality of patients and the public, and their acceptance and responsiveness to information on the overall performance of the system. This approach neglects the more personal and emotional ways in which individuals judge and respond to their interaction with health professionals. As Calnan and Rowe (2005) note, trust can involve using and processing knowledge to reach a judgement, but it can also be more intuitive, based on feelings or emotions:

> Trust has been characterised as a multi-layered concept primarily consisting of a cognitive element (grounded on rational and instrumental judgments) and an affective dimension (grounded on relationships and affective bonds generated through interaction, empathy and identification with others).

The emotional component of healthcare is likely to be quite high, for two reasons. Firstly, it involves intimate personal interventions which have a major impact on personal identity and sense of self (Alaszewski, Alaszewski, and Potter, 2006). Secondly, individuals often have to make 'fateful' life and death decisions in stressful and uncertain situations (Barbalet, 2005). Taylor-Gooby (2006) has argued that recent UK healthcare reforms have tended to neglect the personal and emotional aspects of care, especially the extent to which patients feel that they and their values are respected:

> The current direction of reform leaves affect and emotion out of consideration. There is no sentiment in business, or in a business plan, however good a business plan it happens to be. The appeal is entirely to reason, both in the way the reforms work (through shifting incentives to change the way those involved behave) and in the understanding of people's perceptions of and responses to public sector institutions which is implicit in them.

Taylor-Gooby concludes that concentrating on cognitive rationality is likely to generate a healthcare system which focusses on curing patients, but fails to meet their personal and emotional needs. Such systems do not inspire confidence or trust. Furthermore, they leave the inherent limitations of risk knowledge unexamined. Patients who experience limitations such as those of inductive probabilistic reasoning, discussed in Chapter 4, tend to be less charitable since their lives are at stake.

Conclusion

The development of modern scientific medicine has created a major divide between the evidence base used by experts and lay knowledge. Illness and disease can create major personal threats and challenges. Individuals often have to make fateful decisions under conditions of stress and uncertainty. They may use a variety of strategies for managing this uncertainty, including disregarding the threat, using simplifying heuristics, drawing on the resources of social movements, and relying on an expert agent to make decisions on their behalf. Traditionally, doctors have functioned as expert agents, making decisions for patients without providing full information in order to minimize harm and distress.

By the 1970s, this approach had come to be seen as paternalistic. It was replaced by a partnership model based on informed consent. According to this model, the doctor provides information on the risks and benefit of treatments and the patient takes responsibility for making the required decisions. The reframing of the patient as an active consumer of health care has found expression in the expert patient programme, and in the idea of treatment concordance. At the same time, following a number of scandals and inquiries in the UK, the Government has focussed on the development of a systematic encoded knowledge base as a way of controlling the quality of expert decision-making. This approach aims to reduce harm, improve outcomes, and increase patient and public confidence in the healthcare system.

There are a number of problems with the current reform programme. It is not clear that the investment in evidence-based health services will yield the desired outcomes. Firstly, uncritical 'selling' of evidence-based healthcare underplays the inherent limitations of risk knowledge, rendering its interpretive presuppositions untransparent. Secondly, encoded knowledge is not a sufficient or adequate basis for expert decisions. It needs to be supplemented by professional judgement. Therefore, the goal of controlling expert decisions to minimize risk and maximize health outcomes is likely to remain elusive. Thirdly, a tension exists between decisions based on encoded knowledge and those derived from patient preferences. Policy-makers appear to favour knowledge-based decisions. But disregarding patient preferences conflicts with the rhetoric of a patient-centred service. This neglect is likely to undermine patient confidence in the service, and reduce compliance with treatment. The potential contradictions with the patient-centred approach have not been articulated in official accounts of healthcare strategy.

Chapter 7

Health risks and the media

Monica Shaw

Aim

To explore media constructions and representations of health risks.

Objectives

1. To review the role played by the media in selectively constructing and representing health risks

2. To consider the problems of assessing media influences upon public perceptions of health risks and upon associated changes in behaviour

3. To identify the competing interests which contribute to the selective production of health risk media messages.

Introduction

Health and health risk are subjects of major interest to the media, whether in terms of the latest medical therapies and technical advances, accounts of organizational or personnel failings, human interest stories, or entertainment (Hodgetts and Chamberlain, 2006). Open any newspaper and the chances are that you will find several, often contradictory, health stories. For example, the *Sunday Observer* newspaper on 18th Nov 2007 included two gloomy articles concerning the failure of medicine to combat disease with a full-page spread on *pseudomonas* (as yet a less well publicized hospital-acquired infection) under the headline *Untreatable Bug is Killing Patients*, and a feature on the incurable crippling conditions of older age under the headline *A Longer Life Ignores the Cost of Growing Old*. Conversely the paper reported optimistically on medical progress under the headline *Nature's Tiny Wonders Heal Human Scars: Frogs May Hold the Power to Regenerate Tissue*. The contrast between the progressive image of science and the experience of old age and fallible service delivery typifies oppositions which characterize the representation of health and risk in many media forms (Seale, 2002). The newspaper provided two shorter reports, one relating to Department of Health failings with the headline *MPs Say Consultants are Grossly Overpaid* and one on healthy eating under the headline *School Meals Campaign to Target Teenagers* (*The Observer* newspaper, 18th Nov 2007).

News reports such as those above illustrate common media concerns about the National Health Services (NHS), and their obsessions with health risk and lifestyle, all of which impact upon the public and clinician-patient relationships, although how far and in what ways is only partially understood. In order to map out some of the complex factors involved, the chapter draws on studies of the representation of health risk messages, audience responses to them, and the varying interests which lie behind them. Examples are included from a range of communication channels, including newsprint, television, film, and the Internet, which show some similarities in the way they selectively define health risks. In keeping with the spirit of earlier chapters, readers are asked to critically reflect on the links between media, health, and risk, including how risks come to be constructed by, and within, the media in its various forms. Interesting and potentially useful theoretical frameworks, such as those derived from the social amplification of risk and media framing models, will be considered, along with some of their strengths and weaknesses. Hopefully, the material presented will help to convince readers of the value of a critical and theoretically informed way of studying the media and its role in generating understandings of health risk.

The role of the media in society

From the earliest days of newsprint and public broadcasting, there has been a tension between the informational and democratizing potential of the media and its use as an instrument of propaganda. This tension raises questions about what the proper role of the media should be, and whose interests it should serve (Redley, 2007). One line of argument holds that the media acts as a guard dog for the status quo rather than as a watchdog which challenges it (Durfee, 2006), its purpose being to legitimize the political and social order (McGuigan, 2006). This position suggests that the process of media health risk selection and construction is largely controlled by powerful voices in society, amongst them Government spin doctors, health agency officials, and representatives of clinical drug companies who stand to gain commercially from the promotion of particular risks. However, individuals and groups can from time to time successfully challenge health officials and agencies. For example, rulings on clinical drugs produced by the National Institute of Clinical Excellence (NICE) are often queried through the media. Controversial and contradictory ideas about health risk are reported, a process which may empower the public to contest scientific expertise and medical authority, although it may also make people feel less certain and more anxious about the future (Beck, 1992; Giddens, 1991b). Whether and how far the media increase risk anxiety are open to debate, since news structures are more disposed to report daily events and personal tragedies than to give prolonged coverage to future uncertainty (Eldridge and Reilly, 2003). Nevertheless, the cumulative impact of attention given to certain risks is likely to have some impact, although how much and in what ways is not easy to discern.

From the viewpoint of many Government officials, scientists, health risk managers, and health promoters, the media, old and new, should ideally function to inform the public about risks. With this in mind, media communication is often deemed to fail through putting shock value above accuracy, with potentially detrimental consequences for patients. In the words of a medical columnist for the UK's *Guardian* newspaper:

> Few things can make a doctor's heart sink more in a clinic than a patient brandishing a newspaper clipping. Alongside the best efforts to empower patients, misleading information conveyed with hyperbole is paradoxically disempowering; and it's fair to say that the media don't have an absolutely brilliant track record in faithfully reporting medical news.
>
> (Dr Ben Goldacre, *The Guardian* newspaper, 6th Nov 2007)

Integral to the UK Government's continuing healthcare reforms is its stated concern to better inform, and to improve communication to individuals about health risk (Department of Health, 1999), the central concern of Chapter 6. For many health professionals, like the disconsolate Dr Goldacre quoted above, health campaigners, and policy-makers, getting accurate health information to the public is an essential first step towards informed choice. They are highly critical of what they see as the tendency of the media to distort and mislead (Harrabin, Coote, and Allen, 2003; Cassells, 2007).

Amplification and attenuation effects of media communication

The media are often accused of creating the selective amplification of health risks which, like rumours, grow in telling. Interest in the amplification process contributed to the development of the social amplification of risk framework (SARF) by a group of psychologists in North America. The model was developed to bring together disparate research interests and approaches. The aims were to construct a framework which would integrate understanding of risk perception and communication and would generate more dynamic research into risk perception and social context (Pidgeon, Kasperson, and Slovic, 2003).

SARF does not so much explain what happens as much as it expands awareness of the many complex variables and processes which need to be taken into account when researching risk communication. The mass media is seen as one of a number of social agencies who *generate, receive, interpret and pass on risk signals*, acting as a key primary agent because of its extensive communication role in society (Kasperson *et al.*, 2005).

One of the main objectives of the amplification model is to understand why *hazards and events that experts assess as relatively low in risk become a particular focus of concern and socio-political activity within a society (risk amplification), while other hazards that experts judge to be more serious receive comparatively less attention from society (risk attenuation)* (Kasperson *et al.*, 2005). The high profile of what was labelled 'Mad Cow's Disease' and of genetically modified foods are often cited as examples of amplification compared with risks of disease and death caused by smoking or injuries and deaths arising from car accidents, which are attenuated. An important secondary amplification process is said to occur as the media, acting like a series of relay stations, generate ripple effects such as the fear and risk aversion that followed in the wake of the terrorist attacks in the USA on 11th Sept 2001, and which continue to impact globally on social and economic life (Pidgeon, Simmons, and Henwood, 2006). Similarly the media can help to keep certain health risks or aspects of them at bay, as with *the profound impact of AIDS on culture and social institutions – health care, social services, prisons, and the family* which has been largely ignored (Nelkin, 1996). As argued in Chapter 4, the representation of condomless sex as 'unsafe' in the media and elsewhere has a moral and prescriptive function. It does not merely describe the probability of acquiring a serious sexually transmitted disease (STD) which is very low for the general population of the UK and other rich countries.

One criticism of the amplification model is that it tends to underplay the commercial interests of the media in contributing to such selectivity because the main focus is on communication processes which, like radio waves, become distorted as they radiate outwards. The metaphor is compelling in some respects, but exactly what happens when many interested parties jostle for airspace is not explained (Murdock, Petts, and Horlick-Jones, 2003). Another limitation is that the model takes as its starting point the neutral voice of the expert, a doubtful proposition since experts do not always speak with one voice, and can also use the media to advance their own interests (Horlick-Jones, 2004). In addition, there are many channels of media communication, some more interactional than others, such as the Internet, and it is not yet clear how they might contribute to amplification and attentional effects. Nevertheless, the amplification framework is capable of building in many variables which influence risk selectivity. It thus points to the complex understandings of risk communication and perception which are necessary in order to try to assess media influence.

The 'old' and 'new' mass media

The term mass media covers a vast, differentiated, and fragmented field. It was coined in the 1920s to reflect the arrival of mass circulation newspapers, and magazines and nationwide radio broadcasting. The term refers to channels designed to reach very large audiences. Subsequently, it has encompassed other means of mass communication such as television and increasingly the Internet, reflecting technological advances which increase immediacy and open up global events. The media serve many, varied, and overlapping purposes, including entertainment, education, public relations, campaigning, advertising, and attempting to raise public awareness. Well-being, lifestyle, and health risk have become increasingly popular themes transmitted directly or indirectly through broadcasts, print, film, and photographic images. Media channels of communication continue to expand in the multi-digital age via computers, ipods, and mobile phones. These are collectively referred to as new media in comparison with earlier and more established media channels.

The collective terms 'old' and 'new' media can be misleading since they imply internal coherence in each, and a disjunctive break between two periods of mass communication, with the new often credited as being cutting-edge, progressive, and revolutionary. However, the impact of new media and their relationship with older communication channels has barely begun to be explored (Seale, 2005). Such exploration raises complex issues since the media are segmented into an array of local radio stations, television channels, print forms, and a plethora of Internet websites. Although the media are multi-faceted and diverse, it does not follow that they are conveying complex messages. Some argue that a number of socioeconomic trends, in particular increasing consumerism, have led to uniformity and 'dumbing down' of the media as a whole (Collins, 2007). As is discussed further in the chapter, early optimism about the radical and democratizing promise of the new media in relation to health representation has been somewhat modified since much of its content appears to converge with that conveyed through more established channels (Seale, 2005).

Nevertheless, the Internet opens up multiple information channels for individuals who are interested and able to access them, including websites devoted to health support groups and personal biographies, as well as those promoting 'expert' medical advice of various sorts. How different sources of information, including websites created by 'lay' people, might widen the concept of expertise, create an Internet empowered patient, and change the relationship between health professionals and patients are important questions that are beginning to generate a variety of research interests (Gillet, 2003; Seale, 2005). The somewhat anarchic nature of information production on the Internet has fuelled medical concern about the accuracy and quality of health information about health risk, and stimulated increased attention to the guidance needed for consumers (Gagliardi and Jahad, 2002; Theodosiou and Green, 2003).

Despite concerns about media distortion, health professionals recognize the potential of new media, the Internet in particular, to offer *mass customisation, interactivity and convenience as the new parameters of health communication* (Kivits, 2006). Changes in media consumption in Western societies include the diminishing influence of newspapers and the growing use of new media (Anderson, 2006). Figures have been cited indicating that almost half of Americans and a third of Europeans accessed health information on the internet by the end of 2002 (Theodosiou and Green, 2003), proportions which will have increased substantially since then. Which groups are involved, for what purposes, and how much trust is placed in web-based information remain under-researched questions. Some evidence suggests that 'the worried well' are most likely to be the information seekers and to constitute 'the informed patient' (Kivits, 2006). But they may well be joined by other groups as computer access, literacy, and health consumerism advance. For example, in the USA, a heavily consumerist culture, it is common for people to purchase clinical drugs over the Internet, a trend which is growing in the UK. Extensive advertising of medical products and services on the Internet is a matter of concern to health professionals on both sides of the Atlantic.

Media representation of health risks

Health risk representation in the media has been the subject of extensive research, much of it focussed on newsprint and relying heavily on content analysis (Seale, 2003). This trend reflects the importance attached to news coverage by media researchers, not least because studies confirm that it is accepted by the public as a credible source of information (Durfee, 2006). However, this focus also reflects the relative ease with which content analysis can be conducted on any form of print as compared with other media channels such as film (Murdock, Petts, and Horlick-Jones, 2003). The methods applied to content analysis of media communications are various, some focussed on the deeper sociological meanings of the text, considered later in the chapter. Others concentrate on trying to measure the gap between news reports and the views of experts, as discussed below. Although requiring some adaptation, the methods used to study print media can also be applied to content analysis of websites on the Internet (Seale, 2005).

There is a preoccupation in studies of both old and new media with quality and accuracy (Seale, 2005) and, from the perspective of health professionals, the capacity of inadequate information to mislead an unknowing public (Harrabin, Coote, and Allen, 2003; Thirlaway and Heggs, 2005). From this vantage point the media fails to meet its responsibility to impart neutrally the appropriate 'facts'. To quote Dr Goldacre once more:

> So if anyone is listening, this is the information I want from a newspaper, to help me make decisions about my health: I want to know who you're talking about (e.g. men in their 50s); I want to know what the baseline risk is (e.g. four out of 100 will have a heart attack over 10-years); and I want to know exactly what's causing that increase in risk – an occasional headache pill or daily pain relief for arthritis. Health journalists are perfectly well paid, and the ones I know get paid more than the NHS pays me: it's not too much to ask!'
>
> (Dr. Ben Goldacre, *The Guardian* newspaper, 20th June 2005 see Box 7.1)

As argued by Dr Goldacre, fuller statistical pictures might lead to better under-standing. However, their relative absence cannot necessarily be blamed entirely upon health journalists, and the extent to which they would be absorbed by the public remains uncertain. However, the purposes of news reports do not often include the communication of risks as experts measure them. Rather, like modern equivalents of medieval morality tales, news stories allocate blame, simplify 'causes', and give greater and more protracted coverage to catastrophic events, particularly those which are dramatic, unexpected, and relatively rare, and those which result in serious harm (Singer and Endreny, 1993; Kitzinger, 1999; Anderson, 2006).

To the extent that health websites replicate newspaper reports and television broadcasts, which many do, similar representations of health risk will reap-pear, compounding the concerns of health professionals about misleading information on the Internet (Seale, 2005). Box 7.1, below, provides some examples of the predilections of 'old' media forms for simplification, and for what experts regard as distortion.

Findings, such as those summarized in Box 7.1, suggest that there is often a gap between risk constructions in the media and expert statistical assessments or scientific judgements, particularly through the use of dramatic news headlines and stories designed to make immediate impact. Health professional concern about the potential for harm of misleading information in the 'old' media is just as vigorously expressed about inadequate and erroneous information provided in the 'new', in particular via the Internet.

Box 7.1 The representation of health risks in the 'old' media

Studies of news reports show a tendency to:

♦ *Focus on unusual and dramatic health risks rather than those encountered every day*

A study of the BBC calculated that a story on the health risk of smoking would require, on average, 8 751 smoking related deaths for it to be regarded as newsworthy, whereas only 0.33 deaths from variant CJD would be needed (Harrabin, Coote, and Allen, 2003).

♦ *Highlight catastrophic events associated with harm to a lot of people at once*

It has been calculated that a death from a plane crash is 6 000 times more likely to be front page news than is a death from cancer (Hughes, Kitzinger, and Murdock, 2006).

♦ *Simplify accounts of scientific findings posed in the for and against mode*

A study of North American newspaper accounts of the health benefits of the drug herceptin for breast cancer failed to include any contraindications, specifically the potential risk of cardiac toxicity (Cassells, 2007).

♦ *Provide incomplete statistical information about a health risk*

UK newspapers in 2005 headlined a 24% increased risk between heart attacks and the use of the painkiller ibuprofen, but only a minority gave the frequency as well, i.e. a 1 in 1005 increase (Dr. Ben Goldacre, *The Guardian* newspaper, 20th Jun 2005). (The issue of absolute versus relative risks is discussed in Chapter 5.)

♦ *Project negative images of the NHS suggesting that healthcare delivery is a risky business for patients.*

A study of UK newspaper articles found that negative stories about waiting lists for consultations, operations and treatments were popular news items whereas success stories in these areas were rarely featured (Harrabin *et al.* 2003).

Weak internet regulation and editorial control may exacerbate accuracy problems (Theodosiou and Green, 2003).

According to one critical review of representational studies of the Internet, these have so far been dominated by *the narrowly defined issue of accuracy or quality as defined by medical interests* (Seale, 2005). Box 7.2, below, illustrates these concerns.

Box 7.2 The accuracy of internet health information

- A study of 167 websites providing dietary information found that 76 (45%) made recommendations which deviated from the Canadian national guidelines on nutrition and were really concerned with advertising products (Davison, 1996)

- A study examining information on the management of fever in children found that only four out of 41 web pages gave information to parents which adhered to clinical guidelines (Impicciatore *et al.*, 1997)

- An updated review of websites offering consumers instruments to evaluate health information showed that even when the criteria were specified very few provided instructions on their use and most had not been tested for reliability. The researchers found that most of the 47 rating systems which they had found 4-years earlier were no longer in use. However, they identified 51 new rating instruments, also non-validated and of little help as markers of quality for the consumer (Gagliardi and Jahad, 2002)

- A 2005 study found that most postings to an online breast cancer support group were accurate. Only 0.22% of postings was misleading or false and most were corrected by participants within 4 hrs. The authors conclude that, given a sufficiently active forum, participants can identify and correct most false or misleading statements quickly and reliably without requiring professional review (Esquivel, Meric-Bernstam, and Bernstam, 2006).

In order to counter perceived media misinformation and to gain ascendancy of the information and patient choice agenda, a growing number of official websites have been launched by the NHS and health professional groups such as:

- NHS Direct, initially a phone helpline for the public has launched a website (http://www.nhsdirect.nhs.uk) which the public can use to access advice and information and self-diagnose. For example, under 'Breathing Problems for Adults', clicking on the Yes button produces the advice to make an emergency phone call for an ambulance

- Behind the Medical Headlines (http://www.behindthemedicalheadlines. com/) states that its aim is *to provide the public and health professionals with equitable access to authoritative and independent commentaries from leading medical experts on articles or news items which appear in the media in an attempt to reduce the confusion which can often arise from conflicting, incomplete or misleading media reports.*

These examples reflect official faith in the Internet's potential for expert medical opinion and advice to influence responsible choices on healthy living and health care, given that accurate information is properly provided and controlled by experts. But as indicated in Box 7.2, above, the evidence so far is equivocal about the criteria that relate to accuracy as defined by medical standards on the Internet and some have thought the effort not worthwhile as the range of health information is so variable (Wilson, 2002). What counts as accurate information is a complex matter of judgement for producers and recipients alike, driven by their values and interests, and subject to variation and contradiction. Unravelling the many competing and intricate sources of health information and opinions on the Internet can be a daunting task. It is uncertain whether a system such as quality kite marks would simplify or complicate the task. However, some evidence suggests that the variability of information supplied is more limited than is implied by its sheer quantity and converges with that supplied in the established media (Seale, 2005).

The convergence of 'new' and 'old' health risk representations

Thus far, the discussion of representations of health risk has suggested that concern about accuracy has been the driving force behind many studies which start from a presupposition, conscious or not, that the role of the media is to provide unadulterated information supplied by experts. More critically informed sociological studies have alternatively searched for the deeper moral and political meanings contained in media representations of health risks. The latter perspective is more developed in the study of old than in new media, where the questions of accuracy and quality of information presented on the Internet have somewhat dominated the representational field. One rare study (summarized in Box 7.3, below) sought to correct this bias. The study reviewed Internet sites for breast cancer and prostate cancer in order to compare the content with that provided in newspapers and explore their potential convergence (Seale, 2005).

In addition to documenting convergence, Seale's study sheds light on the ways in which different media representations of health and illness reflect and uphold dominant values of society, in this case, those associated with gender. However, as he pointed out, his study did not investigate the actual search behaviour of Internet site users, or assess what they made of the material they accessed. These aspects of media research are considered later. First, some of the more complex structures of media representation are examined.

Box 7.3 Convergence between 'old' and 'new' media representations of breast and prostate cancer on the internet (Seale, 2005)

Seale's study found that, as with conventional media, new media gave greater coverage to breast than prostate cancer, and that the same few health organizations figured most prominently in newspapers and on the Internet. Their website addresses were referenced in newspaper reports, and the popularity of their websites confirmed by the number of hits. Examination of website content showed that the gender representation of the two cancers followed similar lines to those found in studies of conventional media.

The portrayal of breast cancer on the Internet via information, images, and personal stories demonstrated its definition as a disease requiring emotional management of self and families and identifying the support available to help. Prostate cancer, in contrast, is portrayed in more masculine terms as requiring stoicism and rational control. Coverage rarely deals with emotions or feelings.

Seale concluded that his *case study has shown considerable similarities between old and new media representations of gender and cancer, supporting the hypothesis of media convergence.*

Media framing of health risks

Media reports communicate meaning as much by what is left out as by the content selected for inclusion. A number of overlapping concepts have been developed by social scientists to explain message construction and projected meanings, including framing and the use of anchors, templates, and stereotypes (see Box 7.4, below, for their definition).

The concepts summarized in Box 7.4, although open to varying definitions, are widely employed by media analysts to explain the ways in which the media reflect social categories and values. For example, a study of local television news broadcasts in Los Angeles found a common pattern of selective reporting of deaths and accidents which represented the incidence of these events in ways that grossly diverged from their 'true' frequency (McArthur et al., 2001). Of greater interest was the discovery that a strong link was made between accidents, death, and crime across television channels, suggesting that media constructions reinforce dominant ideologies about risk by framing them in certain common ways (McArthur et al., 2001), as discussed in Box 7.5.

Box 7.4 Definitions of concepts used in media analysis

Framing – Media framing involves classifying an event as instance of X rather than Y which works *at three levels: denotation, connotation, and myth* (Murdoch, Petts, and Horlich-Jones, 2003). For example, health risks may be framed as dangerous and likely to lead to harm or death if not skilfully managed (Alaszewski and Coxon, 2007). (The role of iconography in risk thinking is discussed in Chapter 3.)

Template – Templates bring into play dominant and pervasive past events, reference to which forecloses the meaning of further events with which they are associated, resulting in rigidity of representation. According to Kitzinger, who originally applied this term to media analysis, *templates are defined by their lack of innovation, their status as received wisdom and by their closure* (Kitzinger, 2000, quoted author's emphasis). She compares them to the templates stored on computers which shape documents in a particular way.

Anchoring – Anchoring allows new events to be linked to past ones which are encapsulated in *resonant phrases and images* (Murdoch, Petts, and Horlick-Jones, 2003), grounding reported events in the familiar. Anchors are used particularly when a novel threat emerges, and are therefore highly relevant to risk reporting (Moscovici, 2000). The anchor used may serve to heighten the projected risk, as happened in the media coverage of severe acute respiratory syndrome (SARS). The Black Death and the Spanish Influenza epidemic of 1918 were used as anchors, an association which emphasized the potentially terrible outcomes of a SARS epidemic (Washer, 2004).

Stereotype – A stereotype provides audiences with a grossly simplified, common understanding of a person or group of people. It condenses a wide range of differences into crude assumptions about characteristics possessed by members of social categories defined in terms of attributes such as class, ethnicity, race, gender, sexual orientation, social role, or status. Those who are defined by society to be outsiders, such as people with a mental illness, are particularly prone to being stereotyped (Philo, 1993). Stereotypes can change assumptions into perceived realities. They are often used to uphold the position of those in power and to perpetuate social prejudice and inequality.

Box 7.5 Local TV news reports on deaths and accidents in Los Angeles (McArthur *et al.*, 2001)

The study encompassed nine local television news channels (seven English and two Spanish speaking) located in Los Angeles over a 3-month period in late 1996 and early 1997.

News reports focussed on those events with 'high visual intrigue', such as air crashes and homicides. Deaths due to car crashes and all other deaths were reported in much lower proportions. Injuries due to assault and fire were much more likely to be reported than those from accidental poisoning, falls, and suicide. The researchers found that a heightened risk of death or injury through crime was projected by the way events were reported, and by what was left out. They concluded that:

> The absence of context, supporting information, and education about the noncriminal circumstances surrounding most traumatic events leaves viewers uninformed about critical features, such as their precipitating causes and relative riskiness.

News stories, like those discussed in Box 7.5, strip away complexity, 'home in' on certain aspects whilst leaving others out, and make use of association to impute meaning. Similar trends are found in other media forms such as film and advertising (Gwyn, 2002; Seale, 2003). As illustrated below, such circumscribing effects are clearly seen in the representation of mental illness in print, television, and film. An extensive body of research has uncovered the negative stereotypes which these media forms consistently reproduce (Stout, Villegas, and Jennings, 2004; Klin and Lemish, 2008).

Media framing of mental illness

An early UK study conducted in 1993 over a 1-month period across a range of media, including the press, magazines, and national and local television, concluded that mental illness is framed in a context of violence and harm in all media forms (Philo, 1993). Within this frame, stereotypes are used to reinforce images of the mentally ill as mad, bad, unpredictable, and to be avoided at all costs (Stout, Villegas, and Jennings, 2004). Extensive news coverage is given to the small number of mentally ill patients who commit violent crimes with headlines such as 'Knife maniac freed to kill, mental patient ran amok in the park' (The *Daily Mail* newspaper, 26th Feb 2005) and 'Maniac killed twin sisters' (front page, *London Evening Standard*, newspaper 18th Apr 2005) (Thornicroft, 2006). The mentally ill person is more variably represented in film media, at times depicted as an 'afflicted genius' or an 'eccentric'. However, the stereotype of the 'mad and bad' killer has predominated over the past four decades (Morris, 2006; Thornicroft, 2006). It has been argued that the selective heightened attention given to risk posed by those with a mental illness both reflects and exacerbates the marginal position they occupy in society (Olstead, 2002; Stout, Villegas and Jennings, 2004). Box 7.6 summarizes a study which showed how reports of mental illness in newspapers differed depending on the mentally ill person's class position such that images of poverty reinforce the construction of mental illness as an 'outsider' problem.

Olstead's findings suggest that media reports leave *the reader to surmise a link between mental illness, violence, criminality and poverty, thus creating a distance between the reader and the person with mental illness* (Edney, 2004). This distancing effect is compounded by the absence of reports about risks to the well-being of the mentally ill, the dangers they encounter, and their vulnerability upon release into the community from institutional care (Wahl, 1995; Kelly and McKenna, 2004). Far less media attention is given to acts of violence committed upon a family member than is given to 'stranger' attacks, although the latter are much rarer (Watts and Zimmerman, 2002). This selective risk perception bias (see Chapter 3) reinforces the image of the mentally ill person as unpredictable and to be feared, especially in public spaces.

Although it is difficult to measure media influence on public opinion and behaviour, research suggests that news and entertainment media images are influential in shaping public perceptions of the risks posed by mentally ill people, helping to sustain intolerance and discrimination towards them (Philo, 1993; Endney, 2004). It is probable that public policy has become more draconian as a result, leading to greater coercion and containment instead of rehabilitation in the community, as has increasingly happened in the UK over recent decades (Rose, 1998a).

Box 7.6 Newspaper portrayals of mental illness related to social class

A Canadian study (Olstead, 2002) found that the reporting style for mental illness depended on the person's class position. Reports on those in the lower social classes were much more likely to focus on behaviour such as criminal incidents and dangerousness as well as poverty and homelessness. Moreover, whereas middle class people were likely to be depicted as suffering from depression, those in the lower classes were more likely to be defined as schizophrenic, itself a loaded and much misunderstood condition as portrayed by the media.

Media coverage of the risks posed by the mentally ill substantiates the view that *within individual risk stories, most of the coverage isn't about risk. It is about blame, fear, anger and other nontechnical issues* (Sandman, 1994). This is further illustrated by studies which analyse the structure and meanings inherent in media health risk stories by examining the metaphors and symbols used. Two examples discussed below are concerned with the unfolding story of hospital-acquired infections, and in particular methicillin-resistant *Staphylococcus Aureus* (MRSA), and the media representation of health professionals.

Media framing of MRSA

War, as a metaphor, has been widely used in the media to convey the daunting challenges facing medical science and threatening the public, particularly to represent emerging infectious diseases. 'Killer bugs', such as the Ebola virus have often been framed within a science fiction discourse which heightens their surreal, uncontrollable, and 'other' qualities (Gwyn, 2002; Washer and Joffe, 2006). An impression has been created that the incidence of hospital-acquired infections is increasing, probably as a result of their being officially recognized, made public, and given media attention. The message conveyed in many media accounts is that hospitals are risky places for one's health!

A study of newspaper reports on one of the recurring superbug health scares, MRSA, shows how a hospital-acquired health risk is constructed by the press as *ubiquitous, threatening and unconquerable* (Washer and Joffe, 2006). Washer and Joffe located their study in a wider analysis of the symbolic representations used by the media to construct emerging infectious diseases, the risks they pose and at whose door the blame should be laid, be it the victim or the authorities. They argued that risk is implicit in the term 'superbug' as it signifies *uniqueness (as in supermodel), strength (as in super-power), and/or indestructibility (as in superhero)* (Washer and Joffe, 2006). In seeking to allocate blame, newspaper accounts appear to have shifted blame away from health professionals, the main focus in the early days of MRSA reporting, onto NHS management and the Government where it now tends to rest. Box 7.7 summarizes the changing focus of the MRSA story in newspaper accounts.

One interesting observation made by the authors of the above study (Washer and Joffe, 2006) was that newspapers displayed very little concern about a possible causal link with the over prescription of antibiotics. Some experts have argued that antibiotic resistant germs in general should be the real grounds of concern and ought to be the main media focus (Katz, 2007). According to Washer and Joffe, newspaper reports have focussed instead on locating blame for the spread of MRSA on failures in standards of hygiene in UK hospitals.

Box 7.7 Media framing of MRSA (adapted from Washer and Joffe, 2006)

The historical comparison summarized below is based on the content-analysis of four UK Sunday newspapers (two tabloids and two broadsheets) from 1995 to 2005.

From 1997, MRSA began to be described as:

- A *killer superbug* in the tabloids and a *potentially fatal superbug* in the broadsheets.

- The seriousness of the threat was conveyed by evocations of a *doomsday scenario*, an *impending health crisis* and a *major threat to public health*.

- The potential of MRSA to beat medical advances was emphasized by allusions to *the end of the golden age of antibiotics*.

By 2002 the above themes were embellished with descriptions of MRSA as:

- An *evolving microbe*.

- Increasingly intelligent and evasive, with phrases such as *the clever microbe* referring to its mutation and resistance to even by the most powerful antibiotics.

The MRSA 'doomsday scenario' was however juxtaposed with stories focussing on medical miracles and breakthroughs with headline such as:

Maggots Make our Flesh Crawl, and Heal. (*The Observer* newspaper, 23rd Jul 2000)
The Bug that Kills Bacteria. (*The Sunday Times* newspaper, 9th Jul 2002)
Air Freshener Could Help Beat Superbug. (*Sunday Mirror* newspaper, 5th Oct 2003)

Natural medicines to boost the immune system also featured as a defence via stories about 'tea tree oil', 'MRSA Pure Mix, a blend of anti-MRSA essential oils' or 'probiotic supplements'.

By 2004, media accounts focussed on MRSA as a political issue, with the emphasis placed on attributing blame either to the Government or hospitals for poor hygiene which have been the focus of health targets and action ever since.

The authors argued that hospital hygiene became the symbol for wider concerns about the under-funding and/or poor management of the NHS, particularly during the 2005 UK general election. Thus, they traced how health risk is selectively framed reinforced within a wider socio-political context, although the dominant frame of MRSA as a 'killer bug' persisted alongside other narratives.

A Canadian study (Driedger *et al.*, 2009) concluded that the dominant definitional frame for health risk events may be powerfully established within the first 10 days of media interest. It may endure provided that the risk event remains constant, although different emphases may emerge due to other social and political factors. The comparative content analysis of newspaper reports of two risk events, both portrayed as a search for justice, showed that an outbreak of drinking water contamination by *Escherichia coli* generated an increasing number of mistrust stories as a result of the judicial enquiry which heard testimony that managers had falsified water test results. With respect to the other risk event, the first BSE case in Canada, the initial emphasis on health gave way to a focus on the threat posed to the economy of Alberta. More dramatic shifts in dominant frames can occur if a new salient issue emerges, as happened when BSE crossed the species barrier in the UK and the more terrifying associative anchor of acquired immune deficiency syndrome (AIDS) replaced that of salmonella (Washer, 2004).

Studies of media framing of health risk events or issues reveal how the media can construct a powerful story with elements of horror, uncertain outcomes, attributions of blame, and a range of heroes and villains, including those from the health professions. For example, the research on MRSA discussed above showed that nurses were blamed by the media for failing to observe basic rules of hygiene, and for sloppy or uncaring attitudes. Conversely, they were also praised wholesomely for their dedicated unselfish care, sometimes in the same newspaper articles (Washer and Joffe, 2006). Not unreasonably, the health professions have vociferously blamed the media for misrepresenting them, as discussed below.

Media images of nurses

Since the 1970s, nurses have challenged media stereotyping of their profession which, they argue, leads to poor understanding of their role amongst the public, and damages recruitment and professional identity (Savage, 1987; Gordon, 2005). The main complaints of nurses concern images which render them both as objects of male fantasies and as subservient to doctors, thus diminishing their professional expertise. Doctors, also disapproving about the media stance towards their profession, have a much higher media profile generally than do nurses. Contributions made to the general enterprise of healthcare from nurses and other health professionals are not typically recognized, rendering these professions largely invisible in any progressive portrayals of healthcare (Gordon, 2005). For example, some popular television programmes transfer nursing responsibilities to doctors and portray nurses as peripheral subordinates.

Media depictions of nurses are considered to demean the profession's standing, whether a nurse is depicted as a hard headed battleaxe, sexual temptress, or ministering angel, and to reinforce feelings of powerlessness in the workplace (Savage, 1987; Gordon, 2005). These representations have been popularised in novels, film, and television dramas with some iconic roles epitomizing a particular image, for example Nurse Ratched in 'One Flew Over the Cuckoo's Nest' as dominatrix (Hallam, 2000). A survey of thousands of nurse images on the Internet shows that in the 21st century they continue to be predominantly portrayed as white, middle class, blond, young, attractive women (Kaminski, 2003). The reasons for the pervasiveness of such images run deep and reflect sex, class, and gender structures in society which are echoed in the traditional power and status divide between doctors and nurses.

The framing of nursing as an essentially feminine profession (regardless of men who enter its ranks) inevitably colours media definitions of the nursing role in various risk scenarios. It is relatively rare for nurses to be featured as heroines. But when this happens, emphasis is placed on self-sacrificial acts which reinforce feminine 'angel of mercy' images by giving a badge of honour to women who carry out extraordinary acts of valour in atypical circumstances, as Box 7.8, below, illustrates.

Box 7.8 Media coverage of heroic nurses

- In 2002 the Toronto Star featured a story about a nurse who had set up a teenage clinic to address gaps in adolescent health care with the headline 'Angel in our Midst'. The lead in to the article invited readers to *Meet Nurse Ruth Ewart. She's kind, gentle and a hero to those whose lives she's touched.* (Gordon 2005)

- The heroism of Nurse Clair Bertschinger was highlighted in a BBC Internet story which was issued on the back of her recently published autobiography entitled 'Moving Mountains'. Elliott's story is headlined 'The Nurse who Inspired Live Aid'. It contains a quote from Michael Beurk describing Bertschinger as *one of the true heroines of our times*, referring to her work for the Red Cross in 1984 when the BBC relayed Michael Buerk's influential reports on famine stricken Ethiopia. Bertschinger is applauded for tackling the impossible task of making decisions about which children should enter her feeding station and which were too sick to be saved. This experience, we are told, left her traumatized for two decades. In the piece, Bob Geldof was quoted as saying *In her was vested the power of life and death. She had become God-like and this is unbearable for anyone* (Jane Elliott, BBC News health reported 7th Jul 2005).

Nurses receive occasional media plaudits for heroic acts, but, in general, they attract more attention when perceived as posing a health risk problem, for example where there are shortages in their ranks, or they are threatening industrial action. Negative publicity is most intense when nurses fall from grace, as in cases where a nurse kills a patient either by accident or design (Gordon, 2005). Nurses involved in rare incidents in which patients are deliberately harmed or killed become the catalyst for media hyperbole about the shocking and baffling gender transgression that has occurred. (By extension, this response is also invoked by male nurses who transgress and are seen as members of a female profession.) This process is illustrated by the case of Beverly Allitt (see Box 7.9, on p. 156). Allitt was convicted in 1993 of killing four children aged 7 and 9 weeks, 15-months, and 11-years, and injuring five others after injecting them with insulin or potassium.

Sentenced to life imprisonment in custody in a high-security mental hospital, Allit was defended in court on the basis of the 'personality disorder', Munchausens Syndrome by Proxy (MSbP). This is a controversial condition and some agencies, such as the Department of Health, tend to refer to as a fabricated or induced illness instead. The real and symbolic impact of MSbP as a potential health risk lies in the abuse of trust it exemplifies in a relationship of intimate care, such as nursing and mothering (a significant association), where one party is vulnerable and dependent on the other.

Media depictions of nurses have varied, reflecting historical changes in the role of women in the home and in paid work (see e.g. Hallam, 2000). But nurses complain that sexualised images, such as 'the naughty nurse', are timeless and still prevalent across the developed world (see e.g. www.nursing advocacy.org/ news/ July 2005). Arguably such disempowering representations, combined with non-existent media coverage of the complexities of nursing jobs, diminish respect for the profession and impact on its potential to inform patient safety policy and practice (Gordon, 2005).

Media images of doctors

Like nurses, doctors are critical of the way they are portrayed in the media. Concern has been expressed about the possible impact media representations may have on public perceptions of doctors and upon their views of themselves. For example, a *British Medical Journal* survey of junior doctors found that a number had spontaneously offered complaints like those quoted below (Goldacre, Evans, and Lambert, 2003):

> The media is always portraying doctors in a poor light and constantly 'doctor bashing'
> Media opinion of the medical profession ('blundering doctors') has spilled over on to the wards, and patients question everything we do.

Box 7.9 Media representations of Beverley Allitt (see p. 154)

(see p. 154)

Allit was portrayed as an 'angel of death', 'stalking' and 'haunting' the ward, words which carry with them the idea of a determined and ruthless hunter in search of unsuspecting and vulnerable prey. Although in many respects unique, the resonances of 'the angel of death' story to healthcare risk were secured and amplified by the following:

- *Frame* – The Allitt case provided a media frame for other unrelated errors, misdiagnoses, or mistreatment in British hospitals which occurred in the 1990s (*The Daily Mail* newspaper, 18th Jun 1993; *The Glasgow Herald*, newspaper 14th Jul 1995). The longevity of this frame can be seen in a much more recent report on 175 nurses accused of misconduct but allowed to continue on the wards whilst their cases were being considered. The co-director of the lobby group Patient Concern was quoted as saying, *However unlikely, we want to know if there are any Nurse Shipmans among this group. We have had two already – Beverley Allitt and Benjamin Green* (*The Observer* newspaper, 25th Jun 2005).

- *Association* – Associations have been drawn between Beverly Allitt and other dissimilar cases of serial killers which have served to amplify more specific anxieties, such as the state of the family and of the National Health Service (e.g. *The Guardian* newspaper, 4th Jul 1993; *The Glasgow Herald* newspaper, 15th Oct 1993).

- *Template* – The Allitt case provided a media template for other instances of Munchausen's Syndrome by Proxy (MSbP). She has been cited in over a dozen cases reported in the national press since 1993 in which MSbP was used to explain mothers overdosing their children with salt, or suffocating them (d'Cruse *et al.*, 2006):

   Symbolically the "angel of death" haunted the normatively safe spaces of home and hospital. She could bring harm to people vulnerable through illness and to children at risk from their own mothers.'

The media demonises the medical profession seizing upon the occasional failure (of course they must be addressed) to condemn the entire profession.

Medical scandals such as Alder Hey and the Bristol Infirmary, discussed in Chapters 6 and 8, have provided significant opportunities for the media to engage in what those inside the profession regard as 'doctor bashing', and others consider a welcome questioning of their accountability (Seale, 2002).

It is a common feature of media reports of adverse events in health delivery that they are framed as an individual failing and not as a systems' problem, as if each adverse event were rare, due to personal incompetence, and therefore shocking (see Chapter 9). The Allitt case and those of other nurses who have been involved in killing patients, whether deliberately or otherwise, have been treated in this way, as have doctors like Dr Shipman who have abused public trust and murdered patients. As noted by one commentator on the media coverage of the American Institute of Medicine's own report on medical errors, *much of the news media simply equated medical errors with malpractice – perpetuating the notion that most of the bad stuff going on in medicine can be attributed to the negligence of incompetent professionals* (Dentzer, 2000). The focus on flawed heroes can reach fever pitch in some instances, for example in the treatment meted out to a woman doctor, Marietta Higgs, in England's Cleveland child abuse scandal, summarized in Box 7.10.

The Cleveland case is one of the few medical scandals where gender bias is so obvious in media coverage. No doubt, it is more widespread in portrayals of the health professions and, as has been seen, is deep-seated in relation to nurses.

Box 7.10 The Cleveland sex abuse scandal and media treatment of Dr. Marietta Higgs

A total of 121 children were taken into care in 1987 in the English County of Cleveland as a result of diagnoses of sexual abuse made by two paediatricians. The test they used, the anal reflex dilation test, became discredited. However, it was widely used as a contributory test in the detection of sexual abuse, and was not the only evidence on which the Cleveland diagnoses were made. The families of the children loudly protested their innocence. Most of the children were sent home from care, although some were subject to care orders, not reported by the press. In the media frenzy which accompanied these events, the main storyline which developed was of the battle between innocent families and interfering doctors and social workers who were cast as *over-zealous and incompetent*, or even evil (Seale, 2002). The portrayal of Higgs was *sexist* and at times *positively perverse* (Kitzinger, 2000). She was depicted as an ideologue feminist. Coverage suggested that her foreign origins and broken home had made her psychologically disturbed. By association, the objectivity of her medical practice was called into question (Seale 2002). Her fellow paediatrician, Geoff Wyatt, largely escaped media opprobrium.

Despite such projection of negative views about the medical profession, the standing of doctors portrayed in newspaper reports (Lupton and McLean,1998) and media entertainment such as television soaps remains high. It has been adroitly questioned in sharper comedies such as *Scrubs* but doctors benefit by association from media stories about advances which uphold the progressive force of science and medicine. Television documentaries like the BBC six-part 'Fight for Life', broadcast in July–August 2007, portray the life saving techniques afforded by new technologies and skilful surgeons operating live on seriously ill patients. Such programmes convey a positive image of the profession and medical progress.

Media images of doctors basking in the optimistic light of scientific progress reinforce the message that science will eventually cure all ills. However, when juxtaposed against reports of new diseases, they may serve to underscore a common representational story of health risk as a gruelling battle where the forces of good can never be taken for granted. Whether health professionals are up to the mark is often personalized in the media and research indicates that medical authority and progress receive more ambivalent treatment than they once did (see Chapter 6). As Seale argues, *Like the villain, the professional hero category is no longer a secure category* (Seale, 2003).

Media, health risks, and audiences

Researching the impact of media communications is problematic. Responses to intended messages can only be assessed by making judgements about the purpose(s) of messages, which may be to inform, persuade, or defuse risk perceptions, or simply to tell a compelling risk story. Assessing people's intentions in using and relating to the media is equally challenging. There are problems in finding appropriate methods of investigation since the influence of the media may be indirect and subtle rather than linear and straightforward. Too many studies use students to test responses to media output. Even if samples are more carefully chosen, there remains the problem of gathering responses in somewhat artificial circumstances and in response to a single event/media account. Asking people if they have changed or intend to change their behaviour in response to a risk message assumes, amongst other things, that they understood the message and could access the means to do so (Thirlaway and Heggs, 2005). It assumes that making sense of a health risk is a simple matter of absorbing information and acting rationally in response.

Crucially, researching the audience depends upon how the audience is defined and construed. Media producers, whether of the so-called quality or popular press, are fully aware of the importance of knowing and targeting their various audiences in order to maximize market share. A large market research industry exists to gauge varying public predilections for products and services. It provides the basis for the advertising that bombards us daily, not least in relation to health products. A view of the audience as made up of passive, receptive, and pliant recipients of information tends to underlie these approaches even when they recognize diversity. Such simplistic assumptions are being challenged by the interactive possibilities of the new media, as well as by a body of emerging research which argues for a more complex understanding of audience responses to media health risk communication.

Media influence and alternative models of 'the audience'

The study of the impact of media risk communications on audiences is as yet relatively underdeveloped and under-theorized (Allan, 2002; Seale, 2003; Anderson, 2006; Hodgetts and Chamberlain, 2006). There is a lingering tendency to see media recipients as undiscerning, a position which was characterized by past studies of media effects (Gauntlett, 2005). The notion of audiences as passive sponges is somewhat related to a belief that media distortion of health risk events can produce panic reactions amongst the public, for example in relation to food scares such as BSE or childhood immunization programmes; and, conversely, fails to alert them to others such as the potentially serious effect on health of mobile phones (Allan, 2002; Alazewski, 2006). However, studies of the impact of health panics have produced variable findings about whether people change their attitudes and behaviour. For example, the effect can be short lived as in the case of not eating beef after the BSE crisis, or more prolonged and serious as with the Measles, Mumps, and Rubella (MMR) vaccine. It may be that the influence of prolonged media representations works more insidiously and indirectly. However, social scientists have increasingly argued that what is needed is an analysis of the social dynamics underpinning people's interaction with the media which sheds light on variable responses to communications about health risk (Hughes, Kitzinger, and Murdock, 2006).

An interactive model of the audience takes account of the shared social values and meanings that they bring to their interpretations of media health-risk communications. At the same time, it takes account of the ways in which health risk understandings are modified through everyday conversations with family, friends, and work colleagues (Murdock, Petts, and Horlick-Jones, 2003; Kivits, 2006; Pidgeon, Simmons, and Henwood, 2006). The interactive model challenges 'the rational actor' approach underpinning much representational research and public health policy. This approach assumes that the public would act on information supplied by experts if only the media would refrain from blocking *the flow of knowledge from the knowledgeable doctor to the uninformed patient* (Alaszewski, 2005). Audience responses to risk communications suggest that the 'rational' model is defective for two reasons. It overlooks the complexity and diversity of health risk knowledge, and assumes that the individual is passive, rather than actively engaged in sifting and interpreting media communications.

The active audience and trust

As researchers focus upon the ways in which people make sense of the vast amount of health risk information available through different media channels, a picture is emerging of 'the actively engaged audience'. This was the conclusion of the author of a set of studies looking at audience responses to medical narratives in television programmes which attract large audiences. As is shown in Box 7.11, Davin (2003) found evidence to support the view that *viewers are sophisticated, astute, insightful and media-literate. They produce complex, multi-layered, sometimes contradictory and/or unexpected interpretations.*

Box 7.11 The reception of television medical narratives (Davin, 2003)

Davin compared responses to an American medical drama (*ER*) with the results of her separate follow-up study evaluating responses to the portrayal of a woman being diagnosed with breast cancer in a UK soap opera (*Eastenders*) and in a documentary. Her findings suggest that people are more wary of the documentary form which they perceive to be incomplete and artificial. *ER* was seen as a quality drama, which was both entertaining and a trustworthy source of information on a range of topics concerning the health professions, medical diagnosis and treatments, and social and political aspects of health care. *Eastenders* did not receive the same critical acclaim but was still ahead of the documentary in terms of being trusted as a useful pedagogical tool. One of the key reasons given, as with the *ER* audience, was the emotional information gathering tactics of identification with the characters. Davin argues that such emotional tactics are an important element of response to media narratives about health risk:

> This is especially pertinent to health promotion, because, contrary to the long-held belief that new knowledge directly leads to behaviour modification (i.e. once informed that their conduct may be dangerous, rational listeners will stop/alter it) responses to health messages may have more to do with emotions than cognition.

Davin argued for a perspective on responses to media portrayals of health risks which sees the 'emotional' rather than the 'rational' as key to the ways in which audiences respond to media health risk messages (Davin, 2003). A study exploring how women respond to a specific news risk story reporting on the increased risk of developing breast cancer due to alcohol (Thirlaway and Heggs, 2005) offers supportive evidence for Davin's view that information is filtered by audiences emotionally as well as cognitively. The study is summarized in Box 7.12.

Box 7.12 Women's responses to a news story linking alcohol with risk of breast cancer (Thirlaway and Heggs, 2005)

The study explored the responses of 127 women to a story which appeared in *The Guardian* newspaper in Nov 2002. The article was headlined 'Drinking a single glass of wine a day increases a woman's chance of developing breast cancer by 6%'. Women were asked to address three open-ended questions about the meaning of the figures in the report, how it made them feel, and whether the information would make them change their behaviour.

Analysis of responses showed that only 43 women attempted to quantify the risk, 25 rating it as low and 18 as high. Nevertheless, most women reported feeling anxious or worried as a result of reading the news story. However, only a small minority (20%) said that they would definitely or might change their behaviour as a result. The reasons given by most of the women fell into a range of categories, the largest of which was that they were not at risk as they did not drink enough, even though most reported drinking more than one glass of wine a day. Amongst a wide range of other responses, women referred to personal philosophies and strategies for dealing with this risk, personal experiences of breast cancer scares and of friends who had the disease, and mistrust of experts and the media. Some commented on the confusing statistical estimates of risk in the article.

The researchers concluded that:

> When presented with a risk a small minority of women will attempt an objective risk analysis, only to discover that they do not have the information to do so. A more common response is to focus on the way the risk makes them feel and to attempt to alleviate any negative feelings in the most accessible and effective way. Responses to risk will vary enormously mediated by individual experiences, the way the message is presented and the social environment in which it is received.

Thirlaway and Heggs concluded that people are actively engaged in interpreting health risk media messages in different ways. They argued that risk assessments are filtered by personal philosophies and values, and informed by strategies embedded in social contexts beyond that of their immediate reading of a specific risk message. Because people contextualize media messages differently, there is always more than one audience involved in any media risk communication. However, in the case of the breast cancer article used by Thirlaway and Heggs, incomplete statistical information, contradictory expert opinions, and the moralizing tone of the article seem to have been influential in discrediting its message. The authors considered that *Lack of trust in the risk communication process enables women to dismiss the whole story, effectively alleviating any anxiety caused* (Thirlaway and Heggs, 2005).

Although revealing the difficulties of unravelling the interactions between the content of the media message, its interpretation by the audience, and its ultimate impact, the studies discussed above identify trust as a key dynamic in the mix. Trust has always been an important ingredient in media communication, and has been manipulated in times of uncertainty and war through propaganda (Redley, 2007). In what some define as the current 'age of suspicion' (Bakir and Barlow, 2007), cynicism about experts and media reports on health risks have burgeoned. Issues of trust and distrust will increasingly impact on practitioner-patient relationships (see Chapter 6).

Audiences, trust, and 'the expert'

Trust in the source of a health risk message may be more important than its content, although the content clearly contributes, for example when contradictory messages undermine the notion of expert opinion. With reference to the communicating source, trust may be thought of as having two key components, belief in competence and integrity, i.e. that the source can further your interests and seek to benefit not harm you (Franklin, 1999). Producers of media messages try to enlist the trust of the audience by designing communications which encourage identification in both senses with the source. For example, it has been argued that the portrayal of HIV/AIDS and its effect on one of its key characters and family in the soap opera *Eastenders* did more than official health campaigns of the late 1980s and early 1990s to raise awareness of the condition amongst young adults (Allan, 2002).

Interest is growing in trust as a key mediating influence upon people's interpretation and response to media risk communications. The significance of trust has been enhanced by declining levels of public faith in the Government and other major institutions during the last decades of the 20th century. This decline has been exacerbated by various health scandals and crises (Hughes, Kitzinger, and Murdock, 2006). The growth of new media and the unregulated world it promises to open have also made trust a more significant issue. The potential of the Internet and other digital media to better inform and empower patients is seen by optimists to be a key advantage of new media. But realizing this potential depends in large part on access and use. There may be a role for health professionals, for example nurses in general practitioner (GP) practices, to draw attention to NHS trusted sites for particular health conditions. However, ultimately the patient is responsible for making sense of information gleaned in this as in any other way. The rise of new media also raises the important question of who defines what information can be trusted. The Internet opens up new possibilities for individuals and groups to provide their own health biographies and advice to others. It may thus challenge both the notion of 'the expert' in the field of health risk and the idea of the audience as a passive receptor (Franklin, 1998; Gillet, 2003; Richardson, 2003). Box 7.13 provides a summary of Richardson's study of the discourse of people sharing information and opinions on the Internet about the health risks of handheld mobile phones.

Box 7.13 The health risk of handheld mobile phones: Trust and credibility on the Internet (Richardson, 2003)

The study analysed 93 'threads' of conversation on 45 Internet newsgroups (bulletin boards) and found that contributors used a range of warranting strategies, i.e. methods of establishing credibility in order to secure trust, often tinged with expressions of cynicism about experts and expertise. Newsgroup participants can include experts who volunteer information, but they have no more standing than anyone else. Companies and organizations are not represented. The warranting strategies used by individuals in the interactive dialogues included references to sources such as mass media, science publications, as well as drawing upon personal experience, knowledge of expert persons, and technical expertise. Disclaimers were also used such as *I'm not a scientist or anything special, but ...*, and were another way of showing awareness of the importance of trust and credibility in this virtual discussion of health risk.

Richardson argues that warranting strategies and challenges made to their credibility were necessary because newsgroup participants offering information and opinion *cannot rely upon their reputation or upon any prior introduction to underwrite that information*. However, she concluded that their use reflects a more general ambivalence about expertise and experts found elsewhere.

Richardson's study illustrates how necessary it has become for information providers to offer some assurances of credibility in the more sceptical climate which now surrounds the interpretation and assessment of information on health risks. The study demonstrates the importance of credibility and trust in assessing health risk information, particularly when the expert no longer has a dominant position in the interaction, in this case in the virtual situation of a newsgroup. How this might translate into the real life interactions between health professionals and patients is unclear. Initial research suggests that Internet users who investigate health information sites are not usually seeking to supplant medical advice, although they may see the information supplied by doctors and other health professionals as inadequate in certain respects (Hart, Henwood, and Wyatt, 2004; Kivits, 2006). However, they may turn to other sources when unwilling to accept the information provided by health professionals if it indicates a poor outcome or requires actions they do not want to undertake.

Media impact on audiences can never be ruled out because of its capacity to pervasively promote certain health risk messages over others, although such impact may be not be immediate, linear, or comprehensive. Although in a relatively early stage of development, research on 'the active' or 'interactive' audience indicates that the communicative relationship between user and media is much more complex than most representational research envisages. In contradiction of earlier assumptions that people consume media messages uncritically, this new research indicates that audiences are discerning, and use wider sources to make sense of media communications. Their responses are mediated by the social influences of family, friendship groups, or fellow sufferers with whom they can check understandings and opinions, for example in Internet chat rooms. It is possible that these reference groups hold more sway than experts, at least as experts are portrayed in the media. Research suggests that judgements about the trustworthiness of the communicator are more important than media informational content. The challenge for even the most discerning of users is, however, to be able to assess whose interests and what political forces lie behind the selection of health risk promotion in the media.

The production of media health risk messages

Consideration of the part played by the media in the selective production of health risk messages provides another way of posing questions about the media's role in society. Should media producers such as editors, journalists, and reporters be held accountable for selectively promoting some health risks over others, or are they merely mouthpieces for powerful groups in society whose interests determine the health risk agenda? Representational studies sometimes touch on the political events associated with unfolding health risk stories, as shown in the example of MRSA discussed earlier (Washer and Joffe, 2006). However, the interplay of socio-political forces which lie behind the production of media health risk messages is as yet not well understood (Seale, 2003). The purpose here is to map some of the key aspects which might be usefully considered, whist acknowledging the complexity of the task.

Competing interests and media production of health risks

Studies indicate that Government departments, health care agencies, and senior health professionals all seek to exercise strong influence upon news media definitions of key health risks, and to signal priorities for clinical interventions (Eldridge and Reilly, 2003). As is discussed below, these attempts to exert pressure extend to concerted efforts to control web presence and prominence on the Internet, as well as to 'manage the news' through more conventional channels. Studies indicate that media producers turn to official sources for statements and opinions and therefore are more likely to convey what might be termed 'the party line' on health risks (Hughes, Kitzinger, and Murdock, 2006). Although official accounts can be challenged in subsequent media accounts, as happened with the BSE crisis where Government officials were increasingly put under the media spotlight for having misled the public about the safety of beef, official sources are guaranteed a voice and tend to dominate health risk coverage, at least initially. They become particularly visible when a health crisis occurs (Anderson, 2006), or is predicted, as when the Chief Medical Officer of Health provides statements in relation to such threats as SARS or swine flu. However, the 'official line' may be unclear or strategically absent in cases of extreme uncertainty. In these circumstances, other opinions will be sought by journalists, at least until the story runs cold.

The amplification model (SARF) discussed earlier has been criticized for underestimating the contribution of media interests to the politics of production (Petts *et al.,* 2001; Murdock, Petts, and Horlick-Jones, 2003). From this perspective, the media is more than a transmitting system for the battles of others and is itself engaged in a continuous struggle to retain and expand audiences, a process which colours health risk selection, representation, and production. One extensive study (Petts *et al.,* 2001) of the relevance of the amplification model in the UK context concluded that:

> The media are not transmitters of official information on risk as suggested by the linear SARF framework, but dynamic interpreters and mediators, who seek to respond to and reflect social preferences and concerns and in so doing stake and maintain their

position. The media are highly effective interpreters of public concerns, arguably far more so than Government departments and agencies.

Health risk stories have been shown to be subject to the predilections of campaigning journalists and editors (Critcher, 2007). They are produced in a competitive arena in which media players jostle to gain commercial advantage (Murdock, Petts, and Horlick-Jones, 2003; Anderson, 2006; Kitzinger, 2006). For example, the media are keen on controversies amongst officials, scientists, and medical experts. They may be used to fuel the development of a health risk story to give it added interest and spin (Nelkin, 1996). Disagreements amongst officials and scientists as to the nature and degree of health risk involved in the risk posed by eating potentially contaminated beef helped to stoke up the BSE story when interest was wavering (Eldridge and Reilly, 2003). Contention also became a defining feature of the media's approach to reporting on the MMR controversy. In this case, the journalistic convention of 'balance' (i.e. giving equal coverage to both sides) ironically helped to skew and amplify the risks involved (Critcher, 2007).

The production of the MMR story is instructive in a number of ways since it was affected by a range of competing interests, including those of the media, in particular the *Daily Mail* newspaper, health professionals, and the doubting public (Critcher, 2007). But there were also 'hidden influences', including an undeclared conflict of interest in the research paper published in the *Lancet* which initiated the health scare. The research conducted by Dr Andrew Wakefield and colleagues was funded in part by the Legal Aid Board. The parents of some of the subjects of the investigation were pursing legal action against the manufactures of the vaccine as a result of their contention that it had damaged their children (Theodore Dalyrymple, *The Telegraph* newspaper, 22nd Feb 2004). Thus, the MMR case serves to illuminate the multilayered nature of the selective processes influencing media definitions of health risk, including the potential for scientists themselves to obscure conflicts of interest.

Government leaders and spokespersons, scientific and medical experts, and those who own, control, and work in the media industry are all highly significant players in defining health risk. But research shows that marginal groups can also make their mark (Kitzinger, 2006; Anderson, 2006). For example, individuals successfully campaigned to challenge the NICE ruling on the non-prescription of the drug herceptin for the treatment of early breast cancer, helping to secure its much wider availability in the UK, although not without controversy (Bristow, 2006). The human interest stories at the heart of grassroots campaigns provide good copy for journalists and their editors. In addition, individual women have been proactive in seeking media coverage of their plight. Their predicament in the face of what they see as large faceless, intractable, and inhumane health organizations has all the ingredients for weaving a good health risk story, such as those discussed earlier in the chapter. However, such campaigns are often supported by drug firms who stand to gain by a relaxation of NICE rulings. Thus although the outcome may be a triumph for the 'ordinary person' it may also be meeting less visible, but well orchestrated, commercial interests. According to some accounts, commercial interests have even led to the invention and promotion of diseases in order to sell products. Examples of such 'disease mongering' include female sexual dysfunction and 'restless legs syndrome' (Moynihan, Doran, and Henry, 2008).

The production of health risk information on the Internet may seem more anarchic and therefore less subject to powerful interests than other forms of media. But, as earlier indicated, the voices of the powerful are bolstered to a considerable extent by financial investment and technological 'know how' which ensure permanency and high status for their websites on the most popular search engines. Evidence suggests that Internet users are more likely to look for health information via search engines than through medical portals or medical societies and libraries. Maintaining a leading position on a popular search engine is crucial to controlling health information (Eysenbach and Kohler, 2002). Seale has cogently argued that *the politics of links, combined with the politics of search engines give prominence to already powerful interests – a process familiar to analysts of the conventional media* (Seale, 2005). His view is that institutional interests, such as media conglomerates, shape messages in mainstream media, and are replicated on the Internet by major health organizations who invest in consolidating their web presence. Newspaper links to selected websites, the filtering impact of search technology and the probability that most Internet users go no further than the first page of links on a topic, all help to secure the dominant interests of a few producers (Seale, 2005).

Although questions linger about what Internet users might be searching for when accessing health information, those who want to be its main producers seek this position for a number of related political reasons. As already discussed, the medical profession want to ensure the quality and accuracy of information as medical experts and scientists define it. Their motivation can be viewed in two ways, as a wish to retain traditional power as well as to encourage the development of the informed and thus empowered patient, the often stated reason. Analysis of Department of Health policy documents, amongst those from other Western countries, indicates that the promotion of individual self-management of health and the development of patient agency has much to do with the political imperative of controlling spiralling health costs

(Eysenbach, 2000). However, the Internet enables alternative non-mainstream sites to be developed through which consumers can become the producers and sharers of information about health risk as they see it in specific diseases and chronic conditions, such as HIV/AIDS (e.g. Gillet, 2003) and breast cancer (e.g. Fogel *et al.*, 2002). Thus, specialist and marginal interests can be served, just as they can in some conventional forms of media. However, the evidence obtained so far supports Seale's view that the most powerful voices in society have precedence in media production and that those in control will seek to retain their position (Seale, 2005).

Describing the many interests, including their own, which the media might channel and represent is an easier task than establishing how they interact to bring about particular views of a health risk. Although there are case studies which seek to chronicle the selective development of health risk stories such as BSE and MMR (Eldridge and Riley, 2003; Critcher, 2007), it is as yet difficult to discern generic patterns of risk selection, particularly in the rare cases where stories run on and on. Exactly how competing interests dynamically interact to bring about the production of specific health risk messages is not yet well understood. However, research evidence documents the susceptibility of the media to the voices of officialdom. As Seale and others have argued, those with most power will be more than ready to find ways of retaining their presence even as the new media presents them with fresh challenges (Seale, 2005).

Conclusion

Hopefully the material presented in this chapter has persuaded the reader that an awareness of the theoretical and methodological issues involved can assist health practitioners in thinking more clearly about the complex role that 'old' and 'new' forms of media play in relation to health risk management. Representational studies indicate that all media forms are selective about which risks are highlighted, and how they are portrayed, and that there is some convergence between them. Medical experts may conclude that the media engage in deliberate and irresponsible distortion. But this perspective assumes that the media can and should transmit 'accurate' and 'objective' scientific and medical information which resolves controversy. In any event, how health risk stories are covered varies somewhat in content and style depending on intended audiences (Petts *et al.*, 2001). The media are not an independent social force, and are subject to a range of commercial, social, and moral pressures. The most powerful voices in society appear to speak loudest, but minority interests can also break through, particularly via the Internet. However, in seeking to meet the real or manufactured demands of its publics, the media are well placed to reinforce mainstream cultural and political values, and thus engage in a process of preserving the status quo via their pervasive presence (Philo and Miller, 2000).

Blanket coverage tends to generate fear about selected health risks through amplification effects, whilst attenuating others. Media communication may therefore contribute significantly to the selective public attention to some risks, and the allocation of resources to combat them, for example in relation to prolonged and widespread stereotypes of the mentally ill as dangerous. Some writers have suggested that the selective focus on certain dangers in the media helps to secure a compliant public, especially with regard to managing health risks (McGuigan, 2006). But others have questioned the assumption that the media sets out deliberately to amplify risks or succeeds in raising anxiety levels and affecting behaviour, since people tend to be most concerned about risks that are rooted in personal and shared everyday experiences (Petts *et al.*, 2001; Tulloch and Lupton, 2003). The relationship between audience and media is complex and has to take account of the filtered perceptions and interpretations of members whose cultural group allegiances and influences vary. The issue of trust versus distrust is emerging as an important dynamic in understanding how audiences make sense of the abundance of health risk information available in a media intensive world. Trust is likely to be a defining problem of 21st century healthcare as practitioners and patients chart their way through increasingly complex risk-based models of professional practice.

Chapter 8

The regulation of health risks

Monica Shaw

Aim

To explore the regulation of health risks.

Objectives

1. To examine some of the complex socio-political influences on the development of health risk regulation
2. To critically explore the role and significance of clinical governance in the regulation of health risks
3. To consider the impact of a spiralling relationship between health risk and regulation.

Introduction

Reflecting international trends, such as those emerging in the USA, Canada, and Australia during the closing decade of the 20th century, risk analysis and risk prevention have come to dominate the Government's agenda for transforming health services in the UK (Southgate and Dauphinee, 1998; Vincent, 2006). Since its election in 1997, the Labour Government and devolved administrations throughout the UK have spawned numerous policy initiatives and regulatory quangos under the dual banner of a more dependable and higher quality health service. Such aspirations have been explicitly couched in terms of concern about the harm that has occurred, or might occur, to patients as a result of medical interventions and their by-products such as serious infections. This concern has been combined with a conviction that iatrogenic risks can be prevented.

The present chapter focusses on the evolving UK National Health Service (NHS) regulatory and governance frameworks, within which professionals and healthcare managers are now required to orient their practice. A closely related subsequent chapter will look in further detail at the conceptual and practical problems arising in the implementation of Government policies and guidelines on the management of safety incidents resulting from healthcare interventions.

The regulatory and policy developments discussed in this and the next chapter are based upon the 'scientific-bureaucratic' philosophy which underpins Government thinking on achieving safer, more accountable, and efficient health care (Bilson and White, 2004). This approach to governance is therefore founded on the belief that an evidential knowledge base combined with clearly defined protocols and standards for clinical practice will enable rational control of risks (Harrison, 2004). It assumes that accountability, transparency, and compliance can be made to follow, backed up by explicit internal and external inspection systems. This chapter exposes some of the weaknesses that lie behind such seductive notions of rationality in the regulatory control of health risks.

Building on the first part of the present book, it will be argued that regulation helps to construct health risks even as it endeavours to tame them. For example, it prioritizes the selective control of certain health risks through target setting, performance indicators, and ratings systems. Regulators use a variety of techniques to translate indicators into practice, such as agreed clinical standards and criteria against which to measure and judge professional and managerial performance. However, monitoring is an essentially interpretive and subjective process. Moreover, regulators have vested interests in securing success for their agency mission and for retaining power.

The evolution of health regulation has been significantly influenced by transformations in the economy and political ideology (Moran, 2004), as it has in other sectors of public life. In the process, health regulation has become embroiled with conflicting interests. For example, a power struggle between the state and the medical profession has resulted from attempts to shift from governance working through 'communion' to a system based on 'command' (Harrison, 2004). More will be said about this important shift later in the chapter.

Regulatory frameworks in the modern NHS are subject to constant review and revision. They therefore defy easy summary or description (Bradshaw and Bradshaw, 2004), neither of which are attempted in this chapter. Rather, the purpose is to explore socio-political influences on the development of regulatory frameworks and the possible functions they serve in a modern health service. Three broad areas will be considered. Firstly, the impact of the prevailing inquiry culture on Government policies for increasing the accountability and transparency of healthcare delivery will be reviewed. The central place accorded to clinical governance as the vehicle for bringing about changes designed to deal with identified shortcomings will also be considered. Secondly, key features of the shifting regulatory landscape, including the rise of audit and risk management, are discussed. Thirdly, the escalatory relationship between risk and regulation is explored. It will be argued that regulatory failures trigger tighter controls which, in turn, generate further problems. This self-reinforcing spiral can be seen particularly in relation to medical scandals and apparent service failures to protect vulnerable members of society, such as 'at risk' children. The regulatory state has become a risk state which attempts to build strong protective governance structures for the private and public sectors, and the public now to be shielded against harm (Moran, 2007).

The emergence of an inquiry culture

One important factor leading to the operation of the complex regulatory framework now operating in the NHS, together with the increasing pressure on the health professions to submit to managerial control, was the accumulation of high profile public service disasters from the 1960s onwards. As Alaszewski and Coxon, (2007) put it:

> The development of the regulatory state is heavily influenced by the emergence of an inquiry culture in which accidents are increasingly classified as man-made disasters resulting in a cycle of disaster, inquiry and new safety measures, especially increased regulation.

As a result of several highly publicized health scandals, trust in the expertise of doctors and their ability to self-regulate, the traditional basis of the clinician-patient relationship, was brought under the media and policy microscopes (Flynn, 2002; Alaszewski, 2002). Such cases brought professional conduct under public scrutiny, and generated widespread concern about patient safety, costly litigation, and loss of reputation (Allsop and Saks, 2002; Alaszewski and Coxon, 2007). Similar concerns emerged in other Western countries at around the same time (Vincent, 2006). In the UK, the Bristol Royal Infirmary disaster (see Box 8.1, below) was a seminal instance supporting the case for regulatory changes in the NHS. The Bristol case provided a *defining moment*, not least because it marked *a major change in the Government's relationship with the professions in general and the medical profession in particular* (Alaszewski, 2002). Bristol became a symbol of all that could go wrong. Professionals were deemed to have become inward looking, unreflective, and unwilling to acknowledge failings in service performance (Weick and Sutcliffe, 2003).

The incoming Labour Government drew upon the Bristol case, and on evidence from other high-tech disasters such as errors in cervical and breast screening, to support the urgency of improving the safety and consistency of healthcare treatment and outcomes.

Box 8.1 The Bristol Royal Infirmary

Following the demands of parents in 1996, a public inquiry into children's heart surgery at the Bristol Royal Infirmary was established in 1998 and reported in 2001. It followed the General Medical Council's decision to strike off two cardiac surgeons, and to suspend a third. The inquiry covered events during the period 1984–95. It concluded that children below the age of 1-year undergoing open-heart surgery were exposed to unacceptable risks which resulted in avoidable harm to some. What constitutes an acceptable risk is of course problematic, not least because calculation of the precise harm in each child's case was obscured by the serious nature of the children's illnesses. However, the inquiry found that the mortality rate was double that of other comparable centres in England for 5 of 7 years examined. Concerns about the deaths emerged as early as 1986. Despite being raised by a whistleblower, colleagues, and parents, they were ignored by surgeons who continued to operate. Senior managers and consultants appeared to have been in denial, justifying higher death rates at Bristol than elsewhere on the grounds that the cases were more complex (Alazewski, 2002; Weick and Sutcliffe, 2003).

The inquiry considered events at Bristol to be a story of a paediatric cardiac surgical service where professionals were dedicated and well motivated but where serious failures of insight, communication, leadership, and teamwork occurred:

> The story of the paediatric surgical service in Bristol is ... an account of people who cared greatly about human suffering, and were dedicated and well motivated. Sadly, some lacked insight and their behaviour was flawed. Many failed to communicate with each other, and to work together effectively for the interests of their patients. There was lack of leadership, and of teamwork ... It is an account of a hospital where there was a 'club culture'; an imbalance of power, with too much control in the hands of a few individuals.
>
> (The Bristol Royal Infirmary Inquiry, 2001, synopsis paragraphs 3 and 8)

The Bristol Inquiry findings, provided timely backing supporting arguments for reforms designed to develop a more systematic approach to setting, delivering, and monitoring standards (Department of Health, 1998). Reforms were designed to establish the following:

◆ Clear national standards for services and treatments, through National Service Frameworks and a new National Institute for Clinical Excellence

◆ Local delivery of high quality health care, through clinical governance underpinned by modernized professional self-regulation and extended life-long learning

◆ Effective monitoring of progress through a new Commission of Health Improvement, a Framework for Assessing Performance in the NHS and a new national survey of patient and user experience. (The Commission for Health Improvement (CHI) was replaced in 2004 by the Healthcare Commission which in 2009 became part of the Care Quality Commission (CQC) together with the Commission for Social Care Inspection and the Mental Health Act Commission. These changes illustrate the volatile nature of the regulatory landscape, considered later in the chapter.)

Medical scandals have continued to impact upon the regulation and governance of the NHS, an important example being the Inquiry into the case of the GP Dr. Shipman who murdered over 200 patients, mainly women, in his care over a 15-year period, and was sentenced to life imprisonment in 2000. Despite being found guilty of maladministration of drug offences in 1976, Shipman had been allowed to continue practising, avoiding detection for many years. The Inquiry generated five reports with recommendations for regulatory reform, including the urgent need to revise death and cremation certification. It also found reason to doubt that the culture of medical self-regulation had sufficiently changed, stating that the General Medical Council (GMC) was more interested in protecting doctors than patients (The Shipman Inquiry, 2004).

A number of significant regulatory reforms are slowly emerging in response to the Shipman Inquiry. As a result of regulations which came into force in England in Jan 2007, steps have been taken to improve the management and monitoring of controlled drugs such as diamorphine, the drug prescribed by Shipman to kill his patients (Commission for Healthcare Audit and Inspection, 2008). However, the Commission's report stated that considerable work remained to embed the structures and networks needed to apply the regulations in practice. At the time of writing, a bill which contains proposals for the reform of the inquest system is being considered by the UK parliament. The proposed reforms include the appointment of a national coroner and improved scrutiny of death certificates issued. Two doctors would be required to examine death certificates, and families would be enabled to query them. Changes to the regulation of the medical profession, discussed below, have continued to be implemented through the Health and Social Care Act of 2008. A considered evaluation of the impact of such recent changes is not yet possible. What is evident is that scandals such as the Shipman Inquiry and its aftermath have fuelled continuing debate about the accountability of the health professions, especially doctors.

Accountability

In proposing its quality and standards framework for the NHS, the UK Government expressed its wish to operate in partnership with the public and the clinical professions in a climate where quality and standards improvements would be sensitive to professional self-regulation and would recognize the needs of distinctive services and localities. But the Government made clear that devolution of responsibility for the delivery of healthcare to the constituent elements of the NHS was to be *matched with accountability for performance* in a new climate where failure would not be tolerated (Department of Health, 1998). Thus behind the Government's rhetoric on partnership was a determination to secure firmer control of professional practice and service delivery. The longstanding and extremely powerful position of the medical profession in the NHS was no longer to be tolerated. Protective practices exercised on behalf of members by its self-regulating governing body, the GMC, were to be swept away (Price, 2002; Bradshaw and Bradshaw, 2004).

The GMC, established in 1815, has in recent years begun to respond to political and public pressure to improve its record of dealing with incompetent doctors (Allsop, 2002; Hatch, 2006). The Council articulated performance-standards requirements against which doctors should measure their practice and be judged in 2001 (General Medical Council, 2001). More recent changes include a reduction in the size of the GMC, and an alteration to its composition. There is now enlarged lay participation in its work and on its committees. Fitness to practice panels have been increased in number, and procedures have been streamlined. Attempts have been made to enhance public access to information about the performance of healthcare providers. A White Paper, *Trust, Assurance and Safety* (Department of Health, 2007b), affirmed the GMC's role in defining and assuring standards of practice and its plans to re-licence and re-certificate doctors. The White Paper also confirmed that the GMC will be the sole investigating authority for serious complaints against doctors. However, regulatory reforms emanating from within the profession have been complemented by increased intervention from without via a large number of governmental agencies and bodies set up for the purpose and through the requirements of clinical governance (Price, 2002; Baggott, 2002). Thus it is probable that tensions between the Government and the medical profession will continue.

Clinical governance

As with all public services, regulatory oversight of the NHS has increased notably since the 1980s. It is conducted at arm's length from the Government through a plethora of external bodies. According to Power (2007), these bodies:

> can be increasingly conceptualized as meta-regulators observing the self-regulation of organisations, an approach which represents a radical internalisation of regulatory activity and where the distinction between organising (managing) and regulating is increasingly blurred.

Hutter (2006) has neatly summarized this trend as a *move from government to governance*. A prime example is the central role of clinical governance which relies to a large extent on self-regulation monitored through various audit mechanisms. Through the use of monitoring, the Government, ultimately accountable for the effectiveness and efficiency of health services, *can retain control whilst insulating itself from frontline responsibility* (Flynn, 2004).

The prevalence of audit in modern organizations can be seen as an exemplar of 'governing at a distance' which requires experts and professionals to be more accountable through policing themselves in transparent ways (Rose, 1999). The audit method is intended to both co-opt and empower members, such as health professionals, by enlisting them in the setting of service standards, norms and benchmarks against which performance can be assessed. It is also intended to increase self-reflection amongst individuals and groups (Dean, 1999). At the same time, the audit culture in the NHS, as in other public services, is motivated by a lack of trust in professional self-regulation (Power, 2007). Tensions between generic governance and clinical expertise, although not uniformly felt to the same degree by all of the health professions, are likely to remain.

Although widely employed, clinical governance is a somewhat vague and elastic term that can be used to cover any or all of the complicated links between the constituent parts of the NHS and its regulation. It encompasses a complex and diverse combination of different processes and activities (Alaszewski, 2002; Flynn, 2004; Harrison, 2004). Flynn (2004), tracing the genealogy of the term, argued that one of the features which stands out is the *inherent ambiguity* of the term which has been linked to a *proliferation of mixed metaphors such as umbrella, model, framework, culture and mindset, etc.* As he suggested, this flexibility of meaning can be advantageous with respect to securing acceptance of the concept, but it can lead to misunderstandings and disagreements about what clinical governance means in practice (Flynn, 2004). For example, it is imprecise in specifying the relationship between professional and corporate governance although intending to bring them together through internal audit and risk management systems and committees. In this respect, one analysis has suggested that clinical governance has faltered by being operationalized as an add-on to existing committee structures. This approach may have undermined its effectiveness as a change agent, the role envisaged by the Government (Degeling *et al.*, 2004).

The examples in Box 8.2 illustrate the different emphases contained in governmental definitions of clinical governance in early policy documents which sought to reform and to modernize the NHS. Although imprecise, these definitions brought to the fore the Government's quality assurance aims. Risk thinking played a major role in the policy guidelines and circulars which were subsequently issued. Clinical governance became associated with the development of *new institutions, processes and incentive structures to manage medical quality proactively and minimise risk* (Gray and Harrison, 2004).

The first definition highlights the ambitious if not impossible aim of risk avoidance, with improvements in clinical care mentioned briefly at the end of the specification. As discussed in Chapter 1, the significance of risk avoidance depends upon whether outcome-independent or outcome-contingent risks are being managed. In relation to the latter, enabling people with disabilities to live as independently as possible, for example, should at least be considered.

Box 8.2 UK Government definitions of clinical governance (Adapted from Gray and Harrison, 2004)

The term 'clinical governance' first appeared in the 1997 NHS White Paper (Department of Health, 1997), where it was described as an instrument to:

> assure and improve clinical standards at local level throughout the NHS. This includes action to ensure risks are avoided, adverse events are rapidly detected, openly investigated and lessons learned, good practice is rapidly disseminated and systems are in place to ensure continuous improvements in clinical care.

A later elaboration (Department of Health, 1998) described clinical governance as a:

> framework through which NHS organisations are accountable for continuously improving the quality of their services and safeguarding high standards of care by creating an environment in which excellence in clinical care will flourish.

The second definition focusses explicitly only on excellence in clinical care. Despite their variability of emphasis, both definitions stress the importance of quality assurance systems with respect to achieving safer and improved clinical practice. As such, clinical governance has become an important mantra for the Government's aspirations to modernize the NHS and control the professions (Gray and Harrison, 2004). Effectively, it is intended to shift the onus for managing medical practice to senior managers who have a statutory duty to ensure that all NHS organizations have appropriate quality assurance systems (Flynn, 2002). However, clinical governance is viewed unfavourably by many professionals as a bureaucratic initiative which challenges professional status and autonomy; and as a top-down management device more concerned in practice with meeting externally set performance targets than with enhancing clinical care (Hackett, 1999; Degeling et al., 2004; O'Neil, 2004; Som, 2005).

There is some evidence that nurses, paramedics, and psychologists feel more positive about clinical governance than do doctors, with surgeons least enthusiastic (Walshe et al., 2000). That standard procedures can be valuable when grounded in the work of clinical teams has been demonstrated by Haynes et al. (2009). The research, conducted in eight hospitals, showed that a simple 2-minute checklist used before an operation lowered the incidence of surgical deaths and complications by a third. Surgeons, initially sceptical and reluctant, became more convinced by the outcomes and will be required to implement the procedure for all operations in the UK by 2010. An earlier study of the use of a preoperative team checklist also concluded that it showed promise as a practical tool, perhaps because it promoted effective team communication and cohesion (Lingard et al., 2005).

Although clinical standards can be embedded in practice, and can achieve improvements in care through the use of standardized tools, the development of clinical governance seems so far to have been dominated more by form than substance. This failure may be associated with the top-down nature of its implementation in trusts, and the consequent focus on generic processes which do not inspire its developmental potential or clinical ownership at the level of specialist multidisciplinary teams (Degeling et al., 2004). Some commentators support the view that there is a need to rebalance the managerial focus of clinical governance so that trust in the tacit knowledge of professionals rather than formal procedures per se becomes integral to its operation (Alaszweski and Coxon, 2007).

In summary, the development of clinical governance is intimately bound up with wider regulatory reform. In practice, it has turned into a multi-faceted policy instrument which has generated mixed reactions from health professionals (Flynn, 2004). Clinical governance involves *a fundamental change in medical professionals accountability* and is thus linked to a move towards managerialism in the public services from the 1990s onwards (Flynn, 2004). The design of auditable clinical risk standards is intended to enlist professionals in an explicit and transparent process of self-policing (Power, 2007) which they may resist but cannot entirely ignore. External regulatory agencies play a significant role in shaping, supporting, and controlling the governance activities of healthcare organizations which they are required to establish in an environment of considerable change.

A changing regulatory landscape

The foundations for the modern regulatory state in the UK were forged during the Victorian era, when rapid technological development transformed the organization of economic and social life which arguably made the New World more hazardous (Giddens, 1998; Moran, 2007). Against a backdrop of economic liberalism and industrialization, a network of inspectorates emerged. Protective legislation was passed as factory production raised concerns about worker safety, harm to the environment, and the quality of goods and services. Amongst developments which increased the potential for state provision of welfare services were: a strengthened central state administration; data collection and analysis of population trends, such as birth and mortality rates; and recognition of the needs of the 'deserving poor' (Kemshall, 2006; Moran, 2007). At the same time, patterns of self-governance, in place since the Middle Ages for industry and commerce, were more formally established. In relation to healthcare, new professional groups were formed or reformed so as to consolidate authority and autonomy through self-regulation (Moran, 2007). Through these means 'club management' was established, which has been a source of tension between the health professions, particularly doctors, and successive governments ever since (see Box 8.1).

Lines of debate about who should define and regulate health care began to take hold in the Victorian era. They were brought into sharper relief by the establishment of the NHS in 1945, although the settlement which occurred then with the medical professions preserved their rights to self-regulate for several decades further (Moran, 2004). Since the 1980s, the balances between state control and professional self-regulation, and between central and devolved management structures, have been high on the political agenda, as reflected in the constant restructuring of NHS management and its diverse services.

The modernization of the NHS which was begun in the Thatcher era and carried forwards by the Labour Government has been forged in the context of *a strong (international) deregulatory rhetoric, centring on alleged over-regulation, legalism, inflexibility and an alleged absence of attention being paid to the costs of regulation* (Hutter, 2005). Based on the neo-liberal belief that flexibility and competition were required in contemporary capitalist economies if they were to survive on a global stage, new ideals of less centralized organizational and flatter management structures emerged (Flynn, 2004). Such ideals infiltrated the public sector; they stimulated attempts to establish quasi-markets, and put pressure on traditional hierarchical structures which had flourished in the NHS in 1950s and 1960s. Constant reform of organizational structures, polices, and regulation in health and social services have ensued (Moran, 2007).

The NHS has been the subject of political controversy since its inception and the most recent plan to reconfigure the NHS into foundation trusts with greater autonomy from Whitehall is no exception. Viewed by the Government as *the cutting-edge* of its *commitment to the decentralisation of public services and the creation of a patient-led NHS* (Department of Health, 2005), foundation trusts are seen by critics as paving the way to fragmentation and privatization of health services (Boyle, 2005). By January 2009, there were 113 NHS foundation trusts, half of all eligible acute and mental health trusts, operating in England. Their establishment is seen by the Government as a significant milestone of achievement (Department of Health, 2009).

Foundation trusts are required to be accountable to local people by involving them in governance. They are subject to the full might of NHS regulation, with some duplication by Monitor, a body set up to evaluate the readiness of trusts for foundation status. In effect, Monitor has the role of double checking compliance with NHS standards and targets. However, some doubt has been cast on the concept, operation, and regulation of foundation trusts by two recent damning reports from the Government's 'watchdog', the Healthcare Commission, (subsequently the Care Quality Commission). One report identified significant failures in aspects of care and critical incident reporting at the Birmingham Children's NHS Foundation Trust. The second report (Healthcare Commission, 2009) offered a damning account of emergency care at the Mid Staffordshire NHS Foundation Trust. The investigation of the latter was triggered by a higher than expected mortality rate amongst patients admitted as emergency cases during 2005-08. The report concluded that:

> In the trust's drive to become a foundation trust, it appears to have lost sight of its real priorities. The trust was galvanised into radical action by the imperative to save money and did not properly consider the effect of reductions in staff on the quality of care. It took a decision to significantly reduce staff without adequately assessing the consequences. Its strategic focus was on financial and business matters at a time when the quality of care of its patients admitted as emergencies was well below acceptable standards.

Although dismissed as an aberration by the Health Minister (BBC News 17th Mar 2009, www.news.bbc.co.uk/hi/uk), the Mid Staffordshire case illustrates the collision path that can ensue between meeting financial targets and avoiding placing patients at increased risk. The Healthcare Commission report and the Government put the responsibility for failure on the management of the Mid Staffordshire Trust. But the many operational shortcomings discovered during the investigation appear to have escaped earlier notice by the regulatory bodies (the Healthcare Commission and Monitor). These regulatory failures raise questions about the efficacy of inspection and monitoring systems, a discussion of which is taken up later in the chapter.

Risk management and organizational change

Kemshall (2006) identified *marketization, partnership, and a new managerialism stressing evaluation, accountability, and increased regulation of activities of the workforce,* as key features of the 'new' NHS. Running alongside the 'audit implosion', developed in response to a perceived need to demonstrate transparent forms of self-evaluation and improvement (Power, 2007), has been an increasing use of formal risk-based management approaches in the NHS (see Box 8.3). This change reflects the continuing pressure on public agencies generally to prove their efficacy and efficiency, and to adopt private industry management practices (Hutter, 2005). Use of formal risk management procedures has also been stimulated by a wider strengthening of faith in their importance to the functioning of a well governed organization, *which is internally and externally accountable for how it handles uncertainty* (Power, 2007). Risk management has particularly powerful resonances for health services because of their engagement with life and death issues. Its increasing importance also reflects the wider societal shift towards viewing the world through the lens of risk discussed in the introductory chapter of the book. Power persuasively argues that although risk management of organizations is marketed on the basis of strategy and effective business practice, it has developed as a response to a cultural environment in which *control must be made increasingly publicly visible and ... organisational responsibility must be made transparent* so as to make a convincing public statement that uncertainty is being tackled (Power, 2004).

It is somewhat ironic that the ideology of enterprise risk management, which was intended as the antidote to costly bureaucracy of the past, has generated for the public sector an alternative world of targets, performance indicators, expanding risk registers, and an array of specialist roles in health care such as clinical governance leaders and risk managers. It is difficult to avoid seeing these developments as anything other than bureaucratic. However, risk management in the NHS, and the related emphases on measurable procedures and evidence-based practice, seem to fit well with Courpassen's notion of soft bureaucracy, in which *rigid constraints and structures of domination* coexist with *processes of flexibility and decentralisation* (Courpassen, 2000). It is inevitable that there will be tensions between the two, and professionals may attempt to manoeuvre their way around some of regulatory controls which they see as a brake on their professional autonomy and expertise. Chapter 9 explores this tension further.

Risk management and defensiveness

Regulation through the elaborate forms of audit which now operate in the NHS may serve an important defensive function for organizations. A prime example is the service provided by the NHS Litigation Authority (NHSLA) which was established in 1995 to handle a range of schemes for settling litigation claims, of which the Clinical Negligence Scheme for trusts is one. This scheme administers funds pooled by NHS foundation and primary care trusts in England, all of which are members. Membership is voluntary but strongly advocated by the NHSLA on the grounds that investment in risk management, set out in the risk framework, standards, and guidelines which it provides, will pay dividends in reduced costs for litigation. The NHSLA defines separate risk standards for each type of trust and audits them on an annual, bi-annual, or tri-annual basis depending on achieved levels with respect to the standards under scrutiny. It gives discounts on fees if members are found to comply. As an illustration, the current NHSLA risk standards in use for acute trusts are shown in Box 8.3.

The framework summarized in Box 8.3, on p. 184, contains a number of ambitious aims. Health service organizations are encouraged to comply with external NHS regulatory requirements, to develop internal self-regulation, and to culturally embed risk management. The implementation of the framework requires each institution to put in place a very wide range of processes with substantial supporting documentation which provide evidence for audit. Guidelines and intricate templates are provided for auditors to assess compliance with standards. These can be found on the NHSLA website, www.nhsla.com/home.htm. Demanding procedures do not necessarily produce service improvements such as reduced risks for patients and a number of issues can be raised about this highly formalized approach to organizational risk management.

As is the case with most regulatory bodies, the NHSLA definition of success is bound up with its prescribed mission. It is difficult, therefore, to evaluate the success of the standards framework other than by reference to itself. For example, the increasing litigation costs experienced by the NHS may have more to do with rising claims from a risk aware public and the propensity of evermore complex medical procedures to go wrong than with the outcomes of risk management.

Box 8.3 NHS Litigation Authority (2009) risk standards for acute trusts

The NHSLA standards and assessment process are designed to:

- provide a structured framework within which to focus effective risk-management activities in order to deliver quality improvements in organizational governance, patient care, and the safety of patients, staff, contractors, volunteers, and visitors
- increase awareness and encourage implementation of the national agenda for the NHS
- encourage and support organizations in taking a proactive approach to service improvement
- reflect risk exposure and empower organizations to determine how to manage their own risks
- contribute to embedding risk management into the organization's culture
- cut the cost of litigation by reducing the number of adverse incidents and the likelihood of recurrence
- assist in the management of adverse incidents and claims
- provide quality and safety assurance to the organization, other inspecting bodies, and stakeholders, including patients.

Such observations support the view that a prime purpose of regulatory standards, particularly in the public sector, is to demonstrate that organizations are risk aware, and have adequate systems of defence against adverse events and legal claims (Hutter, 2005). One study has suggested that health professionals see the requirement for them to report patient safety incidents as more concerned with shielding the organization than with improving patient safety (Alaszewski and Coxon, 2007).

Power (2007) refers to the widespread use of formal risk management in public and private organizations as *a new mode of accountability and monitoring in the name of risk*. The adoption of risk management appears to be variable amongst and within sectors. It is unlikely that all health organizations will be immersed in risk management practices to the same degree (Hood, Rothstein, and Baldwin, 2004). Nevertheless, there is considerable pressure upon them to comply with the requirements of regulatory bodies which increasingly look for evidence of risk management as a sign of proper engagement with governmental policies on patient safety. As is illustrated below, this pressure has generated a demanding and continuously spiralling regulatory process.

Recent changes to the regulation of health service delivery

It is not surprising that the regulation of a huge and complex enterprise like the NHS demands regular review. However, the frequency with which agencies are reformed and new bodies created has not made this task any easier (Bradshaw and Bradshaw, 2004). At the time of writing, the UK Government has decided to refocus the work of the National Patient Safety Agency (NPSA). It has created a super-regulator, the Care Quality Commission (CQC), launched in 2009, to bring the Healthcare Commission under one umbrella with the Commission for Social Care Inspection and the Mental Health Act Commission. Constant reconfiguration of regulatory agencies implies government dissatisfaction with the effectiveness of their attempts to monitor and improve health service risk management. This reconfiguration is perhaps motivated by continuing efforts to plug gaps between policy and practice. However, such gaps may be unavoidable in an environment in which professionals focus on delivering care in resource constrained circumstances whilst senior managers concentrate on targets and mergers (Tingle, 2008).

The National Patient Safety Agency (NPSA)

The NSPA was established in 2001. Its two main aims were: firstly, to identify trends and patterns in patient safety problems through its National Reporting and Learning System (NRLS); and secondly, to support staff at the local level to report incidents with a view to ensuring a high national profile to improving patient safety. Subsequently, the agency has undergone several significant changes. In 2005, its remit was expanded to cover safety aspects of hospital design, food and cleanliness, safety issues in research, and support for local performance concerns about individual doctors and dentists through its oversight of the National Clinical Assessment Service. A year later, the NPSA, along with other patient safety agencies and organizations, came under scrutiny following a further review of patient safety commissioned by the Chief Medical Officer for Health (Department of Health, 2006c). The review found that the national profile of patient safety had been raised but that problems remained about the priority given to patient safety locally. Deficiencies in the NPSA's performance were identified, as shown in Box 8.4, below.

Safety First identified national service frameworks and performance targets as competitors to the patient safety agenda which tended to be given less priority. This indicates that co-ordination between different agencies and their collective effect is problematic.

Box 8.4 Excerpts from the 'Safety First' summary statement (Department of Health, 2006c)

Patient safety is not always given the same priority or status as other major issues such as reducing waiting times, implementing national service frameworks and achieving financial balance.

There is little evidence that data collected through the national reporting system are effectively informing patient safety at the local NHS level. Despite the high volume of incident reports collected by the NPSA to date, there are too few examples where these have resulted in actionable learning for local NHS organisations. The National Reporting and Learning System (NRLS) is not yet delivering high quality, routinely available information on patterns, trends and underlying causes of harm to patients.

That financial and performance targets and outcomes move to the top of trust agendas is not surprising since they impact directly on their budgets, and were significant indicators for achieving foundation trust status. The annual star ratings given to each trust from 2001–05 were widely criticized for encouraging them to concentrate on hitting targets, such as cutting waiting times, while neglecting other aspects of their work. Since 2005, star ratings have been superseded by a more comprehensive system for rating performance (Bevan and Hood, 2005), yet another regulatory shift. The Healthcare Commission investigation of the Mid Staffordshire NHS Foundation Trust, discussed earlier, illustrates the potential drawbacks of target driven regimes.

The *Safety First* report concluded that the NPSA's role in harnessing the expertise and commitment of other patient safety bodies was unclear. The agency was required to refocus its objectives, and to refine and simplify its national reporting system which was judged to be failing to fulfil its potential. The NPSA had already been criticized in 2005 by the Public Accounts Committee for not knowing how many patients die per year from medical errors. Its two joint Chief Executives were suspended pending an enquiry into their managerial record (Kmietowicz, 2007). Heading up such agencies is obviously a risky business! The issue of who is held to blame for failures in achieving agency missions is considered later.

In an attempt to reinforce the patient safety agenda, yet another review of the NHS (Department of Health, 2008) demanded increased local self-regulation and accountability, argued for stronger punitive regulatory measures, and spearheaded a plethora of new initiatives. This report, *High Quality For All*, has engendered a National Patient Safety campaign. Borrowing from an American model, the NPSA has designated a list of Never Events such as 'wrong-site' surgery (National Patient Safety Agency, 2009a). With the aim of giving the patient safety agenda more bite, NHS organizations will be punished financially from 2010–11 if patients are harmed by incidents on the Never Events list. Although the Never Events strategy may give the patient safety agenda added symbolic power, it may also spawn a new bureaucracy and have the effect of sidelining other safety issues (Walsh, 2009), as will be discussed in Chapter 9. The revised priorities, targets, and strategies for the NPSA will no doubt be subject to a further cycle of review and reform in this very challenging area of health policy. Whether these constant top-down changes to NHS organizational structures reflect the difficulty of the healthcare risk regulation task, or are themselves part of the problem, remains an open question.

The Care Quality Commission (CQC)

A further important recent change in healthcare regulation has been the creation of the CQC. It was established by the Health and Social Care Act of 2008 to bring together the Healthcare Commission, the Commission for Social Care Inspection and the Mental Health Act Commission, the three former big regulatory guns in the health and adult social care system in England. The creation of a super-agency is intended to overcome barriers between health and social care where the distinctions between their services increasingly blur. Health and social care organizations, including, for the first time, NHS private providers, are required to register with the new regulator in order to provide services.

The CQC is required to adopt a risk-based approach and efficiently target action where it is needed and will have increased powers of enforcement (Department of Health, 2007c; Department of Health, 2008). In relation to governmental efforts to control healthcare associated infections, the CQC will be able to fine hospitals, close wards, suspend services, and increase inspection visits where hygiene requirements are not being met. In the wake of the Mid Staffordshire Trust case, discussed earlier, risk scrutiny is to be strengthened by the establishment of 'risk summits' of inspectors, health watchdogs, and regional NHS chiefs who will vet the safety of every hospital and share information so that patterns in sub-standard care can be identified. Other reforms include faster alert systems to identify trusts with high mortality rates, and risk profiling to identify organizations threatened by management changes and high staff turnover or vacancy rates.

Governmental policy favours decentralized control so long as it is tempered by robust regulation and held in check by performance targets. Whether exacting financial penalties for failure will lead to improvements in patient safety is uncertain. It may have the effect of further weakening the performance of

some organizations and of reinforcing a climate which de-energizes local crea-
tivity in combating patient safety issues. The above examples of agency reform
reveal a dynamic where regulators' missions are subject to constant modification, presenting health organizations and professionals with the difficult task
of managing diverse, overlapping, and expanding requirements. Those below
illustrate the complicated processes underlying the evolution of regulatory
policies as a process of escalation.

Regulation and escalation

The escalation of regulatory requirements for health and social services can be
linked to the paradoxical impact of the contemporary preoccupation with risk
and risk management in society. Rothstein has argued that this concern does
not arise from greater susceptibility to risk and consequent anxiety, as the 'risk
society' thesis (Beck, 1992) suggests. Instead it provides a means for attempting to control the wider world, for example by regulatory bodies who have the
specific role of protecting the public (Rothstein, Humber, and Gaskell, 2006).

Those who promote centrally driven health risk management make the
implicit assumption that orderliness and control of patient safety, can prevail
so long as risks are identified and assessed. But this very activity may help to
generate an *escalating spiral of control and anxiety* which is *a distinctive feature
of contemporary medical culture* (Crawford, 2004). This is nowhere more evident than when critical incidents come to public attention. Regulatory reforms
follow closely in their wake attempting to close the gaps which have been
exposed. Despite problems having arisen with already implemented regulatory
procedures, retrospective tightening of regulation sustains faith in the power
of central authority to control risks. The tragic case of Baby Peter, discussed
below, has been selected to explore this process. Cases of undetected child
abuse which end in their death bring into sharp relief the limitations of risk-
management systems to provide foolproof protection and the impulse to
establish even stronger control of services and professions in response.

Regulatory failure and blame: the case of Baby Peter

Baby Peter died at the age of 17-months in August, 2007 whilst under the protection of Haringey Council in England. The sustained abuse and injuries
which killed him were inflicted whilst he was in the care of his mother, her
partner, and their lodger. Over a period of 8-months, Baby Peter had come
into contact with social workers and health and police agencies on 60 occasions. He was seen by a social worker and a doctor in the last week of his life
(Lord Laming, 2009). The reverberations of Baby Peter's death continue to
impact on the regulation of child services in England generating a wave of

inquires and reviews and far reaching reforms designed to prevent further such deaths (see CommunityCare.com, May 2009 for a time-line résumé). Whether any regulatory and risk management system could ever prevent another such death is a politically unacceptable question, signified by the demands from the media, the public and politicians for increased regulation and punitive measures to address failure.

Seven years before the death of Baby Peter, Victoria Climbié, also under the care of Haringey, died as a result of appalling treatment at the hands of her great-aunt and partner. An independent inquiry into her death led to a highly critical report on the performance of the agencies involved (Lord Laming, 2003). It produced 108 recommendations which brought about a major overhaul of child protection services, including increased regulation and inspection. Lord Laming's second review, after the death of Baby Peter, considered that those reforms had not been properly implemented. The report concluded that implementation had been impeded by the burden of bureaucracy placed on frontline staff, and by ongoing failures of leadership and management (Lord Laming, 2009). His critics have argued that his reforms have themselves fuelled bureaucratic approaches to child protection, resulting in a loss of effective contact with clients (Ferguson and Lavalette, 2009). Laming's second report contained 54 new recommendations, including proposals to enhance the status of social work, increase the number of health visitors, improve the training of managers and GPs, and streamline information management processes, particularly the electronic records system. In addition to recommending these professionally empowering measures, the report advocates punitive disciplinary responses in cases of failure to protect children (Lord Laming, 2009). Laming's suggestion that there should be performance targets for child protection similar to those for education could create further bureaucracy and prove counter-productive.

The reasons for a child slipping through the collective child protective net are complex. Failures generate conflicting perspectives on who is responsible. Douglas (1990) has observed that all societies and social groups apportion blame if norms of behaviour and protective boundaries are breached. When children die from abuse in the home in late modern societies, organizations, and personnel deemed responsible for risk prevention are held to account. The ensuing media 'witch hunt' helps to reinforce a process in which a person or group is marked out for punishment. In the case of Baby Peter, the Head of Children's Services at Haringey, Sharon Shoesmith, was dismissed without compensation. She received death threats and abusive communications from an outraged public, as did members of her family (*The Guardian* newspaper, 2nd Dec 2008). Shoesmith launched a series of legal battles, ongoing at the time of writing, against her dismissal, the manner of her sacking by Haringey Council, and the part played by the Office for Standards in Education (Ofsted) (Peacock, 2009).

Haringey Council has been bombarded by a series of ongoing inquiries, including the joint investigation conducted by Ofsted, the Healthcare Commission, and the police, in the wake of the Baby Peter court case which was heard in late 2008. The ensuing report identified significant management failings, inadequate information collection, and poor collaboration between agencies in Haringey (Ofsted, 2008). The damning tone of the report stands in contradiction to the clean bill of health awarded to Haringey for its child services by an Ofsted inspection only a year before. The Ofsted defence was that Haringey misled the inspectors with false data. But this was contested as having no evidential base (*The Guardian* newspaper, 12th Dec 2008).

Social workers have remained firmly in the media spotlight in relation to the Baby Peter tragedy, but healthcare professionals have not been exempted. Renewed interest in the suspension of the two doctors involved, and in Great Ormond Street Children's Hospital, one of the four trusts implicated, were spurred by a critical review published by the CQC in May 2009. Amongst the systemic failings listed were poor communication between health profession-als and between health and social services, staff not adhering to procedures, staff shortages, poor staff recruitment and training processes, and failings in governance. The CQC found that improvements to child protection systems had occurred, but remained sceptical about the quality of governance since assurances had been given over three consecutive years that the core standards for child protection were being met (Care Quality Commission, 2009). Concern about possible flaws in inspection of the trusts, or in the regulatory framework itself, was deflected by the promise of further inspections of the four hospitals involved. Further investigations of all trusts, designed to see if they were in default of regulations, were also promised.

The regulatory fallout from the Baby Peter case, and the associated spiral of blame and counter-blame is far from spent. Ofsted and the Health Care Commission appear to have side-stepped potential accusations of culpability, perhaps because their claims to control risk management systems effectively are even more vital when the frailty of regulatory regimes becomes so exposed. They have become the ultimate guardians of social order in societies which are organized around attempted risk management. Thus, the escalatory response to the death of Baby Peter is bound up with governmental imperatives to end-lessly try to demonstrate that all doors against uncertainty can ultimately be closed. However, the case also raises questions about the nature of regulation delivered by bodies that are distant from the ground. Limitations to the over-sight which they can realistically achieve remain unacknowledged.

Regulating the regulator: the case of the Nursing and Midwifery Council (NMC)

Although not prompted by a scandal like Bristol or Shipman, and seemingly very different from a critical incident such as the Baby Peter case, an analysis of the process and findings of a performance review of the Nursing and Midwifery Council (NMC) by the Council for Healthcare Regulatory Excellence (CHRE) indicates some similarities concerning the evolution and implementation of regulatory policies. In this case, the spur to investigation was a letter sent privately to the Minister of Health by some members of the NMC in 2007. They complained about *an ingrained culture of racism and bullying* and the poor performance of the NMC which they defined as a *dysfunctioning organisation* (Council for Healthcare Regulatory Excellence, 2008).

The investigative review found no evidence of racism, but confirmed that bullying and sectional interests were features of the NMC's culture. Concerns were expressed about critical safety issues, in particular the process through which cases of professional misconduct and fitness to practice were decided. The NMC subsequently published an action plan for oversight by the CHRE, but an interesting aspect of the initial response was a challenge to the efficacy of the regulator. The NMC expressed disquiet *that today's findings appear to directly contradict CHRE's own performance assessment in March. This is cause for concern* (Nursing and Midwifery Council, 2008). As with the Ofsted inspection of Haringey, the CHRE appears to have missed the crucial evidence the 'first time around'. The initial inspection process might have been inadequately implemented in both cases. The staff whose work was being reviewed might have deliberately or unreflectively misled the inspectors, as is possible whenever evidence relies on testimony. However, these failures of initial regulation may also illustrate the impossible task facing regulators who must act as if they can control risks indirectly. Returning to the case of Baby Peter, the Chief Executive of the Healthcare Commission expressed the difficulties as follows:

> In the health check this year a very high proportion of NHS trusts declared themselves compliant, including the four attended by Baby P. How can they do so when these issues still occur? ... What I think is that boards do have systems in place for safeguarding all children, but they don't always necessarily work all the time in every way. And that of course is what is needed.
>
> (Anne Walker, *The Guardian* newspaper, 11th Dec 2008)

The desire for systems which close off every possible risk and offer foolproof protection to children in care and patients undergoing treatment is understandable. Whether complex systems involving multiple health and social services are fit for purpose must of course be open to scrutiny and debate.

However, when regulatory systems become unwieldy, they may, paradoxically, contribute to the unsafe practices they are trying to control. Moreover, even well designed risk management systems cannot anticipate every possible adverse event.

Conclusion

This chapter was not intended to offer a comprehensive review of NHS regulatory bodies and their missions. Rather, it sought to explore the shifting ground on which they are built and reformed. The chapter has considered some of the wider political and social influences which impact upon the design and modification of such systems. It has illustrated that the governmental agenda for regulating risk and safety in the NHS has not yet generated a comprehensive, cohesive, and stable set of policies. In practice, some policy priorities gain precedence over others as trusts seek to meet performance targets, implement national service frameworks, and achieve financial balance. These priorities can push to one side the requirements of the patient safety agenda. The wide range of regulatory bodies created and reformed since 1997, many with overlapping roles, suggests that central political control of such a large and complex organization as the NHS continues to prove elusive (Bradshaw and Bradshaw, 2004). The effectiveness of the most recent formulation of devolved managerial control and local accountability in foundation trusts, which supposedly provides robust external monitoring combined with punitive measures for failure, has yet to be comprehensively assessed. It would be untenable to have social and health services which were not regulated. However, the limitations of regulatory control need to be recognized. The constant review and reform of regulatory bodies may actually exacerbate gaps between policy and practice.

As the regulatory environment has become more complex, the problems facing those managing risk systems in health organizations have multiplied. The ideal world outlined in governmental policies, and specified by rules, protocols, and standards, is not necessarily valued in the same way by health professionals. Many find it difficult to marry this regulatory regime with their own philosophies of patient care. Health professionals base their practice upon their tacit knowledge as well as protocols (Degeling *et al.*, 2004; Alaszewski and Coxon, 2007). As argued in Chapter 6, it is not even possible to apply 'encoded' knowledge without adapting it to specific cases. Clinical governance is based on an increasingly bureaucratized, rule driven, model of medical professionalism (Harrison, 2004). In consequence, regulation may be experienced as distant and separate from everyday practice. There is some evidence, discussed above, that this barrier may be overcome if protocols and standards are successfully grounded in clinical practice (Haynes *et al.*, 2009). Paradoxically, advances in medicine which have increased its complexity generate new risks of service failure (Gawande, 2008):

> If you had a heart attack in the 1950's, you'd be given some morphine and put on bed rest. If you survived 6 weeks it was a miracle. Today not only do we have 10 different ways to prevent heart attacks, but we have many different treatment options, including stents, clot busters, heart surgery, and medical management. The degree of challenge in applying the ultimate best treatment option for any particular patient is becoming difficult. This puts us at risk for 'failures' that didn't exist in the past.

The next chapter focusses on efforts to avoid 'failures' and safeguard patient safety, themes increasingly viewed through the lens of risk.

Chapter 9

Health risk and the patient safety agenda

Monica Shaw

Aim

To critically review the design and implementation of the UK Government's patient safety agenda.

Objectives

1. To trace the development of the patient safety agenda for the NHS, and to analyse the challenges which it poses

2. To consider efforts to establish a sound evidence base for improving safety in clinical practice

3. To discuss attempts to achieve an open reporting safety culture for the NHS.

Introduction

The previous chapter explored the dynamics of the intricate and turbulent NHS regulatory landscape. It identified the way in which the UK Government's patient safety agenda jostles for attention with financial and other performance targets. This chapter looks in more depth at the UK Government's approach to tackling patient safety, discussing difficulties that arise with respect to developing the evidence base on which it is supposed to depend. The 1997 White Papers for England, Wales, and Scotland established the blueprint for the Labour Government's reforms of the NHS, in which the identification and management of risk were given prominence (Department of Health 1997; Scottish Office 1997). The foundations of the patient safety agenda were put in place, with healthcare organizations required to achieve the following (Department of Health, 1997):

- ◆ Clinical risk reduction programmes of a high standard to be put in place
- ◆ Adverse events and patient complaints to be openly investigated, and lessons learned promptly applied

- ◆ Problems of poor clinical practice to be recognised at an early stage and dealt with to prevent harm to patients.

Subsequent policy documents (Department of Health, 2000c; 2001) set out the Government's critique of current NHS approaches to patient safety, and offered plans for improvement. A world was depicted in which patients were more at risk from adverse events than is generally recognized, and in which recorded cases were likely to be the tip of the iceberg. This alarming analysis of uncertainty drew attention to the importance of collecting evidence on which risk preventive strategies might be based. Policies for improving the safety of healthcare have been predicated on the belief that progress in improving patient safety can be assured, and public confidence in health services restored, so long as it's practice is informed by evidence (Hutter, 2005; Adil, 2008). However, attempts to secure and interpret the appropriate evidence present significant difficulties.

Defining and estimating the scale of the patient safety problem

Vincent (2006) has argued that *the reduction of harm should be the primary aim of patient safety and not the elimination of error*. He made this case on the grounds that harm can result from many factors such as overcrowded hospitals, complications of surgery, and unanticipated adverse drug reactions, whilst, on the other hand, minor errors can be a source of learning (Vincent, 2006). The concept of 'adverse event', widely used to describe harm to patients, is extensively employed in the quantitative risk analysis literature. It was discussed in some detail in the first part of the book, in relation to a critique of the Royal Society (1992) definition of risk. By focussing on consequences, the definition lumps together different causes of adversity, as discussed in Chapter 3. For example, one patient safety policy document defined an adverse event (Department of Health, 2001) as *an event or omission arising during clinical care and causing physical or psychological injury to a patient*. Thus, complications arising from high quality medical interventions, negative outcomes of positive risk-taking, negligence, error, and rare instances of intentional harm are all covered by the term 'adverse event'. A deceptively simple definition, it treats 'events' or 'omissions' as facts to be extracted and counted, obscuring the subjective judgements required to determine their occurrence and significance.

Examples of 'known' adverse events and their impact as identified in the policy document *An Organisation with a Memory* (Department of Health, 2001c) are summarized in Box 9.1.

Box 9.1 Official analysis of adverse events occurring in the NHS (Department of Health, 2000c)

1 Adverse events occur in around 10% of admissions, generating an estimated total of 850 000 per year

2 Adverse events cost approximately £2 billions a year in additional hospital stays alone

3 Around 1 150 people who have been in recent contact with mental health services commit suicide every year

4 400 people die or are seriously injured in adverse events involving medical devices every year

5 The NHS pays out every year around £400 million in settlement of clinical negligence claims .

6 Hospital-acquired infections, about 15% of which may be avoidable, are estimated to cost the NHS nearly £1 billion every year.

Policy documents on patient safety (Department of Health, 2000c; 2001) lamented the failure of the NHS to learn from repeated adverse events, at great cost to patients, their families, and the NHS. Four areas were selected for targeted reduction of risk to patients: spinal injections; obstetrics, gynaecology and midwifery care; the prescribing, dispensing, and administration of medication; and suicides by mental health patients. The importance of meeting these targets was illustrated by the following example. It was estimated that 50% of the NHS litigation bill related to claims concerning brain damaged babies, and that if the targeted 25% reduction in negligent harm cases resulting in litigation were achieved, it would result in a saving of £50 million a year. Risk reduction targets covering major disease and population groups have become central to governmental strategy for improving the quality and safety of healthcare. Like the regulatory structures discussed in Chapter 8, they are continually revised.

The launch of the *Never Events* policy for England in March 2009 (National Patient Safety Agency, 2009a) is the most recent attempt to set patient safety targets in England. Defined by the Chief Executive of the NSPA as *a bold initiative designed to drive measurable improvements in patient safety*, it defines eight core events considered absolutely preventable, including wrong-site surgery, inpatient suicide using non-collapsible rails, and wrong route administration of chemotherapy. The Never Events Framework provides details of the timetable and implementation process for primary care trusts and of the financial penalties for non-compliance. The Framework lists highly specific and selected risks, but is intended to act as a spur to the patient safety agenda as a whole. Is this strategy likely to succeed? There is some evidence to show that targets have brought about positive change in waiting times for inpatients, outpatients in accident and emergency, and for referrals, and a fall in the incidence of the hospital-acquired MRSA (Bevan, 2009). Comparative data indicate that England outshines other countries (Australia, Canada, New Zealand, Wales, and Scotland) for sustained improvements in meeting waiting time targets, which can be interpreted as producing better outcomes for patients (Bevan, 2009). An alternative view is that the wider impact of the target regime is *pernicious* and has sacrificed service development for *measures associated with spin, selection and punishment* and concludes that *targets suit politicians, not patients* (Gubb, 2009). The impact of targets is difficult to establish for a number of reasons. Amongst others, gaming tactics may be used to influence statistical outcomes, and safety issues that are more difficult to measure may slip beneath the radar.

Lying behind the rhetoric on patient safety is the political drive towards achieving greater efficiencies in the delivery of services and avoidance of lost reputation and costly litigation in a context where demand and expectations of high quality care continue to rise (Singh, 2003). The enormous cost to the NHS arising from litigation and hospital-acquired infections is documented in Box 9.1. But the patient safety agenda is also a response to a more risk aware, critical, and vocal public that is willing to challenge medical authority (Donaldson, 2008).

Below the tip of the iceberg: near misses

There is a growing body of research that attempts to quantify iatrogenic health risks to patients (Vincent, 2006). A number of international studies have produced remarkably similar estimates, that one in 10 hospitalized patients will die or be injured as a result of medical interventions (Thomas, *et al.*, 2000; Baker *et al.*, 2004; de Vries, *et al.*, 2008). However, as noted above, adverse outcomes should not be equated with errors. Because the evidence base for treatment efficacy is probabilistic, some individual patients may not benefit from, or be harmed by, an intervention which yields net health gains. This inherent limitation of inductive probabilistic reasoning, which was discussed in Chapter 4, can easily be overlooked.

De Vries *et al.* undertook a systematic review of eight studies published between 1991 and 2006, together covering some 74 000 patient records from the USA, Australia, New Zealand, and UK hospitals. They found a median overall adverse event incidence of 9.2%, with lethal results in 7% of cases. The majority of events related to operations or drugs, and almost half were deemed to be preventable (de Vries *et al.*, 2008). Such estimates have to be treated with caution as the studies on which they are based vary in scope, definition of adverse events and completeness of data. Although not an argument against research into the risk posed by medical interventions, the focus of such studies on negative outcomes obscures the positive effect of developments in healthcare.

It is generally accepted that estimates of adverse event incidence represent only a partial account of the types and frequency of human errors. It is often argued that in reality the problem is one of epidemic proportions. Although not susceptible to treatment in the same way as some epidemics may be, it invokes a similar call to remove human error as if it were a 'plague' (Reason, 2001). Shades of this thinking are apparent in governmental policies that seek to grapple with the dangers lurking beneath the 'official' adverse events figures, and to probe the scale of unreported errors and near misses. The term 'near miss', borrowed from the world of aviation safety, is defined as *an event or omission, or sequence of events or omissions arising during care* which did not develop into an adverse event *whether or not as a result of compensating action* (Department of Health, 2001).

It is likely that near misses in healthcare are more frequent than is known, and may be a normal part of everyday life on busy wards and in General Practitioner (GP) surgeries. Many may simply go unnoticed because their outcomes are inconsequential or unknown. It might also be that near misses exemplify the ability of staff to avoid errors under pressure, their compensating actions constituting valid and creative responses to avoiding poor patient outcomes. An alternative view is that risks can be downgraded as a result of staff accepting everyday organizational defects as events that must be circumvented, the result being that their potential to inform patient safety is wasted (Reason, 2006). This issue is illustrated in Box 9.2, below.

The research findings summarized in Box 9.2 indicate that professionals in NHS organizations, as in many others, may practice forms of risk blind behaviour for a variety of reasons, including pressures on staff time and failures of leadership and management (Tucker and Edmondson, 2003; Vincent, 2006). When risk priorities are externally defined by outcome targets such as reducing waiting times, it is perhaps not surprising that 'quick fix' coping mechanisms can take precedence over proactive learning from errors. Beyond such considerations lie the tricky problems of definition which beset both those charged with analysing data derived from reports about them and those who provide the reports on the ground.

Box 9.2 Coping with organizational deficiencies (Tucker and Edmondson, 2003)

Observational research on 26 nurses working at nine hospitals found that they faced five patient safety critical problem areas on a daily basis. These were:

• Missing or incorrect information

• Missing or broken equipment

• Missing or incorrect supplies

• Waiting for equipment or professional to arrive

• Simultaneous demands on their time

The researchers discovered that on 93% of the observed occasions nurses solved problems on a short-term basis, generating 'quick fixes' in order to get on with the immediate task of caring for patients. On 43% of occasions, nurses sought assistance from someone close to them in status rather than from a more senior member of staff. The majority of nurses who participated in the study felt that they were expected to work through such daily problems on their own unless beyond their capacity to solve. The emerging pattern was for defects to become built-in, and for learning to be lost to the organization about the risks it might be harbouring.

Defining safety risks: errors and outcomes

The NPSA, through its National Reporting and Learning System (NRLS), has responsibility for gathering and analysing information on patient safety incidents provided by the full spectrum of NHS organizations. The NRLS was in place by 2004 and initiated the first analysis of trends and patterns in 2005, mainly based at that point on data from acute hospitals. The system (under review at the time of writing) requires information on *the type of incident, who was involved, the outcome for patients and factors which have contributed to, or helped prevent the impact of the incident* (National Patient Safety Agency, 2005a). The NPSA was reviewed in 2006 and found wanting (see Chapter 8, Box 8.4), not least for failing to deliver *high quality, routinely available information on patterns, trends and underlying causes of harm to patients* (Department of Health, 2006c). An important task now facing the Agency is to refine and simplify its reporting system.

In line with governmental requirements to build a comprehensive evidence base, the NPSA has defined a patient safety incident as *any unintended or unexpected incident that could have or did lead to harm for one or more patients receiving NHS care* (National Patient Safety Agency, 2004). It therefore requires reports of all adverse events and near misses and depends upon the adequacy of reporting systems across NHS organizations for achieving consistent and comparable data. Aware of this challenge the NPSA has developed a range of support tools, including the 2004 *Seven Steps to Patient Safety Guide* (National Patient Safety Agency, 2004), an incident decision tree and training on root-cause analysis. However, one cynical view suggests that they may not be well known by health professionals or taken up in practice (Tingle, 2008).

The first findings from the NRLS indicated difficulties in securing full and consistent data and subsequent analyses show that this trend largely continued, although an upwards trend in reporting has more recently been reported (National Patient Safety Agency, 2009b). Analyses provided by the National Patient Observatory, an off-shoot of the NPSA established to develop appropriate data sets and to gather wider information about health care risks and report on findings, show varying rates of reporting amongst those organizations that provide information and little attention in reports to contributing factors (see National Patient Observatory reports, www.npsa.nhs.uk). The NPSA annual report for 2006/7 (National Patient Safety Agency, 2007) reflected as follows:

> One of our key tasks this year has been a review of our National Reporting and Learning System. Our aim is to develop a process by which we can better involve front-line staff and enable faster local incident reporting and quicker responses back to trusts. Initial research has shown that we have not adequately engaged with local healthcare organisations and not everyone understands the connection between local incident reporting and national incident analysis and response.

In order to understand what issues might arise in the apparently straightforward task of securing better systems for reporting patient safety incidents within a national framework, it is first important to explore more fully the conceptual problems involved in deciding what qualifies as a safety incident, and what errors should be counted. Further complications arising from the response of professionals to the reporting process will be subsequently considered.

Defining and counting errors: a matter of judgement

What counts as an error and where it has occurred in the system of care surrounding a patient case are matters of judgement in relation to both adverse outcomes and near misses. The subjective nature of the process is illustrated by the findings of a Canadian study (Forster *et al.*, 2004). Three reviewers examining the records of patients discharged from hospital varied in the overall proportions of patients they considered to have suffered an adverse event (23% vs. 27% vs. 21%), and agreed unanimously in only 15% of cases.

Difficulties in deciding what constitutes an adverse event arise not only from the detail and completeness of patient records, but also in relation to matters of judgement about whether a case record contains evidence of clinically significant errors. For example, where a patient develops a pneumothorax and dies after having a subclavian line erroneously inserted, it might be deemed that a prior critical illness rather than error is the cause of death (Forster, Shojania, and VanWalraven, 2005).

The tendency of researchers to measure the occurrence of adverse events by poor patient outcomes has been criticized for assuming a causal relationship between the two, and for failing to include an assessment of the degree to which an error contributes to a poor outcome. Reviewers participating in one rare study in which this issue was addressed estimated that only 6% of patients who died as a consequence of clinical error would have been expected to live more than a further 3-months (Forster *et al.*, 2005). However, it must be noted that even a short loss of life may be deeply regretted. Temporal accounting in risk management was discussed in Chapter 5. Furthermore, knowledge that death was caused by clinical error will itself cause distress irrespective of the amount of life lost. Arriving at assessments of the degree to which an error makes a difference to a poor patient outcome requires difficult judgements, which are particularly complex in areas of high risk treatment like heart surgery, as illustrated by the case of the UK John Radcliffe Heart Surgery Unit in Box 9.3.

Whatever the rights and wrongs of the John Radcliffe case, it shows that measuring the impact of an adverse event is not straightforward and that estimates of risks to patients from healthcare interventions are likely to vary considerably according to how adverse events are defined and their outcomes adjusted. Research conducted by *The Guardian* newspaper (16th Mar 2005) exposed fundamental problems of record keeping and risk assessment in individual hospital trusts, problems which made risk statistics from different sites non-comparable. In some cases, a risk adjustment had been made to the figures, whilst in others only raw scores were available. Surgeons disagreed profoundly about how to assess risk and present death rates. As a result of a formal complaint made to the Healthcare Commission by *The Guardian*, the Healthcare Commission and the Society for Cardiothoracic Surgery established a website in April 2006 that published risk-adjusted statistics for all but three hospital trusts in England (*The Guardian* newspaper, 22nd Apr 2006). Some patient groups were reported to be critical of the fact that performance data for individual surgeons was available in only 17 cardiac units,and viewed the unit by unit information as too vague to be of much use (IntheNews.co.uk, 27th Apr 2006). However, a year later, the number of participating units had risen to 29 out of 39 (News for Clinicians from the Healthcare Commission, July 2007).

Box 9.3 Mortality rates related to heart surgery at the Oxford John Radcliffe Surgery Unit 2001–04

In 2005, concerns were raised about the mortality rate of patients undergoing heart surgery at the Oxford John Radcliffe Hospital heart surgery unit. These concerns echo those arising from the earlier case of the Royal Bristol Infirmary, one highly significant outcome of which was that named surgeon data should be published for heart surgery. The mortality rates at the Oxford John Radcliffe heart surgery unit were estimated to be double the national average over three years from 2001–04. The trust defended the record of its heart surgeons by arguing that they did better than expected when the mortality rates were adjusted using a particular scale, the Euroscore scale. However, some experts argue that this scale is 10-years old and significantly better scores should be expected (*The Guardian* newspaper, 9th Dec 2005).

An enquiry by NHS watchdogs into heart surgery at the Radcliffe continued despite the eventual publication of risk-adjusted statistics which showed all units and surgeons to be within or better than the normal range. A local news story reported that surgeons welcomed the Healthcare Commission's decision to provide statistical information on its website but expressed anger at that 'spurious statistics' which had initially been used (*The Oxford Mail* newspaper, 28th May 2006).

The NPSA acknowledges that without an internationally agreed taxonomy for patient safety incidents and more consistency of reporting, comparisons of risk in different parts of the UK health service, and between it and health services abroad, are problematic (National Patient Safety Agency, 2005b). Statistics about errors and their consequences should be interpreted with caution. For professionals, the quality of data relating to their organization will impact upon any review of practice and actions taken. Improvements in this area are unlikely to be effected without cultural changes in NHS organizations which engender a positive learning climate in which incident reporting is encouraged, and there is no fear of blame (Reason, 2006; Alaszewski and Coxon, 2007). Problems involved in achieving a shift of such magnitude are explored below.

Risk and safety: problems in creating open reporting cultures

Clinical governance is officially viewed as a method for promoting reflective cultures in which learning rather than blame and defensiveness predominate

(Berta *et al.*, 2005). The vision is one where patients and staff will be enabled to report errors and guided by this information, local trusts and services will individually and collectively progress through continuous improvement. Organizational culture is difficult to define and assess (Davies, Nutley, and Mannion, 2000) but there is wide agreement that one of the key impediments to openness in NHS institutions is fear of professionally harmful consequences such as loss of job and/or reputation and litigation (Meurier, 2000). Reason (2006) has convincingly argued that the source of such fears lies in the myth that errors are the exception rather than the norm in health care and must therefore be the fault of flawed individuals:

> The notion of infallibility is deeply rooted in the healthcare culture. It leads to the belief that errors, particularly those that have bad outcomes, are manifestations of incompetence, carelessness or recklessness – for which naming and shaming are appropriate responses. This pernicious myth is perhaps the greatest obstacle to improving patient safety.

This deeply ingrained belief system is likely to lead anyone who makes a mistake to experience a range of conflicting emotions. As one medical practitioner (Wu, 2000) put it:

> Virtually every practitioner knows the sickening feeling of making a bad mistake. You feel singled out and exposed – seized by the instinct to see if anyone has noticed. You agonise about what to do, whether to tell anyone, what to say. Later, the event replays itself over and over in your mind. You question your competence but fear being discovered. You know you should confess, but dread the prospect of potential punishment and of the patient's anger.

Fear of blame can lead professionals to draw back from openness, and instead take refuge behind professional lines. For example, an in-depth study of a forensic mental health unit (Shaw *et al.*, 2007) revealed that frontline nurses felt unfairly targeted when patient incidents occurred. As a result, they became less open to new ideas of treatment and to participating confidently in multidisciplinary practice. An insightful observation was made by an occupational therapist about the barriers created by the impact of a blame culture:

> Talking about sort of blame thing, there is something I noticed in the low secure ward … It was sort of set up to be more multidisciplinary. But, since then, there has been a rain [cluster] of incidents [breaches of security]. And, because of the blame culture, the discipline [nursing] is increasingly retreating into themselves. You know, the nurses start being particularly blamed and … it's extremely difficult for them to sort of maintain their prominence and significance in the multidisciplinary team … There is a fear of actually engaging in the multidisciplinary process because that is a potential for further blame (Occupational therapist, multidisciplinary workshop.)

Box 9.4 Maladministration of drugs: Who is to blame? (Anderson and Webster, 2001)

A review of the nursing literature has identified a strong tendency for nurses to be blamed for maladministration of drugs, and to be the focus of attention in finding solutions. The question remains of how appropriate it is to target them as the main source of risk.

The authors of the review argue that repeated publication of the 'golden rules' to stop error year after year in the presence of continuing mistakes in administrating drugs can be seen as evidence of a dogmatic, individual-blaming approach that does not work. Procedures put in place for double checking and triple checking before drugs are administered may either be unrealistic or not wholly effective. Where checking systems exist, they may simply lead other busy nurses to confirm the first nurse's list without further verification, thus compounding an error if it has occurred. Such anti-dotes focus on the nurse as the cause of the problem and ignore the bigger picture. A well designed checking procedure may be an aid to safety, but other factors in the wider system of the drug administration process demand attention. Areas for improvement might include badly written prescriptions, cluttered ward trolleys, poor packaging, and labelling, and confusing colour coding.

As illustrated in Box 9.4, nurses are often targeted when errors occur, in this case in the maladministration of drugs.

The review summarized in Box 9.4 concluded that risk management is likely to be ineffective if blame is attributed to the last practitioner in the chain to interact with the patient. Approaches that refocus attention on the wider antecedents and underlying factors of patient incidents are thought to be more helpful because they avoid prior assumptions of personal blame, promote open reporting, and stimulate learning from mistakes (Vincent, 2006). The Being Open policy (National Patient Safety Agency, 2005b) requires all NHS organizations to establish an infrastructure which facilitate openness between staff and patients and carers following an incident. Research confirms that patients would welcome prompt disclosure and an apology when incidents occur but that doctors fear to use the word 'error' for fear of litigation (Carthey, 2005). Those who argue for a systems approach to tackling patient safety suggest that it is necessary to move away from the myth of errors being rare instances of personal failure, and towards an analysis of underlying conditions which build-in unsafe practices (Reason, 2001; Vincent, 2006).

The systems approach

The systems approach developed by Reason (2001), and adapted by Vincent (2006), draws upon models of accident causation in industry, the military, and transport, particularly aviation. It is based on the premise that errors are consequences rather than causes. The concept of 'root cause' used by the NPSA is somewhat misleading and oversimplified since it implies that there is a single or small number of causes waiting to be unearthed (Vincent, 2004). Systems analysis is seen by its advocates as more dynamic. It extends beyond the active failure of individuals at the sharp end, often those with most direct contact with the patient, to latent failures set in motion by organizational processes and management decisions.

Latent failures, often lying dormant for some time, can set the preparatory conditions for errors to occur, for example through insufficient or inappropriate staffing or inadequate equipment. They can build-in long-lasting design faults such as poor procedures. Central to the approach advocated by Reason is the notion that because all hazardous technologies possess defensive barriers, the real concern should be to understand how they have been breached (Reason, 2000). The case study outlined in Box 9.5, p. 207, illustrates how a systems approach may be applied to understand failure to prevent a patient suicide, for which a ward nurse was blamed. It demonstrates how this approach could help to identify a range of corrective actions, which, with the benefit of hindsight, might secure safer patient care.

Creating a secure reporting culture in which staff openly and willingly participate in such reflection may be harder to achieve than its advocates realize. Limitations are imposed by the amount and quality of information in any particular case and the ability to track latent failures retrospectively, but also crucially by the readiness of managers and all professional groups to become involved. Perhaps the main benefit of trying to do so is that it would encourage 'safety thinking' by making professionals more alert to potential system failures. Ironically, progress is most likely to be made in an organizational culture in which self-reflective learning is already valued, creating a 'chicken and egg' problem. Resistance might be expected to the systems approach as a result of ingrained cultures linked to hierarchical structures which damage trust and create fear of reprisals, as is discussed below.

Impediments to achieving open reporting cultures

It is important to acknowledge the deep-seated cultural and structural factors which impede the development of a safety ethos.

Box 9.5 A patient suicide attempt on an acute medical ward: Retrospective analysis of errors (Meurier, 2000)

A young woman with a history of attempted suicide sustained injuries by jumping out of a toilet window on a medical ward. The more senior F Grade nurse was not yet on duty when the patient was admitted. A student nurse was left to tend the patient who was nursed in a bed out of sight of the central nurse station. The student nurse reported the disturbed state of the patient several times during the night. She was dealing with another patient behind closed curtains when the incident occurred. The Grade F nurse dialled the normal bleep and there was a delay in getting a doctor to the scene.

Potential errors of clinical nursing (active failures):

- The F grade nurse should not have delegated the supervision of the patient to an inexperienced nurse and she should have informed the senior clinical nurse of staffing needs
- The patient's potential suicide intentions should have been considered at an early stage
- The student nurse should have told another nurse when she went behind the curtain to help
- The F grade did not ask a doctor to reassess the patient after her disturbed night, and should have bleeped the emergency medical team.

Potential contributory work conditions

- Inadequate staffing and inexperienced staff
- The F grade had a heavy case load of patients, and could not supervise the inexperienced staff properly
- The design of the ward had the built-in fault that not all patients could be seen, and the toilet windows should have been fixed.

Potential organizational factors (latent failures)

- Staff shortages
- Management perceived to be unsupportive
- Lack of communication between ward staff
- No guidelines on treating self-harm and suicidal patients
- Inadequate staff training.

One alternative or complementary approach which might be more successful locally is that of adopting a learning organizational approach. In terms of this approach, as much might be gleaned from the positive ways in which professionals rescue errors from occurring as would be learnt from listing the events that led to them. Titterton (2005) makes the same point in relation to social care. However, these cultural ideals conflict to some extent with the considerable emphasis now placed on the regulation of practice through the audit of risk management practices in NHS organizations.

Some optimistic policy analysts consider that governmental reforms, made in the interests of safer health services and the protection of the public have promoted a *learning culture based on a systems approach* (Allsop and Saks, 2002). But how far the NHS has actually moved in this direction is questionable. A recent evaluation of cancer care suggests that improvements have been made to the culture of professionals working effectively together across boundaries in order to achieve cancer care targets (National Chemotherapy Advisory Group, 2008). There are examples of local clinical governance initiatives which claim to be making progress in developing reflective cultures (see website www.cgsupport.nhs.uk) but as yet no strong independent body of evaluative research to support this case. However, some studies have suggested that even though some parts of it may be changing, the overall culture of the NHS has not yet undergone a radical shift. For example, a number of studies have indicated that multidisciplinary teamwork, central to improving the quality of healthcare, has proved difficult to achieve because it requires a change in the power dynamics of relationships in circumstances where *turf wars and demotivation of undervalued members of the team are commonplace* (Kavanagh and Cowan, 2004). Nurses in particular perceive medical dominance to be a key impediment to their participation in multidisciplinary teams and to openness in sharing information (Shaw *et al.*, 2007).

Impediments to developing open reporting cultures may also arise from the differing perceptions held by staff about the purpose and value of reporting errors, as was found in an exploratory study of a joint NHS and Social Care Trust providing services for vulnerable adults (Alaszewski and Coxon, 2007). The study was instigated by senior management and concentrated on areas of low error reporting in the trust. The research investigated the perceptions of managers and frontline staff about the reporting system, and found a considerable gap between them as is shown in Box 9.6, below. Alaszewski and Coxon (2007) found few signs of the necessary pre-conditions for a positive reporting culture.

Box 9.6 Perceptions of managers and professionals of error reporting in a joint NHS and Social Care Trust (Adapted from Alaszewski and Coxon, 2007)

Managers

- Saw adverse events as 'self-evident' and their definition unproblematic
- Regarded failure by staff to report as a skills deficit
- Endorsed official trust policy that error reporting was about organizational learning and development
- Thought the system had reasonable ownership amongst staff.

Professionals

- Regarded the definition of an adverse event as problematic and a matter of judgement, and considered the identification of near misses as even more difficult
- Tended to see the purpose in terms of their professional responsibility towards specific clients who might benefit
- Felt that the system was top-down and not widely owned
- Perceived error reporting to be about blame allocation and protecting the Trust from sanctions
- Thought avoidance occurred because of exposure of self and a wish not to expose a colleague
- Thought error reporting could be used to cover individuals' backs
- Felt that the system unfairly privileged doctors who did not comply and applied harsher sanctions to lower status professionals.

They defined these pre-conditions as: consensus over the framing of issues and the purpose of the reporting system; altruism in reporting where there is no reward and possibly something to lose; and a trust-based partnership replacing traditional command and control. For organizational learning to occur, a better balance between authority and trust appears to be required, entailing (Alaszewski and Coxon, 2007):

> recognising and acknowledging [that] the intuitive knowledge of professionals is central to demonstrating they are trusted and without such demonstration they will undermine systems that depend on their active cooperation.

As was concluded in the previous chapter, regulation seems to work best when it is grounded in the practice of collaborative, clinical teams in which tacit knowledge and relevant protocols come together in meaningful synergy.

Conclusion

Reflecting recently on the considerable changes which have taken place in the NHS since its inception in the UK in 1948, the Chief Medical Officer of Health (Donaldson, 2008) argued that *despite the stronger quality and patient safety ethos that exists in the NHS compared with its foundation*, patient safety remains one of the most challenging areas for development in 21st century healthcare. He identified a particular concern with *how actionable learning can reliably flow from adverse event or incident reporting*. The present chapter has considered some of the significant difficulties wrapped up in that aspiration. It has shown that adverse events and safety incidents are complex to define, and their causation and outcomes difficult to track and measure.

Definitional and measurement problems beset researchers who try to estimate the size and shape of the patient safety problem. In addition, the quality of the evidence base on which *actionable learning* might *reliably flow* depends upon reports provided by practitioners who may have good reasons to put up resistance. Their reasons for less than whole hearted collaboration include uncertainty about what counts as an incident, and what is worth reporting, and fear of repercussions for themselves, their profession, or their organization. Governmental policies on clinical governance advocate the empowerment of staff within blame free environments as integral to modern practice. However, the combined impact of audit and risk management contribute to the development of risk averse cultures in the social and health services, and promote defensiveness (Kemshall, 2006).

The recent requirement for the NPSA to refocus its efforts on data analysis and to simplify its reporting system (Kmietowicz, 2007) may have merit in producing better estimates of risk. They may help to identify patterns of risks which can be used to inform national patient safety solutions. Whether this latest change will bring about the safer healthcare which the Government, healthcare professionals and the public want, is not certain. Patient safety targets may yield improvements in selected areas but their wider impact in generating a patient-centred ethos of safety cannot be assumed. The focus on targets may reinforce the trend towards replacing patient need with risk avoidance as the philosophical basis of treatment (Alaszewski, 2002; Singh, 2003). Risk assessment and management appear to have become predominantly concerned with identifying potentially harmful outcomes and minimizing risk instead of generating more potentially empowering approaches. However, without some risk-taking, the service might have to sacrifice progress, and ultimately produce less effective patient interventions (Heyman and Huckle, 1993; Alaszewski, Harrison and Manthorpe, 1998; Titterton, 2005).

A difficult balancing act is required between achieving safer health care and accepting risks where there are good reasons for doing so. Cutting-edge treatments cannot be developed without empowering professionals to take risks. Attempting to avoid adverse events entirely is simply not an option with respect to outcome-contingent risks (Butler, 2008) such as supporting the aspirations of people living with disabilities. The official patient safety agenda has been mainly focused on minimizing outcome-independent risks which should as far as possible be avoided. Such a narrowing of scope may confer a reassuring sense of governmental certainty. But it directs attention away from the more problematic risk management issues which concern service users, carers, and practitioners.

Chapter 10

A case study of swine flu and concluding remarks

Bob Heyman, Monica Shaw, and
Andy Alaszewski

Introduction

The final chapter will review responses to the 2009 swine flu pandemic in order
to draw together themes discussed in the book, including: risk categorization;
the role of values in risk analysis; inductive probabilistic reasoning; the time-
framing of risks; risk management prescriptive encoding; the role of the media
in establishing public understandings about risks; and risk regulation in relation to the safety agenda. Following presentation of the case study, a concluding section will briefly look back at the main issues explored in the book.

The risk management of swine flu

At the time of writing, in mid 2009, the risks associated with swine flu were
receiving intense, if spasmodic, media attention. Readers who have travelled in
time since these words were produced will enjoy the benefit of hindsight, a
perspective not available to the writers. From this later vantage point, the
swine flu pandemic may well have turned out to have generated fairly normal
outcomes, including thousands of worldwide deaths, which are typical of most
outbreaks. In that case, swine flu, like SARS, would be quickly forgotten. It
would be reclassified retrospectively as a false alarm, but not necessarily as an
'unreal' risk. A typical outcome would not disconfirm the truth of the proposition that a larger number of deaths **might** have occurred. However, those
benefitting from hindsight may not retrospectively acknowledge this expired
alternative future, particularly in the febrile political atmosphere of countries
like the UK. On the other hand, it is just possible that the reader, looking
through the retroscope, might know that the swine flu virus mutated into a
virulent form and killed many millions worldwide, affecting younger people
particularly badly. Considering a risk which the reader will know more about

than the writers did at the time of writing may help to illustrate the temporal dynamics affecting the existence of any risk virtual object. This example will be used to draw together the main themes reviewed in the present book.

Some leading scholars, including Castel (1991), Foucault (1991), Beck (1992), and Luhmann (1993) have argued that risk thinking has transformed the organization of societal life. Others, particularly Douglas (1992), have maintained that the lens of risk merely offers old wine in new bottles, a modern label for the traditional notion of danger. In relation to swine flu, anyone comparing governmental, media and societal reactions to the present pandemic with responses to previous outbreaks might sense that a qualitative shift has occurred. But it is not so easy to pin down what, if anything, has changed. Social groups have responded preventatively to the danger of disease throughout historical time. For example, in the Middle Ages, various religiously mediated measures such as the activities of the flagellant movement and persecution of the Jews were adopted in an attempt to mitigate the plague by appeasing God. The flagellants travelled from town to town, encouraging residents to publicly whip themselves as a mark of repentance, thereby inadvertently spreading the epidemic. In addition, quarantine measures were adopted in some affected villages, a measure which makes sense from a current scientific perspective (Scott and Duncan, 2001).

It could be argued that the current response to a pandemic differs from previous efforts only with respect to the greater degree of control now available as a result of scientific and technological advances. The 2009 response to swine flu takes advantage of options which have only recently become available, albeit only in rich countries, particularly antivirals and rapid vaccine development. However, the most distinctive feature of the reaction to swine flu is societal rather than technological. As Power (2007) has pointed out, a new emphasis is now placed on the prospective organization of pre-emptive responses to risks. It is no longer sufficient to manage risks in a localized way. The current version of risk thinking requires anticipatory measures to have been systematically put in place across the entire society in order to anticipate the potentially unlimited class of what **might** happen[1]. Consideration of responses to the pandemic, and the controversy which they gave rise to, provides a useful vehicle for summarizing the issues explored in the present book.

In the UK, the Chief Medical Officer, Sir Liam Donaldson, succeeded in pushing forward the adoption of wide-reaching flu prevention measures, including the stockpiling of antivirals and the implementation of contingency

---

[1] Risk owners can never succeed more than partially in this enterprise because of its potentially infinite scope, as becomes clear in retrospect for adverse outcomes which were not anticipated.

plans designed to enable the National Health Service to cope with the demands of a mass pandemic. These measures had been initiated before swine flu became a global concern, in response to fear that a future pandemic might turn virulent. (However, the roll-out of a flu diagnosis and prescription call-centre and an Internet site were delayed through civil service in-fighting.) Inevitably, any risk management strategy generates new risks. Mass use of antiviral or antibiotic drugs will transmit resistance to the infective agent, both via the bodies of its consumers, and through widespread release into the environment in human waste (Singer *et al.*, 2007). Those who take antivirals, particularly children, face possible increased risk of gastrointestinal disturbance (Shun-Shin *et al.*, 2009), and neuropsychiatric disorders (Maxwell, 2007).

Some randomized controlled trials of the safety and efficacy of antivirals for children aged 12 and under, reviewed by Shun-Shin *et al.* (2009) have been undertaken. These authors concluded that antivirals confer little benefit on children with respect to seasonal flu, and that one form gave rise to an increased risk of nausea. However, in general, only sparse information appertaining specifically to vulnerable groups such as the young, the old, and pregnant women tends to become available. Pre-licensing drug trials often exclude these groups for safety reasons. Once a treatment has been approved, pharmaceutical companies are incentivized to talk up its benefits, to minimize safety issues, and to covertly influence research conclusions, whilst public interest bodies mostly cannot afford to run expensive trials.

Turning now to risk thinking, the collective, usually unreflective, act of conferring real status on a risk requires a complex combination of interpretive steps. These unspoken mental manoeuvres come to be largely taken for granted, whilst remaining constantly vulnerable to challenge. Thinking contingently, a person envisages two or more alternative outcome categories defined so that one and only one must occur. A presently uninfected individual might or might not die from swine flu during the current pandemic, for instance. When contingencies are viewed through the lens of risk, the observer sees at least one of the specified outcome categories as adverse, and believes that their occurrence in individual cases depends partly or wholly on chance. For example, those who wash their hands, keep away from crowds, and avoid becoming pregnant may reduce their probability of dying from swine flu, but cannot realistically rule this possibility out entirely. (If they could do so, then the risk in question would no longer exist as far as they were concerned.)

The imagined outcome categories marked out in a contingency must be simultaneously selected from the infinity of the possible, and, at the same time, recognized as entities, the topic considered in Chapter 2. Categorisation replaces the variety of the real world with simpler homogenous and distinctive packages. These symbolic representations are easily confused with the objects which they stand for. Inevitably, issues will arise about the integrity of the categories, the procedures used to assign individuals to categories, and classification in specific cases. Swine flu viruses vary genetically. They evolve constantly. At the time of writing, they were mostly being treated as homogenous, even though some variants might have been causing more harm than others. If swine flu becomes endemic, sub-strains may eventually be differentiated as has happened with HIV (Davis *et al.*, 2002). In August 2009, an argument erupted about whether seasonal and swine flu should be considered as a single disease entity. The UK Department of Health cast doubt on the relevance of research indicating that antivirals confer little clinical benefit on children exposed to seasonal influenza (Shun-Shin *et al.*, 2009) by arguing that *swine flu behaves differently to seasonal flu* (*The Guardian* newspaper, 11th Aug 2009).

As the social presence of swine flu became established, its status as a real risk was strengthened by some of the consolidation processes outlined in Chapter 2, and illustrated in Chapter 7 in relation to media representation. Swine flu acquired its own iconography, displayed in newspaper pictures of people in China, and then of Western pregnant women, wearing face masks. These images conveyed a sense of looming danger, reminding the public about the pandemic's global reach, and about its unusual propensity to strike at younger people. The risk started to become institutionally embedded, in the UK through the accelerated roll-out of the National Pandemic Flu Service. It became commercially entrenched as multinational pharmaceutical companies stood to make huge profits through rapidly delivering an approved vaccine and large quantities of antivirals. The swine flu risk began to be moralized as the public were enjoined to self-quarantine if they suspected that they might be infected, and to use free antivirals responsibly. Obesity was implicated as a risk factor (MacKenzie, 2009) in an article which advised readers to *fight the flab in order to fend off swine flu.*

Yet, the processes through which this particular risk was selected for a starring role from the infinite set of possible adversity remained mostly unexamined. Liam Donaldson largely succeeded with his campaign to proactively embed responses to flu pandemics in UK healthcare system planning. But he failed in his efforts to reduce risks associated with the marketing of alcohol, and of junk food to children, both serious threats to population health. These two risk-reducing initiatives challenged the financial interests of powerful commercial organizations, whilst the provision of antivirals and vaccines created new lucrative markets. Moreover, members of the public were mostly not prepared to pay more for their drink in order to induce a minority of excessive drinkers to consume less. A second critical issue discussed in Chapter 3, that of combining qualitatively distinctive values linked to multiple consequences of swine flu risk reduction strategies, will be raised below in relation to the encoding of risk knowledge.

As the pandemic travelled from its starting point in Mexico through the USA, and then on to Britain and other countries, attempts were made to assess the probability of death or serious complications from infection. At the time of writing, mass laboratory testing of representative samples of individuals drawn from general populations had not been carried out. In consequence, it was not possible to quantify the risk of an infected person dying because the number of mild cases could not be estimated. However, reasoning inductively from deaths in the USA in relation to known population sizes, relative risks were calculated (MacKenzie, 2009), as discussed in Chapter 4. Obesity, pregnancy, hypertension, and diabetes were identified as risk factors which more or less doubled the very low chance of dying from the disease.

The following example illustrates one of the key issues reviewed in Chapter 4, the potential for multiple probabilities of the same event to be computed from the same data. In July 2009, the UK National Childbirth Trust advised women to consider delaying pregnancy until the pandemic had passed. Professor Steve Field, the chair of the Royal College of General Practitioners dismissed this advice as *scaremongering* (*The Observer* newspaper, 19th Jul 2009). He argued that women should not delay pregnancy because only a small proportion of deaths would occur in this group:

> At its worse, the pandemic will hit 30% of the population, of whom 0.3% might die. The number of pregnant women in this group is tiny.

Although statistically valid in its own terms, this prediction does not provide sensible grounds on which a woman could base her decision as to whether or not to postpone pregnancy. The quotation discusses the chance of a person who has died from swine flu having been a pregnant woman. Because only a small proportion of the population fall into this category, only a tiny percentage of swine flu deaths will be of pregnant women under any foreseeable circumstances. (Similarly, as noted in Chapter 4, most babies with Down's syndrome are born to younger women simply because they make up a large proportion of pregnant women.) However, this way of looking at chance is irrelevant to the circumstances of women thinking about becoming pregnant during the period of the swine flu pandemic. They do not need to know the probability of a person who died from swine flu having been pregnant, but that of a woman who is pregnant dying from swine flu! In the language of Bayesian reasoning, discussed in Chapter 4, the chance of A (pregnancy) **given** B (death from swine flu) should not be confused with that of B (death from swine flu) **given** A (pregnancy).

The statistic discussed by Professor Field is relevant from a public health perspective, but not from that of personal decision-making.

Understanding the quantification of health risks requires the synthesis of medical, statistical, and social scientific perspectives. Those trained primarily in one of these disciplines cannot avoid straying outside their specialist competencies when they make pronouncements about risks. Furthermore, the advice quoted above considers only the impact of swine flu on pregnant women. It spectacularly ignores risks to the child, including possible transmission of virulent influenza across the placenta, infection of the newborn child, side-effects of maternal antivirals on the fetus, and disruption to labour resulting from fever (Rasmussen *et al.*, 2009). The exclusion of impact on the child illustrates the powerful influence of risk selection which foregrounds some contingencies whilst ignoring others. Women taking these considerations into account might still decide not to delay pregnancy until the end of the swine flu epidemic. Nevertheless, this example illustrates the difficulty inherent in trying to facilitate informed decision-making about risks.

Responses to swine flu were suffused with the temporal considerations reviewed in Chapter 5. Those who criticized the measures taken in the UK to deal with the first wave of the pandemic as disproportionate cited the very low death rates observed in Mexico and the USA. Because this wave had struck these countries earlier, it was possible to use observation of its outcomes inductively to estimate what might happen elsewhere, assuming, as always with this form of probabilistic reasoning, that the past provides a good guide to the future. Some doctors concluded from current evidence that the UK (and other) governments were engaging in *over-kill*, a perhaps unfortunate term used by Dr Judith Hooper who was in charge of combating the disease in the Kirklees district of SW Yorkshire (*Huddersfield Daily Express* newspaper, 5th Aug 2009).

The UK authorities adopted a longer temporal perspective, recommended by Liam Donaldson, which emphasized the risk of the virus becoming more virulent during subsequent waves of the pandemic[2]. Some people inferred that becoming infected during the first low virulence phase, and thereby acquiring resistance, might protect them from this greater risk, but this tactic received no official endorsement! Another important temporal consideration concerned the time needed to develop and deliver a vaccine once the virus strain had been identified. Pharmaceutical companies raced to bestow immunity on that proportion of the world's population who could afford to pay for protection

---

[2] A survey published in the New Scientist, 15th Aug 2009, uncovered a similar division of opinion. Half of 60 experts from around the world had taken special measures for their own family, stockpiling antivirals, antibiotics and even food, whilst the remainder considered such measures unnecessary.

before the virus could mutate into a more dangerous form. Time could have been bought by severely restricting travel into and out of infected areas as soon as the pandemic was identified. This drastic course of action was not seriously contemplated. It was not underpinned by an organized international *modus operandi*, and also confronted the 'virtualness' of risk.

When swine flu first affected Mexico, no cases had been identified elsewhere. In the absence of draconian travel restrictions, a quickly spreading global pandemic became inevitable. However, at the time when international spread could have been significantly slowed, this risk existed only as a future problem, not as a material event. Furthermore, the most serious health concern was that the virus would mutate into a virulent form. This outcome was not expected. It merely could not be ruled out. The authorities would have had to impose harsh limitations on Mexican travel, with devastating economic consequences, in order to prevent a possibility. On the other hand, on a longer time frame covering many pandemics, if virus spread is not slowed until a vaccine can be developed, an eventual deadly, unstoppable pandemic, as happened in 1918, is almost inevitable.

In relation to the 2009 flu pandemic, Professor Field, quoted above, also raised the question of temporal boundary-setting for the risks facing pregnant mothers (*The Observer* newspaper, 19th Jul 2009):

> Anyway, pandemics last for two to three years. It is very difficult for people to plan around that, even if they want to.

Decision-making about postponing pregnancy must take into account the length of the time delay which would be required in order to reduce risk to an acceptable level. By extending the anticipated timescale for the epidemic further than have other authoritative commentators, Professor Field bolstered his case for women not to delay pregnancy in response to the swine flu risk. If, for example, the anticipated vaccination programme became effective by spring 2010, then much shorter, and therefore less onerous, pregnancy postponements could be contemplated. The social science of risk should not attempt to adjudicate on such matters of epidemiological science. But it can expose the assumptions upon which particular risk analyses are based, draw attention to alternative constructions, and unpick the reasoning on which they are based. As illustrated above, the rationality of more or less drastic risk-reducing policies depends upon the time frame within which they are viewed.

A cultural shift towards a model of partnership between health professionals and patients, discussed in Chapter 6, has been apparent in organized responses to the swine flu pandemic. The attempt to provide risk-reducing measures for the entire UK population had to rely on self-diagnosis because the health service could not have coped with the magnitude of transactions which would otherwise have been required. Individuals who thought that they might have been infected with swine flu were able to telephone a call-centre, or to follow an online algorithm which took them through a flow chart starting with the presence of fever. Depending upon the outcome, patients were advised to seek medical help, do nothing, or obtain a free supply of antivirals. In the latter case, they were expected to behave responsibly by sending a 'flu friend' to obtain the drug, rather than expose others to risk by collecting it themselves. However, official faith in the public only went so far. Flu friends had to provide proof of identity. Those given antivirals were warned that a second dose would only be offered after medical inquiry, and the possibility of unpleasant side-effects was emphasized. Thus, the authorities attempted to restrain proactive stockpilers and the worried well.

Knowledge encoding, discussed in Chapter 6, plays a crucial intermediary role in the new partnership model of health professional-patient relationships. Behind these efforts to encode best practice lies the assumption that patients will want to follow officially recommended courses. As argued in Chapter 6, this assumption falls foul of patient preferences. For example, some members of the public will obtain antivirals regardless of the recommendations structured into advice algorithms. More fundamentally, responses to the pandemic demonstrate the inherent limitations of encoded prescriptions. These general formulae cannot accommodate the multiple, qualitatively different consequences of any risk management strategy. All the measures proposed to delay the progress of the pandemic until a vaccine could be delivered faced this problem. Closing schools would have held back the education of children, for instance. Attempts to encode recommendations tended to be shot down, as illustrated above with respect to the merits of delaying pregnancy. At the same time, complaints were made that official advice remained unclear. The Royal College of General Practitioners commented that *family doctors also noted that conflicting advice was being provided by different agencies* (*The Guardian* newspaper, 16th Jul 2009), a complaint which they subsequently withdrew. The authorities, who had taken risk ownership of the pandemic upon themselves, thus found themselves trapped in a double bind. Any recommendations they made about how to balance safety with autonomy could be challenged, but they could also be criticized for lack of clarity. Ironically, a campaign promoting better hand hygiene might have yielded greater health gains at smaller cost, whilst avoiding the new risks arising from mass use of antivirals. But this measure was largely overlooked, perhaps because the state had embraced ownership of the swine flu risk.

A debate about gap year students travelling to developing countries in order to do voluntary work well illustrates this dynamic (*The Guardian* newspaper,

11th Aug 2009). Professor Dingwall, a member of the Department of Health Committee on Ethical Aspects of Pandemic Influenza, argued that gap year students should cancel visits to remote areas on the grounds that they would collectively spread the pandemic to populations with little resistance to the disease, and few resources for coping with its effects. However, the companies which organized these trips rejected the above advice, claiming that the benefits of the services provided by volunteers outweighed the risks. The article also noted that students who cancelled on account of the risk they might pose to others, as against actually being ill, would not receive travel insurance compensation for aborted travel. The non-governmental agency Voluntary Services Overseas (VSO) proposed that recipient countries should decide whether to curtail volunteer visits. This example illustrates how difficult it is to encode recommendations for dealing with any health risk.

The media, new and old, played a powerful role in establishing the reality of the swine flu risk, the topic of Chapter 7. Inevitably, the slant taken by different newspapers reflected diverse values and priorities. The right wing, europhobic *Daily Mail* newspaper, for instance, offered front page stories about the alleged demands of publicly funded GPs for huge extra payments (22nd Jul 2009), and about infected British schoolchildren being unsympathetically treated in France (23rd Jul 2009). The headline for the latter read:

UNCLEAN!
French swine flu squad in white suits and masks swoop on terrified English children and send them home in a blacked-out coach

Concerns about media fuelled public panic overwhelming the health service had not materialized by the time of writing. On the whole, most people adopted a calm approach, perhaps because the virus causing the first wave of the pandemic has caused only a small number of deaths, whilst the risk of its mutation to a more dangerous form remained hypothetical. Over 300 000 people received free antivirals via the National Pandemic Flu Service during its first two weeks of operation from 23rd July 2009 (*The Observer* newspaper, 9th Aug 2009). Given the likely overall scale of UK infection, this statistic does not suggest mass panic by a large proportion of the worried well.

As argued in Chapter 7, little is known about the variable impact of media coverage on the attitudes and behaviour of those who are exposed to it. One of the authors heard anecdotal reports that participants at a music festival were snorting cocaine mixed with Tamiflu! Whether true or merely apocryphal, such accounts illustrate the gulfs which can develop between healthcare bureaucracies and social groups who utilize health services on their own terms. Acceptance of information presented in the media depends heavily on levels of trust which, in the UK at least, are generally low. In the case of antivirals, the press has seized upon divisions in expert opinion about their efficacy and potential side-effects. Exposure to these differences may have stimulated a particularly high degree of public mistrust about swine flu risk management policy. Moreover, the authorities and the public are faced by a second double bind at the heart of risk thinking. (The first, a conflict between encoding clear advice and taking into account the variable social contexts for risk management was discussed above.) The organization of responses to a risk defines it as potentially alarm-worthy, even if the decision to select it for preventative effort was taken for merely precautionary reasons. As illustrated in Chapter 8, responses to selected risks may then overwhelm the healthcare systems which invoked them as a cause for concern. These responses generate new risks such as those of side-effects and medical errors. Regulation of health risks then becomes embroiled in escalatory processes which place additional demands on healthcare agencies and professionals.

The National Flu Pandemic Service, and the systematically proactive response to risk which it represents, have not, at the time of writing, existed long enough for more than glimmers of the regulatory and safety issues reviewed in Chapters 8 and 9 to begin to manifest themselves. Regulatory agencies like the Healthcare Commission, now the Care Quality Commission, have focussed on protecting patients from health service shortcomings and errors, rather than on broader questions about the net benefits of risk management policies. Safety issues in this narrow sense emerged remarkably quickly. Newspaper stories about non-medical call-centre staff placing lives at risk by misdiagnosing infections such as meningitis, measles, and pneumonia, as swine flu soon began to appear. A survey of general practitioners showed that nearly 90% were worried about this problem (*The GP* newspaper, 5th Aug 2009).

Concluding remarks

This book offers an introduction to the analysis of health risk thinking. The authors have attempted to unpack this framework from a social science perspective, treating the metaphorical lens of risk as a device for dealing with uncertainty. When science precludes precise prediction in conditions of real world complexity, i.e. almost always, risk thinking provides a potentially useful way of gaining some leverage over the future. But a price has to be paid in terms of accepting simplifications which generate systematic distortions.

Risk thinking can usefully be envisaged as one form of a more universal human tendency to view events as contingent. An observer considers that one out of two or more alternative outcomes might occur, develops expectations about their occurrence, and considers whether to act in ways which might affect what actually happens. Activity initiated in response to a visualized contingency has the potential to change the material world, perhaps making an unwanted outcome less likely or, even bringing it about unintentionally through self-proving prophecy. The sense that alternative future (or past but unknown) outcomes **might** happen originates in the human mind. These multiple possibilities do not exist in nature independently of its intelligent observers. Thinking contingently makes it possible to observe outcomes 'not happening', a form of detection which can only be undertaken in relation to expectations. Risk thinking differs from older ways of viewing events as contingent primarily in its emphasis on the projection of uncertainty onto the world as chance. It is marked by a preoccupation with adversity and the adoption of arbitrary but variable time horizons. As well as enabling the non-occurence of risked events to the 'seen',[3] the metaphorical lens of risks permits its user to conclude that a person, group, or other entity 'might be at risk'. The identification of such double uncertainties requires elegant mental gymnastics, accomplished routinely by those who have learnt to view the world in this way.

The encoding of prescriptive risk management recipes in clinical guidelines, assessment 'tools', care planning protocols, and health promotion advice shifts concern towards procedures, and away from the hypothetical nature of risk virtual objects. Encoding directs organized attention towards a small subset of that which might happen. Encoded recommendations cannot take into account personal preferences, or the contexts in which health risks are managed. In complex 21st century societies, the new and traditional media play a crucial role in communicating beliefs about, and attitudes towards, selected contingencies which trouble their members. Although research has delivered much analysis of media content, little is known about the diverse ways in which the public actually interpret and use information in an age of widespread mistrust. As health services have become more and more elaborate, governments have developed regulatory systems designed to protect the public from risks arising from healthcare itself. However, their adoption raises further difficult risk management issues: about data quality; about how regulatory agencies with limited resources can identify potential service failures proactively in large-scale healthcare systems; and about who should guard the guards, i.e. ensure that regulatory agencies themselves function as intended.

---

[3] Familiarity tends to blunt a sense of wonder about this remarkable human ability to detect what has not, but might have, happened.

Health services have become organized around selected risks such as patients with mental health problems committing suicide, women giving birth to babies with Down's syndrome, or virulent influenza epidemics causing massive numbers of deaths. Risk management now looms large, but not always welcome, in the work of all health professionals. The public can hardly avoid exposure to screening and other risk-oriented systems, but their concerns will not necessarily match up with those which motivate service provision. For better and for worse, heathcare will continue to be viewed through the lens of risk for some time to come. The social sciences can contribute to the practical business of clinical risk management by drawing attention to the unspoken assumptions and concealed emotions without which risks could not exist.

References

All web addresses were live as of 31st July 2009.

Adam B. (1990) *Time and Social Theory*. Cambridge: Polity Press.

Adams J. (1995) *Risk*. London: UCL Press.

Adil M. (2008) Risk-based regulatory system and its effective use in health and social care. *The Journal of the Royal Society for the Promotion of Health*, **128**, 196–201.

Alaszewski A. (2006) Health and Risk. In: P. Taylor-Gooby and J. Zinn (Eds.) *Risk in Social Science: Nursing, Risk, and Decision-Making*. Oxford: Oxford University Press.

Alaszewski A. (2005) Risk communication: Identifying the importance of social context. *Health, Risk, and Society*, **7**, 101–105.

Alaszewski A. (2002) The impact of the Bristol Royal Infirmary disaster and inquiry on public services in the UK. *Journal of Interprofessional Care*, **16**, 371–378.

Alaszewski A., Alaszewski H., Ayer S., and Manthorpe J. (2000) *Managing Risk in Community Practice*. Edinburgh: Ballière Tindall.

Alaszewski A., Alaszewski H., and Potter J. (2006) Risk, uncertainty and life-threatening trauma: Analysing stroke survivors' accounts of life after stroke. *Forum Qualitative Sozialforschung/Forum: Qualitative Social Research* [On-line Journal], 7, Art. 18. Available at: http://www.qualitative-research.net/fqs-texte/1-06/06-1-18-e.htm

Alaszewski A. and Coxon K. (2007) Restructuring health care: Developing systems to identify risk and prevent harm. In I. Wilkinson and A. Petersen (Eds.) *Health, Risk and Vulnerability*. London: Routledge.

Alaszewski A., Harrison L., and Manthorpe J. (1998) *Risk, Health and Welfare*. Buckingham: Open University Press.

Alfirevic Z., Sundberg K., and Brigham, S. (2003) Amniocentesis and chorionic villus sampling for prenatal diagnosis. *Cochrane Database of Systematic Reviews*, **3**, CD003252.

Allan S. (2002) *Media, Risk and Science*. Buckingham: Open University Press.

Allsop J. (2002) Regulation and the medical profession. In J. Allsop and M. Saks (Eds.) *Regulating the Health Professions*. London: Sage.

Allsop J. and Saks M. (2002) The Regulation of Health Professions. In J. Allsop and M. Saks (Eds.) *Regulating the Health Professions*. London: Sage.

Amoah A.G.B. (2003) Hypertension In Ghana: A cross-sectional community prevalence study in Greater Accra. *Ethnicity & Disease*, **13**, 310–315.

Anderson A. (2006) Media and risk. In G. Mythen and S. Walklate (Eds.) *Beyond the Risk Society: Critical Reflections on Risk and Human Security*. Maidenhead: Open University Press.

Anderson D.J. and Webster C.S. (2001) A systems approach to the reduction of medication error on the hospital ward. *Journal of Advanced Nursing*, **35**, 34–41.

Aref-Adib M. Freeman-Wang T., and Ataullah I. (2008) The older obstetric patient. *Obstetrics, Gynaecology & Reproductive Medicine*, **18**, 43–48.

Atherton E. and French S. (1999) Valuing the future: A MADA example involving nuclear waste storage. *Journal of Multi-Criteria Decision Analysis*, **7**, 304–321.

Baggott R. (2002) Regulatory Politics, health professionals, and the public interest. In J. Allsop and M. Saks (Eds.) *Regulating the Health Professions*. Bristol: The Policy Press.

Baker G.R., Norton P.G., Flintoft V., *et al.* (2004) The Canadian adverse events study: The incidence of adverse events among hospital patients in Canada. *Canadian Medical Association Journal*, **170**, 1678–1686.

Bakir V. and Barlow D.M. (2007) The Age of Suspicion. In V. Bakir and D.M. Barlow (Eds.) *Communication in the Age of Suspicion: Trust and the Media*. Basingstoke: Palgrave Macmillan.

Barbalet J. (2005) *Trust and Uncertainty: The Emotional Basis of Rationality*. Paper presented at SCARR Network Trust Conference, London.

Bassett K.L., Lyer N., and Kazanjian A. (2000) Defensive medicine during hospital obstetrical care: A by-product of the technological age. *Social Science & Medicine*, **51**, 523–537.

Beach R. and Reading R. (2005) The importance of acknowledging clinical uncertainty in the diagnosis of epilepsy and non-epileptic events. *Archives of Disease in Childhood*, **90**, 1219–1222.

Beck U. (1998) Politics of risk society. In: J. Franklin (Ed.) *The Politics of Risk Society*. Cambridge: Polity Press.

Beck U. (1992) *Risk Society: Towards a New Modernity*. London: Sage.

Beck-Gernsheim E. (1996) Life as a planning project: In S. Lash, B. Szerszynski and B. Wynne (Eds.) *Risk, Environment & Modernity: Towards a New Ecology*. London: Sage.

Bedford T. and Cooke R. (2001) *Probabilistic Risk Analysis: Foundations and Methods*. Cambridge: Cambridge University Press.

Bernstein P.L. (1996) *Against the Gods: The Remarkable Story of Risk*. New York: John Wiley & Sons.

Berta W., Teare G., Gilbart E., *et al.* (2005) The contingencies of organizational learning in long-term care: Factors that affect innovation adoption. *Health Care Management Review*, **30**, 282–292.

Bevan, G. (2009) Have targets done more harm than good in the English NHS? No. *British Medical Journal*, **338**, a3129.

Bevan G. and Hood C. (2006) Have targets improved performance in the English NHS?. *British Medical Journal*, **332**, 419–422.

Bilson A. and White S. (2004) Limits of governance: Interrogating the tacit dimensions of clinical practice. In A. Gray and S. Harrison (Eds.) *Governing Medicine: Theory and Practice*. Maidenhead: Open University Press.

Bindra R., Heath V., Liao A., Spencer K., and Nicolaides K.H. (2002) One-stop clinic for assessment of risk for trisomy 21 at 11–14 weeks: A prospective study of 15030 pregnancies. *Ultrasound in Obstetrics & Gynecology*, **3**, 219–225.

Binedell J., Soldan J.R., and Harper P.S. (1998) Predictive testing for Huntington's disease: II. Qualitative findings from a study of uptake in South Wales. *Clinical Genetics*, **54**, 489–496.

Blaxter M. and Paterson E. (1982) *Mothers and Daughters: A Three-Generational Study of Health Attitudes and Behaviour*. London: Heinemann Educational.

Boily M.C., Baggaley R.F., Wang L., *et al.* (2009) Heterosexual risk of HIV-1 infection per sexual act: Systematic review and meta-analysis of observational studies. *The Lancet Infectious Diseases*, **9**, 118–129.

Boon S.D. and Holmes J.G. (1991) The dynamics of interpersonal trust: Resolving uncertainty in the face of risk. In R.A. Hinde and J. Groebel (Eds.) *Cooperation and Prosocial Behaviour.* Cambridge: Cambridge University Press.

Booth C.M., Dranitsaris G., Corona Gainford M. *et al.* (2007) External influences and priority-setting for anti-cancer agents: A case study of media coverage in adjuvant trastuzumab for breast cancer. *BMC Cancer*, 7:110. Available at http://ukpmc.ac.uk/picrender.cgi?artid=1038965&blobtype=pdf

Bowker G.C. and Star S.L. (2000) *Sorting Things Out: Classification and its Consequences.* Cambridge, Massachusetts: MIT Press.

Bowles C.J.A., Leicester R., Romaya C., Swarbrick E., Williams C.B., and Epstein O. (2004) A prospective study of colonoscopy practice in the UK today: Are we adequately prepared for national colorectal cancer screening tomorrow? *Gut*, 53, 277–283.

Boyle S. (2005) What foundation trusts mean for the NHS. *LSE Health and Social Care Discussion Paper Number 18.* London: London School of Economics.

Bradfield A. and Wells G.L. (2005) Not the same old hindsight bias: Outcome information distorts a broad range of retrospective judgements. *Memory and Cognition*, 33, 120–130.

Bradshaw P.L. and Bradshaw B. (2004) *Health Policy for Health Care Professionals.* London: Sage.

Brawley O.W. (2001) Prostate cancer screening: A note of caution. In: I.M. Thompson, M.I. Resnick, and E.A. Klein (Eds.) *Prostate Cancer Screening.* New Jersey: Humana Press.

Breakwell G.M. (2007) *The Psychology of Risk.* Cambridge: Cambridge University Press.

Brettell K.M. (1988) Patterns of evaluations of accents among health visitor students. *Journal of Advanced Nursing*, 13, 33–43.

Bristow J. (2006) Herceptin The politics of 'Her Too': The ongoing controversy over the breast cancer 'wonder drug' has become divisive and dangerous. Spiked [On-line Forum]. Available at http://www.spiked-online.com/index.php/site/article/95/

Brook J.S., Whiteman M., and Brook D.W. (1999) Transmission of risk factors across three generations. *Psychological Reports*, 85, 227–241.

Butler V. (2008) *"First Do No Harm" – The Challenge of Safe, Reliable & Effective Service: A Discussion Paper in Support of Strategy and Intention in Regard to Clinical Safety.* Unpublished report: Leeds Partnerships NHS Foundation Trust.

Caballero B. (2007) The global epidemic of obesity: An overview. *Epidemiologic Reviews*, 29, 1–5.

Califano J.A. (2007) Should drugs be decriminalised? No. *British Medical Journal*, 335, 967.

Calnan M. and Rowe R. (2005) *Trust Relations in the NHS.* SCARR Network Trust Conference, London, 2005.

Care Quality Commission (2009) *Review of the Involvement and Action taken by Health Bodies in Relation to the Case of Baby P.* Available at http://www.cqc.org.uk/_db/_documents/Baby_Peter_report_FINAL_12_May_09_(2).pdf

Carr-Hill R.A. (1989) Assumptions of the QALY Procedure. *Social Science & Medicine*, 29, 469–477.

Carrier N., LaPlante J., and Bruneau J. (2005) Exploring the contingent reality of biomedicine: Injecting drug-users, hepatitis C virus and risk. *Health, Risk & Society*, 7, 123–140.

Carthey J. (2005) Being open with patients and their carers following patient safety incidents. *Clinical Governance Bulletin*, **5**, 5.

Cassels A. (2007) The media-medicine mix: Quality concerns in medical reporting. Open Medicine [On-line Journal], **1**, 52–54. Available at http://www.openmedicine.ca/article/viewArticle/54/4

Castel R. (1991) From dangerousness to risk. In: G. Burchell, C. Gordon, and P. Miller (Eds.) *The Foucault Effect: Studies in Governmental Rationality*. London: Harvester Wheatsheaf.

Casti J.L. (1992) *Searching for Certainty: What Science Can Know About the Future*. London: Scribners.

Chan Y.M., Leung T.N., Leung T.Y., Yuen Fung T.Y., Chan L.W., and Lau T.K. (2006) The utility assessment of Chinese pregnant women towards the birth of a baby with Down syndrome compared to a procedure-related miscarriage. *Prenatal Diagnosis*, **26**, 819–824.

Cicourel A.V. (1974) *Cognitive Sociology*. New York: Free Press.

Coghlan A. (2009) Which way to turn on cannabis law? *New Scientist*, 3/01/09.

Collins J. (2007) Risk, advice and trust: How service journalism fails its audience. In: V. Bakir and D.M. Barlow (Eds.) *Communication in the Age of Suspicion: Trust and the Media*. Basingstoke: Palgrave Macmillan.

Commission for Healthcare Audit and Inspection (2009) *The Healthcare Commission 2004-2009: Regulating Healthcare – Experience and Lessons*. London: Healthcare Commission. http://www.nhshistory.net/Healthcare_Commission_legacy_report.pdf

Commission for Healthcare Audit and Inspection (2008) *The Safer Management of Controlled Drugs: Annual Report, 2007*. London: Commission for Healthcare Audit and Inspection. Available at http://collections.europarchive.org/tna/20081211191026/http://healthcarecommission.org.uk/_db/_documents/The_safer_management_of_controlled_drugs_Annual_report_2007.pdf

Council for Healthcare Regulatory Excellence (2008) *Special Report to the Minister of State for Health Services on the Nursing and Midwifery Council*. Available at http://www.chre.org.uk/_img/pics/library/080611NMCFinalReport_1.pdf

Courpassen D. (2000) Managerial strategies of domination: Power in soft bureaucracies. *Organisational Studies*, **21**, 141–161.

Cranor C.F. (2007) Towards a non-consequentialist approach to acceptable risks. In: T. Lewens (Ed.) (2007) *Risk: Philosophical Perspectives*. London: Routledge.

Crawford R. (2004) Risk ritual and the management of control and anxiety in medical culture, health. *Health: An Interdisciplinary Journal for the Social Study of Illness and Medicine*, **8**, 505–528.

Crinson I., Shaw A., Durrant R., de Lusignan S., and Williams B. (2007) Coronary heart disease and the management of risk. *Health, Risk & Society*, **9**, 359–374.

Critcher C. (2007) 'Trust me, I'm a doctor': MMR and the politics of suspicion. In: V. Bakir and D.M. Barlow (Eds.) *Communication in the Age of Suspicion: Trust and the Media*. Basingstoke: Palgrave Macmillan.

Davies H., Nutley S., and Mannion R. (2000) Organisational culture and quality of health care. *Quality Health Care*, **9**, 111–119.

Davin S. (2003) Healthy viewing: The reception of medical narratives. *Sociology of Health and Illness*, **25**, 662–679.

Davis M.D.M., Hart G., Imrie J., Davidson O., Williams I., and Stephenson J. (2002) 'HIV is HIV to me': The meanings of treatment, viral load and reinfection for gay men living with HIV. *Health, Risk & Society*, **4**, 31–43.

Davison C., Davey-Smith G., and Frankel S. (1992) Lay epidemiology and the prevention paradox: The implications of candidacy for health education. *Sociology of Health and Illness*, **13**, 1–19.

Davison K. (1996) The quality of dietary information on the world wide web. *Journal of the Canadian Diet Association*, **57**, 137–141.

d'Cruse S., Walklate S., Pegg S., and Croall H. (2006) *Murder: Social and Historical Approaches to Understanding Murder and Murderers*. Devon: Willan Publishing.

Dean M. (1999) *Governmentality, Power and Rule in Modern Society*. New York: Sage.

Dearnaley D.P., Huddart R.A., and Horwich A. (2001) Managing testicular cancer. *British Medical Journal*, **322**, 1583–1588.

Degeling P.J., Maxwell S., Ledema R., and Hunter D.J. (2004) Making clinical governance work. *British Medical Journal*, **329**, 679–681.

Dentzer S. (2000) Media mistakes in coverage of the Institute of Medicine's error report. *American College of Physician: Effective Clinical Practice Policy Matters* [On-line Journal]. Available at http://www.acponline.org/clinical_information/journals_publications/ecp/novdec00/dentzer.htm

Department of Health (2009) *Background to Foundation Trusts*. Available at http://www.dh.gov.uk/en/Healthcare/Secondarycare/NHSfoundationtrust/DH_4062852

Department of Health (2008) *High Quality Care For All: NHS Next Stage Review Final Report*. London: Department of Health. Available at http://www.dh.gov.uk/en/publicationsandstatistics/publications/publicationspolicyandguidance/DH_085825

Department of Health (2007a) *Best Practice Guidance. Specification for Adult Medium-Secure Services*. London: Department of Health. Available at http://www.dh.gov.uk/en/Publicationsandstatistics/Publications/PublicationsPolicyAndGuidance/DH_078744

Department of Health (2007b) *Trust, Assurance and Safety: The Regulation of Health Professionals*. London: Department of Health. Available at http://www.dh.gov.uk/en/Publicationsandstatistics/Publications/PublicationsPolicyAndGuidance/DH_065946

Department of Health (2007c) *The Future Regulation of Health and Adult Social Care In England: Response to Consultation*. London: Department of Health. Available at http://www.dh.gov.uk/en/Consultations/Closedconsultations/DH_063286

Department of Health (2006a) *Best Research for Best Health: A New National Health Research Strategy*. London: Department of Health. Available at http://www.dh.gov.uk/en/Publicationsandstatistics/Publications/PublicationsPolicyAndGuidance/DH_4127127

Department of Health (2006b) *Choice Matters*. London: Department of Health. Available at http://www.dh.gov.uk/en/Publicationsandstatistics/Publications/PublicationsPolicyAndGuidance/DH_4135541

Department of Health (2006c) *Safety First: A Report for Patients, Clinicians and Healthcare Managers*. London: Department of Health. Available at http://www.dh.gov.uk/en/Publicationsandstatistics/Publications/PublicationsPolicyAndGuidance/DH_062848

Department of Health (2005) *A Short Guide to NHS Foundation Trusts*. London: Department of Health. Available at http://www.dh.gov.uk/en/Publicationsandstatistics/Publications/PublicationsPolicyAndGuidance/DH_4126013

Department of Health (2001) *Building a Safer NHS for Patients: Implementing an Organization with a Memory*. London: Department of Health. Available at http://www.dh.gov.uk/en/Publicationsandstatistics/Publications/PublicationsPolicyAndGuidance/DH_4006525

Department of Health (2000a) *The NHS Plan*. London: Department of Health. Available at http://www.dh.gov.uk/en/Publicationsandstatistics/Publications/PublicationsPolicyAndGuidance/DH_4002960

Department of Health (2000b) *National Service Framework for Coronary Heart Disease*. London: Department of Health. Available at http://www.dh.gov.uk/en/Publicationsandstatistics/Lettersandcirculars/Healthservicecirculars/DH_4094275

Department of Health (2000c) *An Organization with a Memory: Report of an Expert Group on Learning from Adverse Events in the NHS*. London: Department of Health. Available at http://www.dh.gov.uk/en/Publicationsandstatistics/Lettersandcirculars/Dearcolleagueletters/DH_4005264

Department of Health (1999) *Saving Lives: Our Healthier Nation*. London: The Stationery Office. Available at http://www.dh.gov.uk/en/Publicationsandstatistics/Publications/PublicationsPolicyAndGuidance/DH_4008701

Department of Health (1998) A *First Class Service. Quality in the New NHS*. London: Department of Health. Available at http://www.dh.gov.uk/en/Publicationsandstatistics/Publications/PublicationsPolicyAndGuidance/DH_4006902

Department of Health (1997) *The New NHS, Modern Dependable*. London: Department of Health. Available at http://www.dh.gov.uk/en/Publicationsandstatistics/Publications/PublicationsPolicyAndGuidance/DH_4008869

Department of Health, Chief Medical Officer (2006) *The Expert Patients Programme*. London: Department of Health. Available at http://www.dh.gov.uk/en/Aboutus/MinistersandDepartmentLeaders/ChiefMedicalOfficer/ProgressOnPolicy/ProgressBrowsableDocument/DH_4102757

de Vries E.N., Ramrattan M.A., Smorenburg S.M., Gouma D.J., and Boermeester M.A. (2008) The incidence and nature of in-hospital adverse events: A systematic review. *Quality and Safety in Health Care*, **17**, 216–223.

Dixon L., Browne K., and Hamilton-Giachritsis C. (2004) Risk factors of parents abused as children: A mediational analysis of the intergenerational continuity of child maltreatment (Part I). *Journal of Child Psychology and Psychiatry*, **46**, 47–57.

Doll R. and Hill A.B. (1950) Smoking and carcinoma of the lung. *British Medical Journal*, **2**, 739–748.

Donaldson L. (2008) The challenge of quality and safety. *Journal of the Royal Society of Medicine*, **101**, 338–341.

Dormandy E., Michie S., Hooper R., and Marteau T.M. (2005) Low uptake of prenatal screening for Down syndrome in minority ethnic groups and socially deprived groups: A reflection of women's attitudes or a failure to facilitate informed choices? *International Journal of Epidemiology*, **34**, 346–352.

Douglas, M. (1992) *Risk and Blame: Essays in Cultural Theory*. London: Routledge.

Douglas M. (1990) Risk as a forensic resource. *Daedalus*, **119**, 1–16.

Douglas M. (1966) *Purity and Danger: An Analysis of Concepts of Pollution and Taboo*. London: Routledge.

Dragan I., O'Connor D., Green S., and Wilt T. (2007) Screening for prostate cancer: A Cochrane systematic review. *Cancer Causes and Control*, **18**, 279–285.

Driedger S.M., Jardine C.G., Boyd, A.D., and Mistry B. (2009) Do the first 10 days equal a year? Comparing two Canadian public health risk events using the national media. *Health, Risk & Society*, **11**, 39–53.

Durfee J.L. (2006) 'Social change' and status quo framing effects on risk perception: An exploratory experiment. *Science Communication*, 27, 459–495.

Edney D.R. (2004) Mass media and mental illness: A literature review prepared for the Canadian Mental Health Association. Available at www.ontatior.cmha.ca

Eldridge J. and Reilly J. (2003) Risk and relativity: BSE and the British media. In: N. Pidgeon, R.E. Kasperson and P. Slovic (Eds.) *The Social Amplification of Risk*. Cambridge: Cambridge University Press.

Elliott J. (2005) The Nurse who inspired Live Aid. BBC News. Available at news.bbc.co.uk/2/hi/health/4640255.stm

Ericson R.V. and Doyle A. (Eds.)(2003) *Risk and Morality*. Toronto: University of Toronto Press.

Esquivel A., Meric-Bernstam F., and Bernstam E.V. (2006) Accuracy and self correction of information received from an internet breast cancer list: Content analysis of posting content. *British Medical Journal*, **332**, 939–944.

Evans-Pritchard E. E. (1976) *Witchcraft, Oracle and Magic among the Azande*. Oxford: Clarendon Press.

Eysenbach G. (2000) Consumer health informatics. *British Medical Journal*, **320**, 1713–1716.

Eysenbach G. and Kohler C. (2002) How do consumers search for and appraise health information on the world wide web? Qualitative studies using focus groups, usability tests and in-depth Interviews. *British Medical Journal*, **324**, 573–577.

Fenge L.A. (2006) Community care: Assessing needs, risks and rights. In: K. Brown *Vulnerable Adults and Community Care*. Exeter: Learning Matters.

Ferguson I. and Lavalette M.(2009) Social work after "Baby P". *International Socialism* [On-line Journal], 122. Available at www.isj.org.uk/index.php4?id=534&issue=122

Flynn R. (2004) 'Soft bureaucracy', governmentality and clinical governance: Theoretical approaches to emergent policy. In: A. Gray and S. Harrison (Eds.) *Governing Medicine: Theory and Practice*. Maidenhead: Open University Press.

Flynn R. (2002) Clinical governance and governmentality. *Health, Risk & Society*, **4**, 155–173.

Fogel J., Albert S.M., Schnabel F., Ditkoff A., and Neugut A.I. (2002) Use of the internet by women with breast cancer. *Journal of Medical Internet Research*, **4**, e9. Available at http://www.pubmedcentral.nih.gov/articlerender.fcgi?artid=1761930

Forster A.J., Clark H.D., Menard A. *et al.* (2004) Adverse events among medical patients following discharge from hospital. *Canadian Medical Association Journal*, **170**, 345–349.

Forster A.J., Shojania K.G., and van Walraven C. (2005) Commentary: Improving patient safety: Moving beyond the 'hype' of medical errors. *Canadian Medical Association Journal*, **173**, 893–894.

Foucault M. (1991) Governmentality. In: G. Burchell, C. Gordon, and P. Miller (Eds.) *The Foucault Effect*. London: Harvester Wheatsheaf.

Franklin B. (Ed.)(1999) *Social Policy, the Media and Misrepresentation*. London: Routledge.

French S. (Ed.) (1994) *On Equal Terms: Working with Disabled People*. Oxford: Butterworth-Heinemann.

Fries J.F. and Krishnan E. (2004) Equipoise, design bias, and randomized controlled trials: The elusive ethics of new drug development. *Arthritis Research & Therapy*, **6**, R250–R255.

Gagliardi A. and Jahad A. (2002) Examination of instruments used to rate quality of health information on the Internet: Chronicle of a voyage with an unclear destination. *British Medical Journal*, **324**, 569–573.

Galtier-Dereure F., Boegner C., and Bringer J. (2000) Obesity and pregnancy: complications and cost. *American Journal of Clinical Nutrition*, **71**, 1242S–1248S.

Garland D. (2003) The rise of risk. In: R.V. Ericson and A. Doyle (Eds.) *Risk and Morality*. Toronto: University of Toronto Press.

Gauntlett D. (2005) *Moving Experiences, 2nd edition: Media effects and Beyond*. Eastleigh: John Libbey.

Gawande A. (2008) Check lists are critical to improving patient safety: [Online Interview]. Available at www.getbetterhealth.com

General Medical Council (2001) *Good Medical Practice* 3rd edition. London: General Medical Council.

Giddens A. (1998) Risk society: The context of British politics. In: J. Franklin (Ed.) *The Politics of Risk Society*. Cambridge: Polity Press.

Giddens A. (1991a) *Modernity and Self-Identity: Self and Politics in the Late Modern Age*. Cambridge: Polity Press.

Giddens A. (1991b) *The Consequences of Modernity*. Cambridge: Polity Press.

Gigerenzer G. (2002) *Reckoning with Risk: Learning to Live with Uncertainty*. London: Penguin.

Gigerenzer G., Todd P.M., and the ABC Research Group. (1999) *Simple Heuristics that Make us Smart*. Oxford: Oxford University Press.

Gil K.M., Mishel M.H., Belyea M. *et al.* (2004) Triggers of uncertainty about recurrence and long-term treatment side-effects in older African American and Caucasian breast cancer survivors. *Oncology Nursing Forum*, **31**, 633–639.

Gillet J. (2003) Media activism and Internet use by people with HIV/AIDS. *Sociology of Health and Illness*, **25**, 608–624.

Godfrey K.M., Lillycrop K.A., Burdge G.C., Gluckman P.D., and Hanson M.A. (2007) Epigenetic mechanisms and the mismatch concept of the developmental origins of health and disease. *Pediatric Research*, **61**, 5R–10R.

Godin P. (Ed.) (2006) *Risk and Nursing Practice*. Basingstoke: Palgrave Macmillan.

Goizet C., Lesca G., and Dürr A. (2002) Presymptomatic testing in Huntington's disease and autosomal dominant cerebellar ataxias. *Neurology*, **59**, 1330–1336.

Goldacre M., Evans J., and Lambert T. (2003) Media criticism of doctors: Review of UK junior doctors' concerns raised in surveys. *British Medical Journal*, **326**, 629–630.

Golsworthy R. (2004) Counselling psychology and psychiatric classification: Clash or co-existence? *Counselling Psychology Review*, **19**, 23–29.

Gordon S. (2005) *Nursing Against the Odds*. New York: Cornell University Press.

Graham J. and Coghill D. (2008) Adverse effects of pharmacotherapies for attention-deficit hyperactivity disorder: Epidemiology, prevention and management. *Drugs*, **22**, 213–237.

Gray A. and Harrison S. (Eds.) (2004) *Governing Medicine: Theory and Practice.* Maidenhead: Open University Press.

Gronberg H., Damber L., and Damber J. (1998) Total food consumption and body mass index in relation to prostate cancer risk: A case-control study in Sweden with prospectively collected exposure data. *The Journal of Urology*, **155**, 969–974.

Gross S. (2009) What do I have in mind doc? Experts at work in a brain cancer clinic. *Social Science and Medicine*, in press.

Gubb J. (2009) Have targets done more harm than good in the English NHS? Yes. *British Medical Journal*, **338**, a3130.

Gwyn R. (2002) *Communicating Health and Illness.* London: Sage.

Hackett M.C. (1999) Implementing clinical governance in trusts. *International Journal of Health Care Quality Assurance*, **12**, 210–13.

Hacking I. (2003) Risk and dirt. In: R.V. Ericson and A. Doyle (Eds.) *Risk and Morality.* Toronto: University of Toronto Press.

Hacking I. (1975) *The Emergence of Probability: A Philosophical Study of Early Ideas About Probability, Induction and Statistical Inference.* Cambridge: Cambridge University Press.

Hájek A. (2008) A philosopher's guide to probability. In: G. Bammer and M. Smithson, *Uncertainty and Risk: Multidisciplinary Perspectives.* London: Earthscan.

Hallam J. (2000) *Nursing the Image: Media, Culture and Professional Identity.* London: Routledge.

Hann A. and Peckham S. (2010) Cholesterol screening and the gold effect. *Risk, Health & Society*.

Hansson S.O. (2005) Seven myths of risk. *Risk Management: An International Journal*, **7**, 7–17.

Harrabin R., Coote A., and Allen J. (2003) *Health in the News: Risk, Reporting and Media Influence.* London: The Kings Fund.

Harris R. and Lohr K. (2002) Screening for prostate cancer: An update of the evidence for the U.S. Preventive Services Task Force. *Annals of Internal Medicine*, **137**, 917–929.

Harrison S. (2004) Governing medicine: Governance, science and practice. In: A. Gray and S. Harrison (Eds.) *Governing Medicine: Theory and Practice.* Maidenhead: Open University Press.

Hart A., Henwood F., and Wyatt S. (2004) The role of the internet in patient-practitioner relationships: Findings from a qualitative research study. *Journal of Medical Research*, **6**, 1–11.

Hatch D. (2006) Professional self-regulation, revalidation, poor performance and clinical governance. In: M. Lugon and J. Secker-Walker (Eds.) *Clinical Governance in a Changing NHS.* London: Royal Society of Medicine Press.

Haynes A.B., Weiser T.G., Berry W.R. *et al.* (2009) A surgical safety checklist to reduce morbidity and mortality in a global population. *New England Journal of Medicine*, **360**, 491–499.

Hayward R.A., Hofer T.P., and Vijan S. (2006) Narrative review: Lack of evidence for recommended low-density lipoprotein treatment targets: A solvable problem. *Annals of Internal Medicine*, **145**, 520–530.

Hazani E. and Shasha S.M. (2008) Effects of the holocaust on the physical health of the offspring of survivors. *Israeli Medical Association Journal*, **10**, 251–255.

Hazell L. and Shakir S. (2006) Under-reporting of adverse drug reactions: A systematic review. *Drug Safety*, **29**, 385–396.

Healthcare Commission (2009) *Investigation into Mid Staffordshire NHS Foundation Trust.* Care Quality Commission. Available at http://www.rcn.org.uk/__data/assets/pdf_file/0004/234976/Healthcare_Commission_report.pdf

Health Protection Agency (2008) *HIV in the United Kingdom: 2008 report.* Available at www.hpa.org.uk/web/HPAweb&HPAwebStandard/HPAweb_C/1227515299695.

Henriksen M. and Heyman B. (1998) Being old and pregnant. In: B. Heyman (Ed.) *Risk, Health and Health Care: A Qualitative Approach.* London: Edward Arnold.

Heyman B. (Ed.)(1998) *Risk, Health and Health Care: A Qualitative Approach.* London: Edward Arnold.

Heyman B. and Henriksen M. (2001) *Risk, Age and Pregnancy. A Case Study of Prenatal Genetic Screening and Testing.* Basingstoke: Palgrave.

Heyman B., Henriksen M., and Maughan K. (1998) Probabilities and health risks: A qualitative approach. *Social Science & Medicine*, **9**, 1295–1306.

Heyman B. and Huckle S. (1993) Not worth the risk? Attitudes of adults with learning difficulties and their informal and formal carers to the hazards of everyday life. *Social Science & Medicine*, **12**, 1557–1564.

Heyman B., Huckle S., and Handyside E.C. (1998) Freedom of the locality for people with learning difficulties. In: B. Heyman (Ed.) *Risk, Health and Health Care: A Qualitative Approach.* London: Edward Arnold.

Heyman B., Lewando Hundt G., Sandall J. *et al.* (2006) On being at higher risk: A qualitative study of prenatal screening for chromosomal anomalies. *Social Science & Medicine*, **62**, 2360–72.

Heyman B., Shaw M.P., Davies, J.P., Godin, P.M., and Reynolds R. (2004) Forensic mental health services as a health risk escalator: A case study of ideals and practice. In: B. Heyman (Ed.) *Special edition on Risk and Mental Health. Health, Risk & Society*, **6**, 307–325.

Hilgartner S. (1992) The social construction of risk objects: Or how to pry open networks of risk. In: J. Short and I. Clarke (Eds.) *Organizations, Uncertainties and Risks.* Boulder, CO: Westview Press.

HM Government (2008) *Government Response to the Recommendations Made by the Advisory Council on the Misuse of Drugs in its Report Cannabis: Classification and Public Health.* London: HM Government. Available at http://drugs.homeoffice.gov.uk/publication-search/cannabis/acmd-cannabisreclassification?view=Binary

Hodgetts D. and Chamberlin K. (2006) Developing a critical media research agenda for health psychology. *Journal of Health Psychology*, **11**, 317–327.

Holick M.F. (2004) Sunlight and vitamin D for bone health and prevention of autoimmune diseases, cancers, and cardiovascular disease. *The American Journal of Clinical Nutrition*, **80**, 1678S–1688S.

Holland, J. C. (2002) History of psycho-oncology: Overcoming attitudinal and conceptual barriers. *Psychosomatic Medicine*, **64**, 206–221.

Holzl E. and Kirchler E. (2005) Causal attribution and hindsight bias for economic developments. *Journal of Applied Psychology*, **90**, 167–174.

Home Office/Department of Health and Social Security (1975) *Report of the Committee on Mentally Disordered Offenders*. London: HMSO.

Hood C., Rothstein H., and Baldwin R. (2004) *The Government of Risk: Understanding Risk Regulation Regimes*. Oxford: Oxford University Press.

Hopkins, P.N. and Williams, R.R. (1981) A survey of 246 suggested coronary risk factors. *Atherosclerosis*, **40**, 1–52.

Horlick-Jones T. (2004) Experts in risk? Do they exist?. *Health Risk & Society*, **6**, 107–114.

Huang Z., Hankinson S.E., Colditz G.A. *et al.* (1997) Dual effects of weight and weight gain on breast cancer risk. *Journal of the American Medical Association*, **278**, 1407–1411.

Hughes E., Kitzinger J., and Murdock G. (2006) The media and risk. In: P. Taylor-Gooby and J. Zinn. (Eds.) *Risk in Social Science*. Oxford: Oxford University Press.

Human Genome Project Information (n.d.) *Genome Project 5-Year Research Goals, 1998–2003*. Available at http://www.ornl.gov/sci/techresources/Human_Genome/hg5yp/goal.shtml

Hunt A. (2003) Risk and moralization in everyday life. In: R.V. Ericson and A. Doyle (Eds.) *Risk and Morality*. Toronto: University of Toronto Press.

Hutter B.M. (2006) Risk, regulation, and management. In: P. Taylor-Gooby and J. Zinn (Eds.) *Risk In Social Science*. Oxford: Oxford University Press.

Hutter B.M. (2005) The attractions of risk-based regulation: Accounting for the emergence of risk ideas in regulation. *CARR Discussion paper*. Centre for Analysis of Risk and Regulation at the London School of Economics and Political Science, **33**. Available at http://www.lse.ac.uk/collections/CARR/pdf/DPs/Disspaper33.pdf

Ilkka, N. (2002) *Critical Social Realism*. Oxford: Oxford University Press.

Impicciatore P., Pandolfini C., Casella N., and Bonati M. (1997) Reliability of health information for the public on the world wide web: Systematic survey of advice on managing fever in children at home. *British Medical Journal*, **314**, 1875–1879.

Janssen I., Katzmarzyk P.T., and Ross R. (2004) Waist circumference and not body mass index explains obesity related health risk. *American Journal of Clinical Nutrition*, **79**, 379–384.

Japp K.P. and Kusche I. (2008) Systems theory and risk. In: J.O. Zinn (Ed.) *Social Theories of Risk and Uncertainty*. Oxford: Blackwell.

Jefferson T., Di Pietrantonj C., Debalini M.G., Rivetti A. and Demichell, V. (2009) Relation of study quality, concordance, take home message, funding, and impact in studies of influenza vaccines: Systematic review. *British Medical Journal*, **338**, b354. Available at http://www.pubmedcentral.nih.gov/articlerender.fcgi?artid=2643439

Johanson R., Newburn M., and Macfarlane A. (2002) Has the medicalisation of childbirth gone too far? *British Medical Journal*, **324**, 892–895.

Jung R.T. (1997) Obesity as a disease. *British Medical Bulletin*, **53**, 307–321.

Kahneman D., Slovik P., and Tversky A.E. (Eds.) (1982) *Judgements under Uncertainty: Heuristics and Biases*. Cambridge: Cambridge University Press.

Kaminski J. (2003) The in/visibility of nurses in cyberspace *Canadian Nursing Informatics Journal*, **1**, 15–26.

Kasperson J.K., Kasperson R.E., Pidgeon N., and Slovik P. (2005) The social amplification of risk: Assessing 15 years of research and theory. In: J.K. Kasperson and R.E. Kasperson (Eds.) *The Social Contours of Risk: Publics, Risk Communication & the Social Amplification of Risk*. London: Earthscan.

Katz D. L. (2007) Meeting the menace of MRSA. *New York Times*. Available at www.davidkatzmd.com

Kavanagh S. and Cowan J. (2004) Reducing risk in healthcare teams: An overview. *Clinical Governance: An International Journal*, **9**, 200–204.

Kelly S. and McKenna H.P. (2004) Risks to mental health patients discharged into the community. *Health, Risk & Society*, **6**, 377–386.

Kemshall H. (2006) Social policy and risk. In: G. Mythen and S. Walkgate (Eds.) *Beyond the Risk Society: Critical Reflections on Risk and Human Security*. Maidenhead: Open University Press.

Klin A. and Lemish D. (2008) Mental disorders stigma in the media: Review of studies on production, content, and Influences. *Journal of Health Communication*, **13**, 434–449.

Kingham M. (1998) Risk imagery and the AIDS epidemic. In: B. Heyman (Ed.) *Risk, Health and Health Care: A Qualitative Approach*. London: Edward Arnold.

Kinloch-de Loës S. and Perneger T.V. (1997) Primary HIV infection: Follow-up of patients initially randomized to zidovudine or placebo. *Journal of Infection*, **35**, 111–116.

Kiortsis D., Filippatos T., Mikhailidis D., Elisaf M., and Liberopoulos E. (2007) Statin-associated adverse effects beyond muscle and liver toxicity. *Atherosclerosis*, **195**, 7–16.

Kitzinger J. (2000) Media templates: Media patterns of association and the (re)construction of meaning over time. *Media, Culture and Society*, **22**, 61–84.

Kitzinger J. (1999) Researching risk and the media. *Health, Risk & Society*, **1**, 55–69.

Kiviat N.B., Hawes S.E., and Feng Q. (2008) Screening for cervical cancer in the era of the HPV vaccine: The urgent need for both new screening guidelines and new biomarkers, *Journal of the National Cancer Institute*, **100**, 290–291.

Kmietowicz Z. (2007) Safety agency must simplify reporting of patient incidents. *British Medical Journal*, **334**, 12.

Knight F. (1921) *Risk, Uncertainty and Profit*. Boston: Houghton Mifflin.

Krimsky S. and Golding D. (Eds.) (1992) *Social Theories of Risk*. Westport CT: Praeger.

Laing R.D. (1959) *The Divided Self: An Existential Study in Sanity and Madness*. London: Tavistock.

Lakoff G. (1987) *Women, Fire and Dangerous Things: What Categories Reveal About the Mind*. Chicago: University of Chicago Press.

Lambert W.E., Frankle H., and Tucker G.R. (1966) Judging personality through speech: A French-Canadian example. *Journal of Communication*, **16**, 305–321.

Law J. (1996) Organisation and semiotics: Technology, agency and representation. In: R. Munro and J. Mauritsen (Eds.) *Accountability, Power and Ethos*. London: Chapman and Hall.

Leake C.D. (Ed.) (1927) *Percival's Medical Ethics*. Baltimore: Williams and Wilkins of Medicine.

Lee E.J. (2007) Infant feeding in risk society. *Health, Risk & Society*, **9**, 295–309.

Lewens T. (Ed.) (2007) *Risk: Philosophical Perspectives*. London: Routledge.

Lingard L., Espin S., Rubin B. *et al.* (2005) Getting teams to talk: Development and pilot implementation of a checklist to promote interprofessional communication in the OR. *Quality and Safety in Health Care*, **14**, 340–346.

Link B.C. and Phelan J. (2004) Social conditions as fundamental causes of disease. In: G. Scambler (Ed.) *Medical Sociology Volume 2 (Major Themes in Health and Social Welfare)*. London: Routledge.

Lippman A. (1999) Embodied knowledge and making sense of prenatal diagnosis. *Journal of Genetic Counselling*, **8**, 224–274.

Lloyd A.J. (2001) The extent of patients' understanding of the risk of treatments. *Quality in Health Care*, **10**, i14–i18.

Locker D. (2003) Living with chronic illness. In: G. Scambler (Ed.) *Sociology as Applied to Medicine*. Edinburgh: Saunders.

London Borough of Brent (1985) *A Child in Trust: The Report of the Panel of Inquiry into the Circumstances Surrounding the Death of Jasmine Beckford*. Wembley, Middlesex: London Borough of Brent.

Lord Laming (2009) *The Protection of Children in England: A Progress Report*. London: The Stationery Office. Available online at http://publications.everychildmatters.gov.uk/eOrderingDownload/HC-330.pdf

Lord Laming (2003) *The Victoria Climbié Inquiry: Report of an inquiry by Lord Laming*. London: The Stationery Office. Available online at http://www.victoria-climbie-inquiry.org.uk/finreport/finreport.htm

Luhmann N. (1993) *Risk: A Sociological Theory*. New Brunswick: Aldine Transaction.

Luke B. and Brown M.B. (2007) Elevated risks of pregnancy complications and adverse outcomes with increasing maternal age. *Human Reproduction*, **22**, 1264–1272.

Lupton D. and McLean J. (1998) Representing doctors: Discourses and images in the Australian press. *Social Science and Medicine*, **46**, 947–958.

Lyall J. (2006) The prognosis so far. In Cancer care in the UK: The social implications, Guardian Supplement, *The Guardian*, 8th Apr 2006, 1–2.

MacIntyre C.R., Goebel K., Brown G.V., Skull S., Starr M., and Fullinfaw R.O. (2003) A randomised controlled clinical trial of the efficacy of family-based direct observation of anti-tuberculosis treatment in an urban, developed country setting. *International Journal of Tuberculosis and Lung Disorders*, **7**, 848–854.

MacKenzie D. (2009) Fight the flab to fend off swine flu. *New Scientist*, **203**, 12.

Maher, D., Uplekar, M., Blanc, L., and Raviglione, M. (2003) Treatment of tuberculosis, *British Medical Journal*, **327**, 822–823.

Manning N. (2000) Psychiatric diagnosis under conditions of uncertainty: Personality disorder, science and professional legitimacy. *Sociology of Health & Illness*, **22**, 621–639.

Marinker M., Blenkinsopp, A., Bond, C. *et al.* (Eds.)(1997) *From Compliance to Concordance: Achieving Shared Goals in Medicines Taking*. London: Royal Pharmaceutical Society of Great Britain.

Marinker M., and Shaw J. (2003) Not to be taken as directed: Putting concordance for taking medicines into practice, *British Medical Journal*, **326**, 348–349.

Maxwell S.R.J. (2007) Tamiflu and neuropsychiatric disturbance in adolescents. *British Medical Journal*, **334**, 1232-1233.

McArthur D.L., Magana D., Peek-Asa C., and Kraus J.F. (2001) Local television news coverage of traumatic deaths and Injuries. *West Journal of Medicine*, **175**, 380–384.

McCormack J.P., Levine M., and Rangno R.E. (1997) Primary prevention of heart disease and stroke: A simplified approach to estimating risk of events and making drug treatment decisions. *Canadian Medical Association Journal*, **157**, 422–428.

McGarrigle C.A., Cliffe S., Copas A.J. *et al.* (2006) Estimating adult HIV prevalence in the UK in 2003: The direct method of estimation. *Sexually Transmitted Infections*, **82**, 78–86.

McGuigan J. (2006) Culture and risk. In: G. Mythen and S. Walklate (Eds.) *Beyond the Risk Society: Critical Reflections on Risk and Human Security.* Buckingham: Open University Press.

McGuire A., Henderson J., and Mooney G. (1988) *The Economics of Health Care: An Introductory Text.* London: Routledge.

McNeil B.J., Weichselbaum R., and Pauker S.G. (1978) Fallacy of the five-year survival in lung cancer. *New England Journal of Medicine,* **299,** 1397–1401.

Medicines Partnership (2006) *Connecting Prescribers,* Issue 4, available at http://www.npc. co.uk/med_partnership

Menzel P., Dolan P., Richardson J., and Olsen J.A. (2002) The role of adaptation to disability and disease in health state valuation: A preliminary normative analysis. *Social Science & Medicine,* **55,** 2149–2158.

Meurier C.E. (2000) Understanding the nature of errors in nursing: Using a model to analyze critical incident reports of errors which had resulted in an adverse or potentially adverse event. *Journal of Advanced Nursing,* **32,** 202–207.

Middleton D. and Curnock D. (1995) Talk of uncertainty: Doubt as an organisational resource for co-ordinating multi-disciplinary activity in neonatal intensive care. Paper presented at the ESRC *Risk in Organisational Settings Conference,* May 1995.

Miller J. (1978) *The Body in Question.* London: Jonathan Cape.

Mitchell T.R. and Kalb L.S. (1981) Effects of outcome knowledge and outcome valence on supervisors' evaluations. *Journal of Applied Psychology,* **66,** 604–612.

Montori V.M., Devereaux P.J., Adhikari N.K.J. *et al.* (2005) Randomized trials stopped early for benefit: A systematic review. *Journal of American Medical Association,* **294,** 2203–2209.

Moran M. (2007) T*he British Regulatory State: High Modernism and Hyper- Innovation.* Oxford: Oxford University Press.

Moran M. (2004) Governing doctors in the British regulatory state. In: A. Gray and S. Harrison (Eds.) *Governing Medicine: Theory and Practice.* Maidenhead: Open University Press

Moran M. (2003) *The British Regulatory State: High Modernism and Hyper-Inflation.* Oxford: Oxford University Press.

Morgan M. (2003) The doctor-patient relationship. In: G. Scambler (Ed.) *Sociology as Applied to Medicine.* Edinburgh: Saunders.

Morris G. (2006) *Mental Health Issues and the Media: An Introduction for Health Professionals.* Oxford: Routledge.

Moscovici S. (2000) *Social Representations: Explorations in Social Psychology.* Cambridge: Polity Press.

Mosholder A.D., Gelperin K., Hammad T.A., Phelan K., and Johann-Liang R. (2009) Hallucinations and other psychotic symptoms associated with the use of attention-deficit/hyperactivity disorder drugs in children. *Pediatrics,* **123,** 611–616.

Moynihan R., Doran E., and Henry D. (2008) Disease mongering is now part of the global health debate. *Public Library of Science Medicine* [On-line Journal], **5.** Available at www. plosmedicIne.org.

Mrowietz U., Elder J.T., and Barker J. (2006) The importance of disease associations and concomitant therapy for the long-term management of psoriasis patients. *Archives of Dermatological Research,* **298,** 309–319.

Murdock G., Petts J., and Horlick-Jones T. (2003) After amplification: Rethinking the role of the media in risk communication. In: N. Pidgeon, R.E. Kasperson, and P. Slovic (Eds.) *The Social Amplification of Risk*. Cambridge: Cambridge University Press.

Mythen G. and Walklate S. (Eds.) (2006) *Beyond the Risk Society: Critical Reflections on Risk in Human Society*. Maidenhead, UK: Open University Press.

National Chemotherapy Advisory Group (2008) *Chemotherapy Services in England: Ensuring Quality and Safety*. Available at www.b-s-h.org.uk/upload/20081119141254Chemotherapy report.pdf

National Institute for Health and Clinical Excellence (2009) *About NICE*. Available at www.nice.org.uk/aboutNICE

National Patient Safety Agency (2009a) *Never Events Framework 2009/10*. Available at www.npsa.nhs.uk/nrls/improvingpatientsafety/neverevents

National Patient Safety Agency (2009b) *The Organisation Patient Safety Incident Reports*. Available at www.npsa.nhs.uk/nrls/patient-safety-incident-data/organisation-reports/

National Patient Safety Agency (2007) The Year In Review: National Patient Safety Agency Summary Annual Report for 2006/07. Available at www.npsa.nhs.uk

National Patient Safety Agency (2005a) *Building a Memory: Preventing Harm, Reducing Risk and Improving Patient Safety*. Available at www.npsa.nhs.uk/EasySiteWeb/GatewayLink.aspx?alId=5532

National Patient Safety Agency (2005b) *Being Open When Patients are Harmed*. Available at www.npsa.nhs.uk/nrls/alerts-and-directives/notices/disclosure/

National Patient Safety Agency (2004) *Seven Steps to Patient Safety: An Overview Guide for NHS Staff*. Available at http://www.npsa.nhs.uk/nrls/improvingpatientsafety/patient-safety-tools-and-guidance/7steps/

National Patient Safety Agency (2001) *Doing Less Harm*. London: Stationery Office. Available at http://www.health.vic.gov.au/clinrisk/downloads/nhsrisk.pdf

Nelkin D. (1996) An uneasy relationship: the tensions between medicine and the media. *The Lancet*, **347**, 1600–1603.

Neville N. (1996) *The Decline of Deference: Canadian Value Change in Cross-Sectional Perspective*. Peterborough, Ontario, Canada: Bradview Press.

NHS Executive (1999) *Clinical Governance: Quality in the New NHS*. Health Service Circular, HSC 1999/065. Leeds: Department of Health.

NHS Litigation Authority (2009) *Risk Management Standards for Acute Trusts Primary Care Trusts and Independent Sector Providers of NHS Care 2009/10*. London: Stationery Office. Available at http://www.clingov.nscsha.nhs.uk/Default.aspx?aid=4502

Nord E. (2005) Concerns for the worse off: Fair innings versus severity. *Social Science & Medicine*, **60**, 257–263.

Nord E. (1999) *Cost–Value Analysis in Health Care: Making Sense out of QALYS*. Cambridge: Cambridge University Press.

Nriagu J.O. (1983) Saturnine gout among Roman aristocrats: Did lead poisoning contribute to the fall of the empire? *New England Journal of Medicine*, **308**, 660–663.

Nursing and Midwifery Council (2008) NMC *responds to CHRE's expanded performance review*. Available at www.nmc-uk.org/aArticle.aspx?ArticleID=3199

Nutt D., King L.A., Saulsbury W., and Blakemore C. (2007) Development of a rational scale to assess the harm of drugs of potential misuse. *The Lancet*, **369**, 1047–1053.

O'Hara L. and Gregg J. (2006) The war on obesity: A social determinant of health. *Health Promotion Journal of Australia*, **17**, 262–263.

O'Malley P. (2008) Governmentality and risk. In: J.O. Zinn (Ed.) *Social Theories of Risk and Uncertainty*. Oxford: Blackwell.

O' Neil O. (2004) Accountability, trust and informed consent in medical practice and research. *Clinical Medicine*, **4**, 269–276.

Ofsted (2008) *Haringey Children's Services Authority Area Joint Area Review*. London: Ofsted.

Olstead R. (2002) Contesting the text: Canadian media depictions of the conflation of mental illness and criminality. *Sociology of Health and Illness*, **24**, 621–643.

Ormerod L. P. (2005) Multidrug-resistant tuberculosis (MDR-TB): Epidemiology, prevention and treatment. *British Medical Bulletin*, **73–74**, 17–24.

Oulton K.L. and Heyman B. (2009) Devoted protection: How parents of children with severe learning disabilities manage risks. *Health, Risk and Society*, **11**, 313–319.

Paling J. (2006) *Helping Patients Understand Risks*. Gainesville, Florida: The Risk Communication Institute.

Papagrigoriadis S. and Heyman B. (2004) Patients' views on follow-up of colorectal cancer: Implications for risk communication and decision-making. *Postgraduate Medical Journal*, **79**, 403–407.

Parker G. and Hickie I. (2007) Is depression overdiagnosed?. *British Medical Journal*, **335**, 328–329.

Parsloe P. (1999) *Risk Assessment in Social Care and Social Work*. London: Jessica Kingsley.

Patient Opinion (2006) *Patient Opinion*. Available at http://www.patientopinion.org.uk.

Peacock L. (2009) Shoesmith adds sex discrimination to tribunal claims against Haringey. *Personnel Today*. Available at http://www.perosnneltoday.com

Petersen A. and Wilkinson I. (2008) *Health, Risk and Vulnerability*. London: Routledge.

Peterson M. (2007) On multi-attribute risk analysis. In: T. Lewens (Ed.) *Risk: Philosophical Perspectives*. Abingdon Oxford: Routledge.

Peto R. (1994) Smoking and death: The past 40 years and the next 40. *British Medical Journal*, **309**, 937–939.

Petts J., Horlick-Jones T., Murdock G., Hargreaves D., McLachlan S., and Lofstedt R. (2001) *Social Amplification of Risk: The Media and the Public: Contract Research Report 329*. Health and Safety Executive. Available at http://www.cert.bham.ac.uk/research/risk/HSEWorkshopReport.pdf

Phillips L.N., Bridgeman J., and Ferguson-Smith M.A. (2000) *The BSE Inquiry*. Available at http://www.bseinquiry.gov.uk/

Philo G. (1993) *Mass Media Representations of Mental Health: A Study of Media Content*. Glasgow: Glasgow University Media Group

Philo G. and Miller D. (2000) Cultural compliance and critical media studies. *Media Culture and Society*, **22**, 831–839.

Piaget J. (1965) *The Moral Judgement of the Child*. Cambridge: The Free Press.

Pidgeon N., Kasperson R., and Slovik P. (Eds.) (2003) *The Social Amplification of Risk*. Cambridge: Cambridge University Press.

Pidgeon N., Simmons P., and Henwood K. (2006) Risk, Environment and Technology. In: P. Taylor-Gooby and J. Zinn (Eds.) *Risk in Social Science*. Oxford: Oxford University Press.

Power M. (2007) *Organized Uncertainty: Designing a World of Risk Management.* Oxford: Oxford University Press.

Power M. (2005) Organizational responses to risk: The rise of the chief risk officer. In: B. Hutter and M. Power (Eds.) *Organisational Encounters with Risk.* Cambridge: Cambridge University Press.

Power M. (2004) *The Risk Management of Everything: Rethinking the Politics of Uncertainty.* London: Demos.

Price D. (2002) Legal aspects of the regulation of the health professions. In: J. M. J. Allsop and M. Saks (Eds.) *Regulating the Health Professions.* London: Sage.

Prior L., Wood F., Gray J., Pill R., and Hughes D. (2002) Making risk visible: The role of images in the assessment of (cancer) genetic risk. *Health, Risk & Society,* **4,** 241–258.

Procter S. (2002) Whose evidence? Agenda setting in multi-professional research: Observations from a case study. *Health, Risk & Society,* **4,** 45–59.

Rasmussen S.A., Jamieson D.J., MacFarlane K. *et al.* (2009) Pandemic influenza and pregnant women: Summary of a meeting of experts. *American Journal of Public Health,* **99.** Available at http://www.ajph.org/cgi/reprint/AJPH.2008.152900v2

Reason J. (2006) Resisting cultural change. In: M. Lugon and J. Secker-Walker (Eds.) *Clinical Governance in a Changing NHS.* London: Royal Society of Medicine Press.

Reason J. (2001) Understanding adverse events: Human factors. In: C. Vincent (Ed.) *Clinical Risk Management: Enhancing Patient Safety.* London: British Medical Association.

Reason J. (2000) Human error: Models and management. *British Medical Journal,* **320,** 768–770.

Redfern M., Keeling J., and Powell E. (2001) *The Royal Liverpool Children's Inquiry Report.* London: HMSO.

Redley M. (2007) Origins of the problem of trust: Propaganda during the First World War. In: V. Bakir and D.M. Barlow (Eds.) *Communication in the Age of Suspicion: Trust and the Media.* Basingstoke UK: Palgrave Macmillan.

Renn O. (2008) *Risk Governance: Coping with Uncertainty in a Complex World.* London: Earthscan.

Rescher N. (1983) *Risk: A Philosophical Introduction.* Washington: University Press of America.

Rexrode K.M., Hennekens C.H., Willett W.C. *et al.* (1997) A prospective study of body mass index, weight change, and risk of stroke in women. *Journal of the American Medical Association,* **277,** 1539–1545.

Richardson K.P. (2003) Health risks on the Internet: Establishing credibility on line. *Health, Risk & Society,* **5,** 171–184.

Roberts C.G.P., Guallar E., and Rodriguez A. (2007) Efficacy and safety of statin monotherapy in older adults: A meta-analysis. *The Journals of Gerontology Series A: Biological Sciences and Medical Sciences,* **62,** 879–887.

Robertson M. (2008) The loss of sadness: How psychiatry transformed normal sorrow into depressive disorder. *Acta Neuropsychiatrica,* **20,** 168–169.

Robinson J. and Bickley K. (2004) The role of the national confidential inquiry in relation to suicide prevention. In: D. Duffy and T. Ryan (Eds.) *New Approaches to Preventing Suicide.* London: Jessica Kingsley.

Rosa E.A. (2003) The logical structure of the social amplification of risk framework (SARF): Metatheoretical foundations and policy implications. In: N.F. Pidgeon, R.E. Kasperson, and P. Slovic (Eds.) *The Social Amplification of Risk*. Cambridge: Cambridge University Press.

Rose D. (1998a) Television, madness and community care. *Journal of Community and Applied Social Psychology*, **8**, 213–228.

Rose N. (1999) *Powers of Freedom: Reframing Political Thought*. Cambridge: Cambridge University Press.

Rose N. (1998b) Governing risky individuals: The role of psychiatry in new regimes of control. *Psychiatry, Psychology and Law*, **5**, 177–195.

Rosenhan D.L. (1973) On being sane in insane places. *Science*, **179**, 250–258.

Rothstein H., Huber M., and Gaskell G. (2006) A theory of risk colonisation: The spiralling regulatory logics of societal and institutional risk. *Economy and Society*, **35**, 91–112.

Ruston A. (2006) Interpreting and managing risk in a machine bureaucracy: Professional decision-making in NHS Direct. *Health, Risk, and Society*, **8**, 257–271.

Ruston A. and Clayton J. (2002) Coronary heart disease: Women's assessment of risk: A qualitative study. *Health, Risk & Society*, **4**, 125–137.

Ruston A., Clayton J., and Allen C. (2003) *Call Management and Delivery in NHS Direct: Explaining Variations in Practice*. University of Greenwich, London: Centre for Health Services Research.

Samanta A. (2006) Medical experts, the law and professional regulation. *Journal of the Royal Society of Medicine*, **99**, 217–218.

Sandman P.M. (1994) Mass media and environmental risk: Seven principles. *Risk: Health, Safety, and Environment*, **5**, 251–260.

Sassi F. (2006) Calculating QALYs, comparing QALY and DALY calculations. *Health Policy and Planning*, **21**, 402–408.

Savage J. (1987) *Nurses, Gender and Sexuality*. London: Heinemann.

Schmid G. (2006) Social risk management through transitional labour markets: Theory and practice related to European experiences. *Socio-Economic Review*, **4**, 1–33.

Schutz A. (1962) *Collected Papers Volume 1: The Problem of Social Reality*. The Hague: Martins Nijhoff.

Schwartz M.B., O'Neal Chambliss H., Brownell K.D., Blair S.N., and Billington C. (2003) Weight bias among health professionals specializing in obesity. *Obesity Research*, **11**, 1033–1039.

Scott S. and Duncan C.J. (2001) *Biology of Plagues: Evidence from Historical Populations*. Cambridge: Cambridge University Press.

Scottish Office (1997) *Designed to Care: Renewing the National Health Service in Scotland*. Available at http://www.archive.official-documents.co.uk/document/scotoff/nhscare/scotnhs.htm

Seale C. (2005) New directions for critical internet health studies: Representing cancer experience on the web. *Sociology of Health and Illness*, **27**, 515–540.

Seale C. (2003) Health and media: an overview. *Sociology of Health and Illness*, **25**, 513–531.

Seale C. (2002) *Media and Health*. London: Sage.

Shaw J.E., Zimmet P.Z., McCarty D., and de Courten M. (2000) Type 2 diabetes worldwide according to the new classification and criteria. *Diabetes Care*, **23**, Supplement 2: B5–10.

Shaw M., Heyman B., Reynolds L., Davies J., and Godin P. (2007) Multidisciplinary teamwork in a UK regional secure mental health unit: A matter for negotiation?. *Social Theory and Health*, **5**, 356–375.

Shelko K., Van Wart J., and Francis C. (2009) Social aspects of the food industry. In: C.J. Baldwin (Ed.) *Sustainability in the Food Industry*. Ames, Iowa: Wiley-Blackwell and the Institute of Food Technologists.

Shun-Shin M., Thompson, M., Heneghan C., Perera R., Harnden A.,and Mant D. (2009) Neuraminidase inhibitors for treatment and prophylaxis of influenza in children: Systematic review and meta-analysis of randomised controlled trials. *British Medical Journal*, **339**. Available at http://www.bmj.com/cgi/reprint/339/aug10_1/b3172

Singer E. and Endreny P.M. (1993) *Reporting on Risk: How the Media Portray Accidents, Diseases, Disasters, and other Hazards*. New York: Russell Sage.

Singh B. (2003) Why clinical governance is important: An approach to the resolution of managerial and professional conflict in mental health. *Australasian Psychiatry*, **11**, 412–417.

Skala J.A., and Freedland K.E. (2004) Postponing death: Death takes a raincheck. *Psychosomatic Medicine*, **66**, 382–386.

Skolbekken J. (1995) The risk epidemic in medical journals. *Social Science and Medicine*, **40**, 291–305.

Slovic P. (2000) *The Perception of Risk*. London: Earthscan.

Smalley S. (2008) Reframing ADHD in the genomic era. *Psychiatric Times*, **25**, 1st Jun 2008.

Smith D.E. (2005) *Institutional Ethnography: A Sociology for People*. Oxford: AltaMira Press.

Smith G. and Charlton R. (2000) New-variant Creutzfeldt-Jakob disease. *British Journal of General Practice*, **50**, 611–612.

Som C.V. (2005) Nothing seems to have changed, nothing seems to be changing and perhaps nothing will change in the NHS: Doctor's response to clinical governance. *International Journal of Public Sector Management*, **18**, 463–477.

Southgate L. and Dauphinee D. (1998) Maintaining standards in British and Canadian medicine: The developing role of the regulatory body. *British Medical Journal*, **316**, 697–700.

South West London Strategic Health Authority (2006) *The Independent Inquiry into the Care and Treatment of John Barrett*. London: South West London Strategic Health Authority.

Spencer K. (2001) Age-related detection and false positive rates when screening for Down's syndrome in the first trimester using fetal nuchal translucency and maternal serum free beta-hCG and PAPP-A. *The British Journal of Obstetrics & Gynaecology*, **108**, 1043–1046.

Spitzer W.O. (1997) The 1995 pill scare revisited: Anatomy of a non-epidemic. *Human Reproduction*, **12**, 2347–2357.

Stahlberg D. and Maass A. (1998) Hindsight bias: Impaired memory or biased reconstruction? In W. Stroebe and M. Hewstone (Eds.) *European Review of Social Psychology*, **8**, 105–132, Chichester, UK: Wiley.

Stolzer J. (2005) ADHD in America: A bioecological analysis. *Ethical Human Psychology and Psychiatry*, **7**, 65–75.

Stout P.A., Villegas J., and Jennings N.J. (2004) Images of mental illness in the media: Identifying gaps in the research. *Schizophrenia Bulletin*, **30**, 543–561.

Súilleabháin C.B.Ó., Menezes N., McKay C.J., Carter C.R., and Imrie C.W. (1997) Minimally invasive thoracoscopic splanchnicectomy (MITS) for pain secondary to chronic pancreatitis: A prospective audit. *British Journal of Surgery*, **89(s1)**, 63.

Suppes P. (1994) Qualitative theory of subjective probability. In: G. Wright and P. Ayton (Eds.) *Subjective Probability*. Chichester: John Wiley.

Sutton S. R. (1999) How accurate are smokers' perceptions of risk? *Health, Risk & Society*, **1**, 223–230.

Sweeting M.J., De Angelis D., Hickman M., and Ades A.E. (2008) Estimating hepatitis C prevalence in England and Wales by synthesizing evidence from multiple data sources: Assessing data conflict and model fit. *Biostatistics*, **9**, 715–734.

Taylor-Gooby P. (2006) Trust, risk and health care reform. *Health, Risk, and Society*, **8**, 97–103.

Taylor-Gooby P. (2000) Risk and Welfare. In: P. Taylor-Gooby (Ed.) *Risk, Trust and Welfare*. London: Macmillan.

The American College of Obstetricians and Gynecologists (2004) *Ethics in Obstetrics and Gynecology*. Washington, DC: The American College of Obstetricians and Gynecologists.

The Bristol Royal Infirmary Inquiry (2001) *Learning from Bristol: The Report of the Public Inquiry into Children's Heart Surgery at the Bristol Royal Infirmary 1984–1995*, (Chairman, Sir Ian Kennedy). Available at http://www.bristol-inquiry.org.uk/final_report/index.htm

The Cochrane Collaboration (2009) Home Page. Available at http://www.cochrane.org

The NHS Information Centre (2008) *Statistics on NHS Stop Smoking Services in England April 2007–December 2007 (Q3 – Quarterly Report)*. Available at http://www.ic.nhs.uk/statistics-and-data-collections/health-and-lifestyles/nhs-stop-smoking-services/statistics-on-nhs-stop-smoking-services-in-england-april-2007–december-2007-q3–quarterly-report

The Royal Society (1992) *Risk: Analysis, Perception and Management. Report of a Royal Society Study Group*. London: The Royal Society.

The Shipman Inquiry (2004) *Safeguarding Patients: Lessons from the Past – Proposals for the Future*, Fifth Report, 1. Available at http://www.the-shipman-inquiry.org.uk/reports.asp

The UK CRC Screening Pilot Evaluation Team (2003) *Evaluation of the UK Colorectal Cancer Screening Pilot*. Available at http://www.cancerscreening.nhs.uk/bowel/pilot-evaluation.html.

Theodosiou L. and Green J. (2003) Emerging challenges in using health information from the Internet. *Advances in Psychiatric Treatment*, **9**, 387–396.

Thirlaway K.J. and Heggs D. A. (2005) Interpreting risk messages: Women's responses to a health story. *Health, Risk & Society*, **7**, 107–121.

Thomas E.J., Studdert D.M, Runciman T. *et al.* (2000) A comparison of iatrogenic injury studies in Australia and the USA: Context, methods, case mix, population, patient and hospital characteristics. *International Journal for Quality in Health Care*, **12**, 371–378.

Thornicroft G. (2006) *Shunned: Discrimination against People with Mental Illness*. Oxford: Oxford University Press.

Tingle J. (2008) Tackling patient safety. *British Journal of Nursing*, **17**, 1075.

Titterton M. (2005) *Risk and Risk Taking in Health and Social Welfare*. London: Jessica Kingsley.

Trotta F., Apolone G., Garattini S., and Tafuri G. (2008) Stopping a trial early in oncology: For patients or for industry? *Annals of Oncology*, **19**, 1347–1353.

Tucker A.L. and Edmondson A. (2003) Why hospitals don't learn from failures: Organisational and psychological dynamics that inhibit system change. *California Management Review*, **45**, 55–72.

Tulloch J. and Lupton D. (2003) *Risk and Everyday Life*. London: Sage.

Ubel P.A. (1999) How stable are people's preferences for giving priority to severely ill patients?. *Social Science & Medicine*, **49**, 895–903.

Van Loon J. (2002) *Risk and Technological Culture: Towards a Sociology of Virulence*. London: Routledge.

Vandelli C., Renzo F., Romanò L. *et al.* (2004) Lack of evidence of sexual transmission of hepatitis C among monogamous couples: Results of a 10 year prospective follow-up study. *The American Journal of Gastroenterology*, **99**, 855–859.

Vincent C. (2006) *Patient Safety*. London: Elsevier.

Vincent C. (2004) Analysis of clinical incidents: A window on the system not a search for root causes. *Quality and Safety in Health Care*, **13**, 242–243.

Viscusi W.K. (1992) *Fatal Tradeoffs: Public and Private Responsibilities for Risk*. New York: Oxford University Press.

Wahl O. F. (1995) *Media Madness: Public Images of Mental Illness*. Piscataway, New Jersey: Rutgers University Press.

Walley J.D., Khan M.A., Newell J.N., and Khan M.H. (2001) Effectiveness of the direct observation component of DOTS for tuberculosis: A randomised controlled trial in Pakistan. *Lancet*, **357**, 664–669.

Walsh P. (2009) Does making NHS organisations pay for mistakes improve patient safety? *The AvMA Medical and Legal Journal* 15 [On-line Journal]. Available at www.jcn.co.uk/journal.asp?MonthNum=07&YearNum=2002&Type=backissue&ArticleID=479

Walshe K., Freeman T., Latham L., Surgeon P., and Wallace L. (2000) Clinical governance: Scope to improve. *Health Service Journal*, **110**, 30–32.

Wardle J., Carnell S., Haworth C.M.A., and Plomin R. (2008) Evidence for a strong genetic influence on childhood adiposity despite the force of the obesogenic environment. *American Journal of Clinical Nutrition*, **87**, 398–404.

Washer P. (2004) Representations of SARS in the UK newspapers. *Social Science & Medicine*, **59**, 2561–2571.

Washer P. and Joffe H. (2006) The Hospital 'Superbug': Social representations of MRSA. *Social Science & Medicine*, **63**, 2141–2152.

Watson B. and Heyman B. (1998) Risk and coping with diabetes. In B. Heyman (Ed.) *Risk, Health and Health Care: A Qualitative Approach*. London: Edward Arnold.

Watts C. and Zimmerman C. (2002) Violence against women: Global scope and magnitude. *The Lancet*, **359**, 1232–1237.

Webster (1988) *Problems of Health Care: The National Health Service Before 1957*. London: HMSO.

Weick K. and Sutcliffe K. (2003) Hospitals as cultures of entrapment: A re-analysis of the Bristol Royal Infirmary. *California Management Review*, **45**, 73–84.

Which? (2006) Which? Campaigns. Available at http://www.which.co.uk/portals/P/campaigns/index.jsp

Willett W.C., Manson J.E., Stampfer M.J. *et al.* (1995) Weight, weight change, and coronary heart disease in women. Risk within the 'normal' weight range. *Journal of the American Medical Association*, **273**, 461–465.

Williams A. (1997) Intergenerational equity: An exploration of the "fair innings" argument. *Health Economics*, **6**, 117–132.

Williams A. and Sibbald B. (1999) Changing roles and identities in primary health care: Exploring a culture of uncertainty. *Journal of Advanced Nursing*, **29**, 737–745.

Williams T.A., Dobb G.J., Finn J.C., and Webb S.A.R. (2005) Long-term survival from intensive care: A review. *Intensive Care Medicine*, **31**, 1306–1315.

Wilson D.P., Law M.G., Grulich A.E., Cooper D.A., and Kaldor J.M. (2008) Relation between HIV viral load and infectiousness: A model-based analysis. *Lancet*, **372**, 314–320.

Wilson P. (2002) How to find the good and avoid the bad and ugly: A short guide to tools for rating quality of health information on the internet. *British Medical Journal*, **324**, 598–602.

Winkler R.L. (1996) Uncertainty in probabilistic risk assessment. *Reliability Engineering and System Safety*, **54**, 127–132.

Wolff J. (2007) What is the value of preventing a fatality? In: T. Lewens (Ed.) *Risk: Philosophical Perspectives*. London: Routledge.

Wright R.J. (2007) Prenatal maternal stress and early caregiving experiences: Implications for childhood asthma risk. *Paediatric & Perinatal Epidemiology*, **21 S3**, 8–14.

Wroe A.L., Bhan A., Salkovskis P., and Bedford H. (2005) Feeling bad about immunising our children. *Vaccine*, **23**, 1428–1433.

Wu A. (2000) Medical error – the second victim: The doctor who made a mistake needs help too. *British Medical Journal*, **320**, 726–727.

Wynder E. L. and Graham E. A. (1950) Tobacco smoking as a possible etiological factor in bronchogenic carcinoma. *JAMA*, **143**, 329–336.

Wynne B. (1996) May the sheep safely graze? A reflexive view of the expert-lay knowledge divide. In: S. Lash, B. Szerszynski and B. Wynne (Eds.) *Risk, Environment & Modernity: Towards a New Ecology*. London: Sage.

Yaphe J., Edman R., Knishkowky B., and Herman J. (2001) The association between funding by commercial interests and study outcome in randomized controlled drug trials. *Family Practice*, **18**, 565–568.

Yeide H. and Lifton R.J. (1987) Killing in the name of healing. *Medical Humanities Review*, **1**, 43–46.

Yudkin P., Hey K., Roberts S., Welch S., Murphy M., and Walton R. (2003) Abstinence from smoking eight years after participation in randomised controlled trial of nicotine patch. *British Medical Journal*, **327**, 28–29.

Yusuf S., Hawken S., Ôunpuu S. *et al.* (2005) Obesity and the risk of myocardial infarction in 27 000 participants from 52 countries: A case-control study. *The Lancet*, **366**, 1640–1649.

Zammit S., Allebeck P., Andreasson S., Lundberg I. and Lewis G. (2002) Self-reported cannabis use as a risk factor for schizophrenia in Swedish conscripts of 1969: Historical cohort study. *British Medical Journal*, 325, 1199–1123.

Zinn J.O. (Ed.)(2008) *Social Theories of Risk and Uncertainty*. Oxford: Blackwell.

Author Index

Adam B. 108
Adams J. 7, 29
Ades A.E. 49
Adil M. 196
Alaszewski A. 46, 50, 123, 135, 148, 160, 173, 177, 184, 192, 203, 208, 209, 210, 211, 213
Alaszewski H. 46, 50, 135
Albert S.M. 168
Alfirevic Z. 71
Allan S. 159, 162
Allebeck P. 47
Allen J. 139, 143, 144
Allsop J. 173, 176, 208
Amoah A.G.B. 53
Anderson A. 142, 143, 159, 165, 166
Anderson D.J. 205
Andreasson S. 47
Apolone G. 113
Aref-Adib M. 57
Ataullah I. 57
Atherton E. 109
Ayer S. 45, 50

Baggaley R.F. 49
Baggott R. 176
Baker G.R. 128, 198
Bakir V. 162
Baldwin R. 184
Barbalet J. 135
Barker J. 83
Barlow D.M. 162
Bassett K.L. 121
Beach R. 28
Beck U. 7, 80, 81, 110, 125, 139, 188, 214
Beck-Gernsheim E. 110
Bedford H. 71
Bedford T. 88
Belyea M. 111
Bernstam E.V. 145
Bernstein P.L. 19
Berry W.R. 179, 193
Berta W. 204
Bevan G. 80, 186, 198
Bhan A. 71
Bickley K. 110
Billington C. 56
Bilson A. 172
Bindra R. 94, 95, 96, 97, 114
Binedell J. 100
Blair S.N. 56
Blakemore C. 78, 79

Blanc L. 132
Blaxter M. 128
Blenkinsopp A. 132
Boegner C. 102
Boermeester M.A. 198, 199
Boily M.C. 49
Bonati M. 145
Bond C. 132
Boon S.D. 126
Booth C.M. 79
Bowker G.C. 40, 42, 44
Bowles C.J.A. 118
Boyd A.D. 152
Boyle S. 181
Bradfield A. 119
Bradshaw B. 172, 176, 185, 192
Bradshaw P.L. 172, 176, 185, 192
Brawley O.W. 111
Breakwell G.M. 8, 76, 97
Brettell K.M. 61
Bridgeman J. 124
Brigham S. 71
Bringer J. 102
Bristow J. 166
Brook D.W. 110
Brook J.S. 110
Brown G.V. 117
Brown M.B. 95
Browne K. 110
Brownell K.D. 56
Bruneau J. 126
Burdge G.C. 110
Butler V. 20, 23, 211

Caballero B. 102
Califano J.A. 105
Calnan M. 135
Carnell S. 46
Carr-Hill R.A. 66
Carrier N. 126
Carter C.R. 111
Carthey J. 205
Casella N. 145
Castel R. 18, 26, 27, 214
Casti J.L. 88
Chamberlin K. 137, 159
Chan L.W. 71
Chan Y.M. 71
Charlton R. 41
Cicourel A.V. 41
Clark H.D. 90

Clayton J. 125
Cliffe S. 49
Coghill D. 55
Coghlan A. 78
Colditz G.A. 102
Collins J. 141
Cooke R. 88
Cooper D.A. 49
Coote A. 139, 143, 144
Copas A.J. 49
Corona Gainford M. 79
Courpassen D. 182, 183
Cowan J. 208
Coxon K. 148, 173, 179, 184, 192, 203, 208, 209
Cranor C.F. 73
Crawford R. 188
Crinson I. 53, 133
Critcher C. 166, 168
Croall H. 156
Curnock D. 28

Durr A. 100
Damber J. 102
Damber L. 102
Dauphinee D. 171
Davey-Smith G. 102
Davidson O. 41, 216
Davies H. 204
Davies J. 33, 82, 104, 204, 208
Davin S. 160, 161
Davis M.D.M. 41, 216
Davison C. 102
Davison K. 145
d'Cruse S. 156
de Courten M. 53
de Lusignan S. 53, 133
de Vries E.N. 198, 199
De Angelis D. 49
Dean M. 7, 177
Dearnaley D.P. 111
Debalini M.G. 54
Degeling P.J. 178, 179, 192
Demichell V. 54
Dentzer S. 157
Di Pietrantonj C. 54
Ditkoff A. 168
Dixon L. 110
Dobb G.J. 111
Dolan P. 72
Doll R. 125
Donaldson L. 198, 210, 214, 216, 218
Doran E. 167
Dormandy E. 99
Douglas M. 7, 18, 25, 26, 76, 80, 97, 189, 214
Doyle A. 8, 74
Dragan I. 113
Dranitsaris G. 79
Driedger S.M. 152

Duncan C.J. 214
Durfee J.L. 138, 142
Durrant R. 53, 133

Edman R. 54
Edmondson A. 199, 200
Edney D.R. 150
Elder J.T. 83
Eldridge J. 139, 165, 166, 168
Elisaf M. 2
Elliott J. 154
Endreny P.M. 143
Epstein O. 118
Ericson R.V. 8
Espin S. 179
Esquivel A. 145
Evans J. 124, 155
Evans-Pritchard E.E. 124
Eysenbach G. 167, 168

Feng Q. 105
Fenge L.A. 25
Ferguson I. 124, 189
Ferguson-Smith M.A. 124
Filippatos T. 2
Finn J.C. 111
Flintoft V. 83
Flynn R. 173, 177, 178, 179, 180, 181
Fogel J. 168
Forster A.J. 201, 202
Foucault M. 7, 81, 214
Frankel S. 102
Frankle H. 61
Franklin B. 162, 163
Freedland K.E. 117
Freeman T. 179
Freeman-Wang T. 57
French S. 60, 63, 74, 109, 221
Fries J.F. 75
Fullinfaw R.O. 117

Gagliardi A. 142, 145
Galtier-Dereure F. 102
Garattini S. 113
Garland D. 16
Gaskell G. 188
Gauntlett D. 159
Gawande A. 193
Gelperin K. 55
Giddens A. 108, 126, 139, 180
Gigerenzer G. 7, 8, 97
Gil K.M. 111
Gilbart E. 204
Gillet J. 142, 163, 168
Gluckman P.D. 110
Godfrey K.M. 110
Godin P. 8, 33, 82, 104, 204, 208
Goebel K. 117
Goizet C. 100

Goldacre M. 139, 143, 144, 155
Golding D. 7
Golsworthy R. 40
Gordon S. 153, 154, 155
Gouma D.J. 198, 199
Graham E.A. 125
Graham J. 55
Gray A. 178, 179
Gray J. 178, 179
Green J. 142, 144
Green S. 113
Gregg J. 56
Gronberg H. 102
Gross S. 41
Grulich A.E. 49
Guallar E. 2
Gubb J. 198
Gwyn R. 149, 151

Hájek A. 86
Hackett M.C. 179
Hacking I. 7, 28, 76, 79, 87, 88
Hallam J. 154, 155
Hamilton-Giachritsis C. 110
Hammad T.A. 55
Handyside E.C. 5, 20
Hankinson S.E. 102
Hann A. 53
Hanson M.A. 110
Hansson S.O. 17
Hargreaves D. 165, 166, 168, 169
Harnden A. 215, 216
Harper P.S. 100
Harrabin R. 139, 143, 144
Harris R. 109
Harrison L. 211
Harrison S. 172, 177, 178, 179,
     192, 211
Hart A. 164
Hart G. 164
Hatch D. 176
Hawes S.E. 105
Hawken S. 103
Haworth C.M.A. 46
Haynes A.B. 179, 192
Hayward R.A. 53
Hazani E. 110
Hazell L. 54
Heath V. 94, 95, 96, 97, 115
Heggs D.A. 143, 158, 161, 162
Henderson J. 126
Heneghan C. 215, 216
Hennekens C.H. 102
Henriksen M. 21, 43, 51, 55, 56, 57, 64, 89,
     98, 100, 101, 114, 116
Henry D. 167
Henwood F. 164
Henwood K. 140, 159
Herman J. 54

Hey K. 130, 156
Heyman B. 1, 5, 10, 15, 20, 21, 27, 33, 37, 43,
     51, 52, 55, 56, 57, 59, 63, 64, 69, 72, 85,
     89, 98, 100, 101, 104, 107, 114, 115, 116,
     211, 213
Hickie I. 40
Hickman M. 49
Hilgartner S. 23, 45
Hill A.B. 66, 125
Hodgetts D. 137, 159
Hofer T.P. 53
Holick M.F. 46
Holland J.C. 127
Holmes J.G. 126
Holzl E. 119
Hood C. 80, 184, 186
Hooper R. 218
Hopkins P.N. 45
Horlick-Jones T. 140, 142, 148, 159, 165, 166
Horwich A. 111
Huang Z. 102
Huber M. 188
Huckle S. 5, 20, 27, 33, 211
Huddart R.A. 111
Hughes D. 134
Hughes E. 144, 159, 162, 165
Hunt A. 3, 93
Hunter D.J. 178, 179, 192
Hutter B.M. 177, 181, 182, 184, 196

Ilkka N. 125
Impicciatore P. 145
Imrie C.W. 111
Imrie J. 41, 216

Jahad A. 142, 145
Jamieson D.J. 218
Janssen I. 103
Japp K.P. 81
Jardine C.G. 152
Jefferson T. 54
Jennings N.J. 149, 150
Joffe H. 151, 152, 153, 165
Johann-Liang R. 55
Johanson R. 120
Jung R.T. 102

Kahneman D. 7
Kalb L.S. 119
Kaldor J.M. 49
Kaminski J. 154
Kasperson J.K. 140
Kasperson R. 139
Kasperson R.E. 140
Katz D.L. 151
Katzmarzyk P.T. 103
Kavanagh S. 208
Kazanjian A. 121
Kelly S. 47, 50, 150

Kemshall H. 180, 182, 210
Khan M.A. 201
Khan M.H. 201
King L.A. 78, 79
Kingham M. 55
Kinloch-de Loës S. 113
Kiortsis D. 2
Kirchler E. 119
Kitzinger J. 143, 144, 148, 157, 159, 162, 165, 166
Kiviat N.B. 105
Klin A. 149
Kmietowicz Z. 186, 210
Knight F. 7
Knishkowky B. 54
Kohler C. 167
Kraus J.F. 147, 149
Krimsky S. 7
Krishnan E. 75
Kusche I. 81

LaPlante J. 126
Laing R.D. 63
Lakoff G. 42
Lambert T. 61, 155
Lambert W.E. 61, 155
Latham L. 179
Lau T.K. 71
Lavalette M. 189
Law J. 22, 43
Law M.G. 49
Leake C.D. 127
Ledema R. 178, 179, 192
Lee E.J. 133
Leicester R. 118
Lemish D. 149
Lesca G. 100
Leung T.N. 71
Leung T.Y. 71
Levine M. 2
Lewando Hundt G. 10, 51, 52, 64
Lewens T. 8, 17
Lewis G. 47
Liao A. 94, 95, 96, 97, 115
Liberopoulos E. 2
Lifton R.J. 129
Lillycrop K.A. 110
Lingard L. 179
Link B.C. 45
Lippman A. 115
Lloyd A.J. 98
Locker D. 124
Lofstedt R. 165, 166, 168, 169
Lohr K. 109
Lord L. 8, 189
Luhmann N. 7, 17, 18, 22, 26, 27, 29, 81, 83, 92, 93, 108, 214
Luke B. 95

Lundberg I. 47
Lupton D. 8, 158, 169
Lyall J. 123
Lyer N. 121

Maass A. 119
MacFarlane K. 218
MacIntyre C.R. 117
MacKenzie D. 216, 217
Macfarlane A. 120
Magana D. 147, 149
Maher D. 132
Manning N. 40
Mannion R. 204
Manson J.E. 102
Mant D. 215, 216
Manthorpe J. 211
Marinker M. 132
Marteau T.M. 99
Maughan K. 21, 89
Maxwell S. 178, 179, 192
Maxwell S.R.J. 215
McArthur D.L. 147, 149
McCarty D. 53
McCormack J.P. 2
McGarrigle C.A. 49
McGuigan J. 138, 169
McGuire A. 126
McKay C.J. 110
McKenna H.P. 47, 50, 150
McLachlan S. 165, 166, 168, 169
McLean J. 158
McNeil B.J. 117
Menard A. 201, 202
Menezes N. 110
Menzel P. 72
Meric-Bernstam F. 145
Meurier C.E. 204, 207
Michie S. 99
Middleton D. 28
Mikhailidis D. 2
Miller D. 169
Miller J. 125
Mishel M.H. 111
Mistry B. 152
Mitchell T.R. 119
Montori V.M. 113
Mooney G. 126
Moran M. 124, 172, 173, 180, 181
Morgan M. 126
Morris G. 150
Moscovici S. 148
Mosholder A.D. 55
Moynihan R. 167
Mrowietz U. 83
Murdock G. 140, 142, 144, 159, 162, 165, 166
Murphy M. 112
Mythen G. 8

Nelkin D. 140, 166
Neugut A.I. 168
Neville N. 128
Newburn M. 120
Newell J.N. 201
Nicolaides K.H. 94, 95, 96, 97, 115
Nord E. 65, 71, 72, 74, 75, 76
Norton P.G. 82
Nriagu J.O. 30
Nutley S. 204
Nutt D. 78, 79

O'Neil O. 179
O'Connor D. 113
O'Hara L. 56
O'Malley P. 42, 81
O'Neal Chambliss H. 56
Ofsted 190, 191
Olsen J.A. 72
Olstead R. 150
Ormerod L.P. 71
Oulton K.L. 63
Ôunpuu S. 103

Paling J. 9
Pandolfini C. 145
Papagrigoriadis S. 72
Parker G. 40
Parsloe P. 8
Paterson E. 128
Pauker S.G. 117
Peacock L. 190
Peckham S. 53
Peek-Asa C. 147, 149
Pegg S. 156
Perera R. 215, 216
Perneger T.V. 113
Peterson M. 67, 68, 72
Peto R. 125
Petts J. 140, 142, 148, 159, 165, 166, 168, 169
Phelan J. 45
Phelan K. 55
Phillips L.N. 124
Philo G. 148, 149, 150, 169
Piaget J. 73
Pidgeon N. 139, 140, 159
Pill R. 134
Plomin R. 46
Potter J. 135
Power M. 5, 8, 16, 32, 81, 137, 177, 180, 182, 184, 214
Price D. 176
Prior L. 134
Procter S. 134

Ramrattan M.A. 198, 199
Rangno R.E. 2
Rasmussen S.A. 218

Raviglione M. 132
Reading R. 28, 56
Reason J. 199, 203, 204, 205, 206
Redfern M. 130
Redley M. 138, 162
Reilly J. 139, 165, 166
Renn O. 8, 17, 18, 22, 73
Renzo F. 50
Rescher N. 62
Rexrode K.M. 102
Reynolds L. 33, 82, 204, 208
Reynolds R. 104
Richardson J. 163, 164
Richardson K.P. 163, 164
Rivetti A. 54
Roberts C.G.P. 2
Roberts S. 112
Robertson M. 21
Robinson J. 110
Rodriguez A. 2
Romanò L. 50
Romaya C. 118
Rosa E.A. 17, 20, 62
Rose D. 151
Rose N. 3, 177
Rosenhan D.L. 39
Ross R. 103
Rothstein H. 184, 188
Rowe R. 135
Rubin B. 179
Runciman T. 198
Ruston A. 125, 134

Saks M. 173, 208
Salkovskis P. 71
Samanta A. 91
Sandall J. 10, 51, 52, 64
Sandman P.M. 151
Sassi F. 65
Saulsbury W. 78, 79
Savage J. 153, 154
Schmid G. 60
Schnabel F. 168
Schutz A. 21
Schwartz M.B. 56
Scott S. 214
Seale C. 137, 141, 142, 143, 144, 146, 147, 149, 156, 157, 158, 159, 165, 167, 168
Shakir S. 54
Shasha S.M. 110
Shaw A. 53, 133
Shaw J. 132
Shaw J.E. 53
Shaw M. 33, 82, 104, 137, 171, 195, 204, 208, 213
Shojania K.G. 202
Shun-Shin M. 215, 216
Sibbald B. 28

Simmons P. 140, 159
Singer E. 143, 215
Singh B. 198, 210
Skala J.A. 117
Skolbekken J. 3, 4, 25
Skull S. 117
Slovic P. 7, 98, 139, 140, 159
Smalley S. 55
Smith D.E. 38
Smith G. 41, 102
Smorenburg S.M. 198, 199
Social Security 7, 10, 17, 23, 34, 81, 97, 110, 175, 185, 187, 190, 208, 209, 214
Soldan J.R. 100
Som C.V. 179
Southgate L. 171
Spencer K. 99
Spitzer W.O. 46
Stahlberg D. 119
Stampfer M.J. 102
Star S.L. 40, 42, 44, 154
Starr M. 117
Stephenson J. 41, 216
Stolzer J. 55
Stout P.A. 149, 150
Studdert D.M. 198
Súilleabháin C.B.Ó 111
Sundberg K. 71
Suppes P. 19, 89
Surgeon P. 179
Sutcliffe K. 173, 174
Sutton S.R. 125
Swarbrick E. 118
Sweeting M.J. 49

Tafuri G. 113
Taylor-Gooby P. 123, 135
Teare G. 204
Theodosiou L. 142, 144
Thirlaway K.J. 143, 158, 161, 162
Thomas E.J. 89, 127, 198
Thompson M. 215, 216
Thornicroft G. 149, 150
Tingle J. 185, 201
Titterton M. 1, 5, 8, 20, 31, 59, 67, 68, 208, 211
Todd P.M. 7
Trotta F. 113
Tucker A.L. 199, 200
Tucker G.R. 61
Tulloch J. 8, 169
Tversky A.E. 7

Ubel P.A. 72
Uplekar M. 132

Van Loon J. 22, 23, 76, 83
Vandelli C. 50
Vijan S. 53

Villegas J. 149, 150
Vincent C. 25, 171, 173, 196, 198, 199, 205, 206
Viscusi W.K. 116
van Walraven C. 202

Wahl O.F. 150
Walklate S. 8
Wallace L. 179
Walley J.D. 117
Walsh P. 187
Walshe K. 179
Walton R. 112
Wang L. 57
Wardle J. 46
Washer P. 148, 151, 152, 153, 165
Watson B. 69, 115
Watts C. 150
Webb S.A.R. 111
Webster 126
Webster C.S. 205
Weichselbaum R 117
Weick K. 173, 174
Weiser T.G. 179, 193
Welch S. 112
Wells G.L. 119
White S. 131, 172, 176, 178, 195
Whiteman M. 110
Willett W.C. 102
Williams A. 28, 75
Williams B. 53, 133
Williams C.B. 118
Williams I. 41, 216
Williams R.R. 45
Williams T.A. 111
Wilson D.P. 49
Wilson P. 49
Wilt T. 113
Winkler R.L. 88
Wolff J. 66, 76
Wood F. 134
Wright R.J. 116
Wroe A.L. 71
Wu A. 204
Wyatt S. 157, 164
Wynder E.L. 125
Wynne B. 33

Yaphe J. 54
Yeide H. 129
Yudkin P. 112
Yuen Fung T.Y. 71
Yusuf S. 103

Zammit S. 47
Zimmerman C. 150
Zimmet P.Z. 53
Zinn J.O. 8

Subject Index

accountability 10, 30, 33–5, 110, 156, 172, 176, 180, 182, 184, 186, 192
adverse drug reactions (ADRs) 54
adverse events 10, 12, 24–5, 62–3, 110, 113, 157, 178, 184, 196–7, 199, 201–2, 209–11
adversity foregrounding 46–9, 50
agency 127, 138, 167, 172, 185–8, 221
aggregation 23
Alder Hey Hospital Inquiry 130
aleatory probabilities 88
Allitt, Beverly 155, 156–7
anal cancer 69–70
anchoring 148
antibiotic resistance 81
anxiety 116, 123, 126, 139, 162, 169, 188
arthritis 74, 143
attention deficit/hyperactivity disorder (ADHD) 54–5
attenuation model 139–41
attributable positive predictive gain 94, 97
audit 155, 173, 177–8, 180, 182–3, 208, 210
availability heuristic 98
Azande 124–5

Baby Peter case 188–9, 190
base rate 94, 95, 101
Bayesian statistics 89
Behind the Medical Headlines 145
Being Open Policy 205
belief systems 81, 124–5, 204
Bertschinger, Clair 155
binary cut-offs 49–51, 89
blame culture 188–90, 204–5
body mass index (BMI) 103–4
bottle-feeding 133
breast cancer, media representation 147, 160–2, 166–7, 168
Bristol Royal Infirmary 130, 173–4
Bovine Spongiform Encephalitis (BSE) 41, 124, 153, 159, 165–6, 168
Butler Report 23

Caesarean section 120
campaigning journalists 166
cancer
    classification 41
    consequences 65, 69–70, 73
    cosmology 63
    5-year survival 111
    informed consent 127

media representations 146–7, 160–2, 166–7, 168
multidisciplinary teamwork 208
screening 52, 65, 105, 111, 113, 117–18
temporal accounting 116
cannabis, schizophrenia risk 46–7
Care Quality Commission (CQC) 175, 181,185, 187–8, 222
categorization 2, 38, 39–43, 44
    counting 42
    homogenization 38, 39–43
    simplification 44
    transparency 44
cervical cancer screening and vaccination 106
chance 87–9; see also randomness and probability
    roulette computers 88
child protection 188–90
child sex abuse scandal, Cleveland 157
choice 129, 132–3
chromosomal anomalies screening 50, 51, 64–5, 71–2, 89, 94–7, 99–100, 101–2, 114–116
Clark, Sally 90
classification 38, 39–43, 44; see also categorization
Cleveland sex-abuse scandal 157
Climbié, Victoria 189
clinical decision making 131
clinical governance 5, 32, 127, 130, 171–2, 182, 175–9, 208, 210
Clinical Negligence Scheme 183
clinical trials, premature termination 113–114
clinical standards 134, 172, 178, 179
club culture 130, 174, 180
Cochrane Collaboration 131
colonoscopy 118
colorectal cancer
    screening 118
    surgery 73
colostomy 69–70
commercial entrenchment 53–4
commercial interests 167
concordance model 132
conditional probabilities 93–7
confidence intervals 94, 95
consequences, multiple 59, 60, 65
consequentialism 74–6
consumer movement 128–9

content analysis 142–3
contingencies 19, 22–4, 27–8, 31–2, 38–9,
    43–4, 67–8, 121, 215, 218, 223
contingency tables 93
coronary heart disease 1–2, 133
cost–benefit analysis 65–7
cost-effectiveness 111
cot death 90–1
cross-generational risk 110
culture
    risk selection bias 81
    value differences 62

danger 3, 5, 15, 18, 25–9, 34, 48, 50, 63, 127,
    134, 148, 150, 160, 169, 199, 214, 216,
    219, 221
deafness 63
defensiveness 183–5, 203, 210
deference 128
deletion 23, 43
die throwing 87, 88, 89–90
differentiation
    risks 27, 33–4, 38, 57, 81–2
    roles 82
direct observation of treatment 117
disability 72, 238
discount rate 116–117
doctor-patient relationships 126–7, 129
doctors, media images 155–8
double-blind randomized controlled
    trials 54
Down's syndrome screening 42–3, 50, 54–5,
    65, 71–2, 89, 94–7, 99–100, 101–2, 114–116
drugs
    adverse drug reactions (ADRs) 53
    classification 47, 78–9
    maladministration 175, 205

ecological fallacy 92–3, 103
ecological prevention paradox 102, 106
elderly primigravida 57
emotional aspects of care 135
encoded knowledge 123, 134, 136
epidemiology 125
epigenetics 110
epistemic probabilities 88
evidence-based practice 132–3
expected value 59–60, 65–8, 70, 73, 75–7, 79,
    83–4, 108
Expert Patient Programme 129, 136
experts 29, 33, 78, 97–8, 124–6, 135, 140,
    142–3, 145–6, 151, 159, 161–4, 166–8,
    177, 203

'fair innings' 75
false negative rate 97
false positive rate 96–7
fear of blame 203

fecal occult blood test (FOBt) 118
food scares 124, 159
forensic mental health services 68
foundation trusts 181, 192
framing health risks 147–58
future intentions 108, 117

General Medical Council (GMC) 175–6
genetic transmission 110
governmentality 7, 50, 81
Haringey Council 188–90
hepatitis C 48, 49–50, 126
herceptin 144, 166
heuristics 97–106
Higgs, Marietta 157
High Quality For All 186–7
hindsight bias 119–21, 122
HIV 41–2, 48, 55, 113, 162, 168, 216
Human immunodeficiency virus see HIV
Huntington's disease 100–1

iconography of risk 55–6
identity 63, 135, 153, 220
immunization 71, 159
inductive prevention paradox 100, 103–4,
    106, 112, 119–121
inductive probabilistic reasoning 9, 35, 85–6,
    91–3, 100–1, 102, 105–6, 213
inflammatory bowel disease (IBD) 104–5
information about health risks 123–36
informed consent 127–8, 130, 136
institutional embedding 52–3
interactive model of media audiences 159–60
Internet 138, 140–2, 143, 144–6, 147, 154,
    163–4, 167–8, 215

John Radcliffe Hospital, Oxford 203

Laming Report 189
lead-time bias 111
learning disability 63–4
learning organization approach 206, 208
legal issues 127–8
lens of risk 1, 3, 5, 8, 19, 22–4, 32, 35, 37, 45,
    60, 62, 84, 89–90, 121, 182, 193,
    214–15, 222–4
lung cancer surgery 117

maladministration of drugs 204–5
managerialism 180, 182
matched guise paradigm 60–1
may be at risk' 51
Meadows, Professor Sir Roy 90
Measles Mumps Rubella vaccination see MMR
media 137–69
    amplification and attenuation of
        risk 139–41, 165–6
    audiences 141, 148, 158–64, 168–9

framing health risks 147–58
  new 141–2, 143–6, 147, 159, 162, 168
  old media 141, 143–4
  production of health risk
    messages 164–8
  representation of health risk 142–68
  societal role 138–41
  templates 148
medical errors 25, 157, 186
  open reporting 203–10
medical intervention time-framing 110–111
medical scandals 129–30, 156–7, 173–5
Medicines Partnership 132
mental disorders
  classification 39–40
  media framing 149–51
Mid Staffordshire Trust 181–2, 186
MMR vaccination 159
mobile phones 141, 159, 163
Monitor 181
MRSA, media framing 151–3
multidisciplinary teams 12, 179, 208
multiple probabilities paradox 100–2
multivariate statistics 45
Munchausen's Syndrome by Proxy
  (MSbP) 154–5, 156

National Institute for Health and Clinical
  Excellence see NICE
National Patient Observatory 201
National Patient Safety Agency
  (NPSA) 185–7, 200–1
National Reporting and Learning System
  (NRLS) 185, 186, 200–1, 203, 206, 210
national service frameworks 15,186,192
natural attitude to risk 21
Nazi medical experiments 75, 129
near misses 198–200
negative predictive value 94, 97
negative valuing 19
Never Events 20, 187, 197–8
new media 141–2, 143–6, 147, 159, 162, 168
newspapers, see media
National Health Service (NHS)
  modernization 180
  patient relations 131–5
  regulation 130–1, 171–93
  trust in 127, 128, 134–5, 173, 177, 179
NHS Direct 134, 145
NHS Litigation Authority (NHSLA) 183–4
NICE 131, 138, 166
nurses
  blame for drug maladministration 204–5
  media images 153–5, 156
Nursing and Midwifery Council (NMC) 191

obesity 46, 56, 103, 110, 216–7
official inquiries 120, 173–6

Ofsted 190
old media 141, 143–4
open reporting culture 203–10
organizational change 182–92
organizational culture 203–10
outcome-contingent risks 20, 178
overweight 102
ownership of risk 33–4
Oxford John Radcliffe Hospital 203

paternalism 127
patient choice 129, 132–3
patient safety 3, 25, 32, 35, 46, 134, 155, 173,
  184–8, 193, 195–211
Patient's Charter 128
performance targets 179, 185, 189, 192
personal identity 135
personalized medicine 89
personal time-framing 114–116
pesticide residues 77
pharmaceutical company interests 53–4
pollution 81
pregnancy
  chromosomal anomalies screening 50, 51,
    64–5, 71–2, 89, 94–7, 99–100, 101–2,
    114–116
  elderly primigravida 56
preoperative checklists 179
prevention 52–3, 102–6, 171, 189, 214
probability 27–8, 86–7
  and value 73–4
  aleatory 88
  Bayesian statistics 89
  conditional 93–7
  contingency tables 94
  epistemic 88
  heuristics 97–106
  imprecision 87, 88
  inductive probabilistic reasoning 91–3
  multiple probabilities paradox 100–2
  positive predictive value 94, 96–7
  probabilistic reasoning 2, 85–107
prostate cancer 109
  consequences of surgery 65
  media representation 147
  screening 111, 112–113
psychiatric illnesses, see mental
  disorders
psychotropic substances 78–9

quality-adjusted life years (QALYs) 65, 73,
  74, 75, 76, 116
quality assurance 130, 178–9

randomized controlled trials 45, 53, 75
  double-blind 53
  equipoise 75
  premature termination 113–114

randomness 19, 87–8, 89–91; *see also* chance and probability
rational actor approach 134, 159–60
regulation of risks 3, 130–1, 171–93
 light-touch approach 82
religion and contingency 63, 124–5
reporting errors 203–10
retrospection 118–21
risk
 being at risk 11, 15–16, 29–31, 34
 communication 9, 25, 27, 82–3, 132, 138–143, 158–60, 162, 164, 169, 174, 189–90, 207
 concept of risk 15–35, 60, 62
 consolidation 38, 43–56
 definition 16–21, 31, 34, 62, 86, 107, 119, 196
 derivation 60
 differentiation 27, 33, 38, 39–43
 epidemic 3–4
 environmental factors 110
 factor–outcome fusion 45–6
 homogenization 38, 39–43
 iconography 54–5
 individualization 51
 interpretive processes 21, 131
 knowledge 123–6, 29, 132, 134–5
 language 3, 7, 25–8, 60
 legal issues 127–8
 lens of risk 3, 5, 8, 19, 22–4, 32, 35, 37, 45, 60, 62, 84, 89–91, 121, 182, 193, 211, 214–15, 222–4
 literacy 6, 13
 management 3, 5–13, 16, 21, 24, 31–2, 182–92
 managers 32–3, 43, 56, 60, 73, 77, 113–4, 118–21, 174
 'might be at risk' 45, 52, 58, 73, 223
 moral issues 55–6, 74–6
 moralization 55–6
 natural attitude 21
 ownership 33–4
 prevention linkage 52
 projection 20–1, 89
 regulation 3, 118, 130–1, 171–93
 retrospection 118–21
 selection 2, 77–83, 164–5, 168, 218
 social construction 37–57
 social science of 7–8, 17–21, 80–3
 society thesis (Beck) 81, 125, 188, 214
 study of risk/risks 10–11
 systems theory 82–3
 'taking a risk' 16, 29–31
 thinking 3, 5–11, 15–17, 19–21, 30, 35, 37–8, 42, 50, 58–60, 79, 81–5, 89, 108, 121–2, 178, 214
 threshold setting 49–51
role differentiation 82

Safety First 185–6
safety of patients 3, 195–211
 systems approach 205–6, 207
SARF 139–40, 165–6
schizophrenia
 antipsychiatry movement 63
 cannabis link 46–7
science-based societies 26, 81
scientific-bureaucratic philosophy 172
scientific knowledge 19, 88, 123–6
screening
 cancer 106, 111, 112–113, 118
 chromosomal anomalies 50, 51, 64–5, 71–2, 89, 94–7, 99–100, 101–2, 114–116
 false negative rate 94, 97
 false positive rate 94, 96–7
 lead-time bias 111
 negative predictive value 94, 97
 prostate cancer 111, 112–113
 selectivity 94, 96
 sensitivity 94, 96
 threshold setting 50
 time-framing 112–113
 two-stages 118
self-governance 180
self-management 129
self-regulation 173, 176, 180
Seven Steps to Patient Safety Guide 201
sex abuse scandal, Cleveland 157
sexually transmitted disease (STDs) 49, 140
Shipman Inquiry 175
Shoesmith, Sharon, 189–90
smoking cessation 111, 112, 121
soap operas 158, 160, 162
social amplification of risk framework (SARF) 139–40, 165–6
social construction of health risks 37–57
social power 81
social science of risk 7–8, 17–21, 83, 131, 219
standard gamble 71–2
statins 1, 2, 53, 58, 113
statistical independence 89–91
stereotypes 61, 148
stoma 69–70
subjective value measurement 71
suicide 90, 110, 149, 207, 224
superbugs, media framing 151–3
supernatural systems 124–5
systems theory of risks 82–3

technology, side effects 81
television programmes 158, 160, 162; *see also* media
temporal accounting 116–117
threshold setting for risks 49–51
time-framing 2, 107–22
 collective 109–14
 personal 114–116

timid prosperity 123–4
transparency of categorizations 44
trust
  definition 126
  in the media 160–4
  in the NHS 127, 128, 134–5
Trust, Assurance and Safety 176
Tuberculosis (TB) treatment 71, 117–118

uncertainty 27–8, 87–9, 123–4, 126–7
unsafe sex 47–9

values 2, 59–84
  ascribed 62
  dynamics 72–3
  expected 65–76

externalization 62–5
fuzziness 71–2
moral dimension 76
multiple consequences 65–76
negative valuing 19
probability and 73–4
risk selection 77–83
standard gamble 71–2
subjective value measurement 71
surveys 72
variant CJD (vCJD) 41, 42
virtual objects 22–4

waist circumference 103–4
web-based information 141–2, 143, 144–6,
  147, 163–4, 167–8